Challenging Cases in
Pediatric Ophthalmology

David B. Granet, MD, FAAP, FACS, FAAO
Shira L. Robbins, MD, FAAP, FAAO
Leslie Julia Baber, MD

American Academy of Pediatrics
141 Northwest Point Blvd
Elk Grove Village, IL 60007-1019

American Academy of Pediatrics Department of Marketing and Publications

Maureen DeRosa, MPA, Director, Department of Marketing and Publications

Mark Grimes, Director, Division of Product Development

Martha Cook, Senior Product Development Editor

Eileen Glasstetter, MS, Manager, Product Development

Carrie Peters, Editorial Assistant

Sandi King, MS, Director, Division of Publishing and Production Services

Shannan Martin, Publishing and Production Services Specialist

Jason Crase, Editorial Specialist

Linda Diamond, Manager, Art Direction and Production

Linda Smessaert, MSIMC, Manager, Clinical and Professional Publications Marketing

Library of Congress Control Number: 2011904327
ISBN: 978-1-58110-305-2
eISBN: 978-1-58110-621-3
MA0449

The recommendations in this publication do not indicate an exclusive course of treatment or serve as a standard of medical care. Variations, taking into account individual circumstances, may be appropriate.

The publishers have made every effort to trace the copyright holders for borrowed material. If they have inadvertently overlooked any, they will be pleased to make the necessary arrangements at the first opportunity.

Products are mentioned for informational purposes only. Inclusion in this publication does not imply endorsement by the American Academy of Pediatrics. The American Academy of Pediatrics is not responsible for the content of the resources mentioned in this publication. Web site addresses are as current as possible, but may change at any time.

Every effort has been made to ensure that the drug selection and dosage set forth in this text are in accordance with the current recommendations and practice at the time of publication. It is the responsibility of the health care provider to check the package insert of each drug for any change in indications and dosage and for added warnings and precautions.

Printed in China.
9-327

1 2 3 4 5 6 7 8 9 10

Contributors

Robert W. Arnold, MD, FAAP
Pediatric Ophthalmologist
Alaska Blind Child Discovery
  Project, Ophthalmic Associates
Anchorage, AK
85: Failed Vision Screen

Leslie Julia Baber, MD[†]
1: Neonatal Conjunctivitis
2: Adenoviral Conjunctivitis
3: Bacterial Conjunctivitis

Jennifer Bernabe-Ko, MD
Fellow, Cornea Refractive Surgery
University of California San Diego
San Diego, CA
11: Corneal Abrasion
12: Corneal Foreign Body

Gil Binenbaum, MD, MSCE
Attending Surgeon
The Children's Hospital of
  Philadelphia
Assistant Professor of
  Ophthalmology
University of Pennsylvania
Philadelphia, PA
76: Juvenile Xanthogranuloma

**Chantal Boisvert, OD, MD,
  FAAP, FAAO**
Assistant Professor of
  Ophthalmology
Director, Pediatric Ophthalmology
  Service
The University of New Mexico
Albuquerque, NM
62: Brown Syndrome
67: Refractive Error

Erick D. Bothun, MD, FAAP
Associate Professor
Departments of Ophthalmology and
  Pediatrics
University of Minnesota
Minneapolis, MN
5: Molluscum Conjunctivitis With
  Associated Conjunctivitis

Yasmin Bradfield, MD, FAAP
Associate Professor, Pediatric
  Ophthalmology and Adult
  Strabismus
Department of Ophthalmology
  and Visual Sciences
University of Wisconsin–Madison
Madison, WI
83: Toxoplasmosis Chorioretinitis

Edward W. Brown, MD
Ophthalmologist, Children's
  Eye Center
San Diego, CA
56: Accommodative Esotropia

Elysa A. Brown, MD, MS
Resident, Ophthalmology
Wake Forest University Eye Center
Winston Salem, NC
56: Accommodative Esotropia

Angela N. Buffenn, MD, MPH
Assistant Professor of Clinical
  Ophthalmology
The Vision Center, Children's
  Hospital of Los Angeles
University of Southern California
  Keck School of Medicine
Los Angeles, CA
23: Dermoid Cyst

Jane C. Burns, MD
Professor, Department of Pediatrics
University of California San Diego
  School of Medicine
Rady Children's Hospital San Diego
La Jolla, CA
9: Kawasaki Disease

Carl B. Camras, MD, PhD†
15: Congenital Glaucoma

Ruben Carmona, BS
University of California San Diego
La Jolla, CA
68: Non-proliferative Diabetic
  Retinopathy

Edel M. Cosgrave, FRCOphth
Fellow in Pediatric Ophthalmology
Manchester Royal Eye Hospital
Manchester, United Kingdom
70: Neurofibromatosis
77: Sturge-Weber Syndrome
88: Venous Sinus Thrombosis

Fay Charmaine Cruz, MD, DPBO
Diplomate, Philippine Board of
  Ophthalmology
The Medical City, Pasig City
Medical Specialist I, Department of
  Health Eye Center, East Avenue
  Medical Center
Assistant Professor, University of
  the East Ramon Magsaysay Medical
  Memorial Hospital
Manila, Philippines
81: Marfan Syndrome

Tinny T. Dinh, MD, MS
Ophthalmologist
Glendale, CA
18: Ptosis

Arlene V. Drack, MD
Ronald V. Keech Associate Professor
  of Pediatric Genetic Eye Disease
Department of Ophthalmology
Department of Pediatrics
University of Iowa
Iowa City, IA
44: Traumatic Iritis

K. David Epley, MD, FAAP
Pediatric Ophthalmology
Children's Eye Care, PLLC
Evergreen Hospital Medical Center
Kirkland, WA
Swedish Hospital and Medical Center
Seattle, WA
20: Epiblepharon

Henry A. Ferreyra, MD
Assistant Clinical Professor
University of California San Diego,
  Shiley Eye Center
Staff Physician, Veterans Affairs
  San Diego Healthcare System
La Jolla, CA
34: Normal Retinal Variants
38: Retinitis Pigmentosa

Brian J. Forbes, MD, PhD
Associate Professor of
  Ophthalmology
University of Pennsylvania
The Children's Hospital of
  Philadelphia
Philadelphia, PA
76: Juvenile Xanthogranuloma

David B. Granet, MD, FAAP,
   FACS, FAAO
Anne F. Ratner Professor of
   Ophthalmology and Pediatrics
Director, Divisions of Pediatric
   Ophthalmology and Eye
   Alignment Disorders
Anne F. and Abraham Ratner
   Children's Eye Center
University of California San Diego
La Jolla, CA
4: Allergic Conjunctivitis
52: Abusive Head Trauma
57: Intermittent Exotropia
84: Developmental Delay of
   Reading Skills

Christopher W. Heichel, MD
Associate Clinical Professor
University of California San Diego,
   Shiley Eye Center
La Jolla, CA
10: Herpes Simplex Virus Keratitis

Richard W. Hertle, MD, FAAP,
   FAAO, FACS
Chief of Pediatric Ophthalmology,
   Director, Children's Vision Center
Akron Children's Hospital
Professor, Department of Surgery,
   College of Medicine
Northeast Ohio Medical College
Akron, OH
61: Nystagmus
65: Amblyopia
86: Congenital Nystagmus

Irene Hsu-Dresden, MD
Pediatric Ophthalmologist
Peninsula Eye Physicians
San Mateo, CA
32: Peters Anomaly

Amy K. Hutchinson, MD
Associate Professor of Ophthalmology
Emory University School of Medicine
Atlanta, GA
47: Retinal Detachment

John T. Z. Kanegaye, MD, FAAP,
   FACEP
Attending Physician, Emergency
   Care Center
Rady Children's Hospital San Diego
Clinical Professor, Department of
   Pediatrics
University of California San Diego
   School of Medicine
La Jolla, CA
9: Kawasaki Disease

Daniel J. Karr, MD, FAAP, FAAO
Oregon Elks Professor of
   Ophthalmology
Associate Professor of Ophthalmology
   and Pediatrics
Director, Elks Children's Eye Clinic
Director, Pediatric Ophthalmology
   and Strabismus Fellowship Program
Casey Eye Institute
Oregon Health and Science University
Portland, OR
19: Chalazion/Hordeolum
26: Persistent Fetal Vasculature
28: Iris Coloboma

Daniel Kasuga, MD
University of California San Diego
La Jolla, CA
68: Non-proliferative Diabetic
   Retinopathy

Salma Khayali, MD
Pediatric Ophthalmologist
Fellow, University of California
  San Diego
San Diego, CA
69: Facioauriculovertebral Spectrum

Don O. Kikkawa, MD
Professor and Division Chief
Division of Oculofacial Plastic and
  Reconstructive Surgery
University of California San Diego
  Department of Ophthalmology
La Jolla, CA
14: Congenital Nasolacrimal Duct
  Obstruction
17: Periocular Capillary
  Hemangioma
45: Trapdoor Orbital Fracture
51: Canalicular Laceration
69: Facioauriculovertebral Spectrum

Myoung Joon Kim, MD
Associate Professor
Department of Ophthalmology,
  University of Ulsan College
  of Medicine
Asan Medical Center
Seoul, Korea
11: Corneal Abrasion
12: Corneal Foreign Body

Bobby S. Korn, MD, PhD, FACS
Associate Professor of
  Ophthalmology
University of California San Diego,
  Department of Ophthalmology
Division of Oculofacial Plastic and
  Reconstructive Surgery

La Jolla, CA
14: Congenital Nasolacrimal Duct
  Obstruction
17: Periocular Capillary
  Hemangioma
45: Trapdoor Orbital Fracture
51: Canalicular Laceration
69: Facioauriculovertebral Spectrum

Igor Kozak, MD, PhD
Assistant Clinical Professor
University of California San Diego,
  Shiley Eye Center
La Jolla, CA
64: Intermediate Uveitis

G. Robert LaRoche, MD, FRCSC
Professor, Department of
  Ophthalmology and Visual
  Sciences
Dalhousie University
Halifax, Nova Scotia
Canada
41: Optic Nerve Drusen

Janet Lee, BS
University of California San Diego
La Jolla, CA
68: Non-proliferative Diabetic
  Retinopathy

**Sharon S. Lehman, MD, FAAP,
  FAAO**
Chief of Ophthalmology
Nemours Alfred I. duPont Hospital
  for Children
Wilmington, DE
Robison D. Harley MD Endowed
  Chair of Pediatric Ophthalmology

Clinical Professor of Ophthalmology
and Pediatrics
Jefferson Medical College
Philadelphia, PA
Assistant Surgeon
Wills Eye Hospital
Philadelphia, PA
80: Stevens-Johnson Syndrome/
Toxic Epidermal Necrolysis

Alex V. Levin, MD, MHSc, FAAP
Chief, Pediatric Ophthalmology
and Ocular Genetics
Wills Eye Institute
Professor, Department of
Ophthalmology, Department
of Pediatrics
Philadelphia, PA
52: Abusive Head Trauma
75: Sickle Cell Retinopathy

**Steven J. Lichtenstein, MD, FAAP,
FACS, FAAO**
Associate Professor of Clinical
Surgery and Pediatrics
University of Illinois College of
Medicine at Peoria and Chicago
Pediatric Ophthalmology, Illinois
Eye Center
Peoria, IL
31: Corneal Ulcer

**I. Christopher Lloyd, MB, BS, DO,
FRCS, FRCOphth**
Consultant Pediatric
Ophthalmologist
Manchester Royal Eye Hospital

Honorary Senior Lecturer,
University of Manchester
Manchester, United Kindgom
88: Venous Sinus Thrombosis

Jena Mills, BA
Medical Student
Keck School of Medicine at
University of Southern California
Los Angeles, CA
6: Chronic Blepharitis With
Associated Conjunctivitis

Monte Dean Mills, MD
Director, Division of Ophthalmology
Children's Hospital of Philadelphia
Associate Professor, University of
Pennsylvania School of Medicine
Philadelphia, PA
7: Acute Anterior Uveitis Iritis

Andrea D. Molinari, MD
Pediatric Ophthalmology
Hospital Metropolitano
Quito, Ecuador
South America
53: Traumatic Periorbital
Ecchymosis

Will Moore, BSC, FRCOphth
Consultant Paediatric
Ophthalmologist
Great Ormand Street Hospital for
Children NHS Foundation Trust
London, United Kingdom
30: Anisocoria

Jenille M. Narvaez
Medical Student
University of California San
  Francisco
San Francisco, CA
33: Aniridia

Lynnelle Smith Newell, MD
Associate Physician
Kaiser Permanente
Bakersfield, CA
17: Periocular Capillary
  Hemangioma
45: Trapdoor Orbital Fracture

Ken K. Nischal, FRCOphth
Professor of Ophthalmology,
  University of Pittsburgh School
  of Medicine
UPMC Eye Center, Children's
  Hospital of Pittsburgh of UPMC
Director, Pediatric Ophthalmology
  Strabismus and Adult Motility
Pittsburgh, PA
Honorary Consultant
Great Ormand Street Hospital
  for Children
Honorary Senior Lecturer
Developmental Biology
Institute of Child Health
London, United Kingdom
30: Anisocoria

Mary O'Hara, MD, FAAP
Professor, Departments of
  Ophthalmology and Pediatrics
University of California, Davis
Sacramento, CA
22: Rhabdomyosarcoma

Christina M. Ohnsman, MD
Department of Ophthalmology
The Reading Hospital and Medical Center
Reading, PA
16: Orbital Cellulitis

Scott E. Olitsky, MD
Professor of Ophthalmology
Children's Mercy Hospitals and Clinics
University of Missouri–Kansas City
  School of Medicine
Kansas City, MO
82: Leukemia

Cameron F. Parsa, MD
Associate Professor of Ophthalmology
Department of Ophthalmology
  and Visual Sciences
University of Wisconsin School of
  Medicine and Public Health–Madison
Madison, WI
42: Papillorenal Syndrome

David A. Plager, MD, FAAP
Professor and Director
Section of Pediatric Ophthalmology
Indiana University Medical Center
Indianapolis, IN
21: Neuroblastoma

Zane F. Pollard, MD
Pediatric Ophthalmology and Strabismus
Eye Consultants of Atlanta, PC
Atlanta, GA
43: Ocular Toxocariasis

Michael X. Repka, MD, MBA
Professor of Ophthalmology
Professor of Pediatrics
The Johns Hopkins University
Baltimore, MD
37: Pseudotumor Cerebri

Ronald Antonio N. Reyna, MD
Pediatric Ophthalmology
St. Luke's Medical Center, Philippines
University of the East Ramon
 Magsaysay Memorial Medical
 Center, Philippines
Clinica Henson, Philippines
71: Familial Dysautonomia/
 Riley-Day Syndrome
72: Ocular Albinism

**Adele Marie Mediano Roa, MD,
 DPBO**
Staff Physician, Pediatric
 Ophthalmology and Strabismus
Chong Hua Eye Institute, Chong Hua
 Hospital, Cebu City, Philippines
Fellow, University of California
 San Diego
La Jolla, CA
54: Pseudoesotropia
57: Intermittent Exotropia
58: Third Cranial Nerve Palsy
59: Congenital Fourth Cranial
 Nerve Palsy

Shira L. Robbins, MD, FAAP, FAAO
Associate Clinical Professor
Division of Pediatric Ophthalmology
 and Eye Alignment Disorders
Anne F. and Abraham Ratner
 Children's Eye Center
University of California San Diego
La Jolla, CA
1: Neonatal Conjunctivitis
2: Adenoviral Conjunctivitis
6: Chronic Blepharitis With
 Associated Conjunctivitis
14: Congenital Nasolacrimal Duct
 Obstruction

15: Congenital Glaucoma
33: Aniridia
39: Retinopathy of Prematurity
54: Pseudoesotropia
55: Infantile Esotropia
57: Intermittent Exotropia
58: Third Cranial Nerve Palsy
59: Congenital Fourth Cranial
 Nerve Palsy
69: Facioauriculovertebral Spectrum

Arthur L. Rosenbaum, MD[†]
Brindell and Milton Gottlieb
Professor of Pediatric Ophthalmology
Vice-Chairman, Department of
 Ophthalmology
Chief, Pediatric Ophthalmology
 and Strabismus Division
David Geffen School of Medicine
 at University of California
 Los Angeles
Department of Ophthalmology
Jules Stein Eye Institute,
 University of California Los Angeles
Los Angeles, CA
63: Duane Syndrome

James B. Ruben, MD, FAAP
Pediatric Ophthalmologist
The Permanente Medical Group
Roseville, CA
Clinical Professor of Ophthalmology,
 University of California, Davis
Sacramento, CA
25: Congenital Cataracts

Tina Rutar, MD
Assistant Professor
University of California San Francisco
San Francisco, CA
50: Ruptured Globe

Donald P. Sauberan, MD
Pediatric Ophthalmologist
Eye Surgical Associates
Lincoln, NE
82: Leukemia

David J. Schanzlin, MD
Gordon-Weiss-Schanzlin Vision
   Institute
San Diego, CA
11: Corneal Abrasion
12: Corneal Foreign Body

Terry Schwartz, MD
Professor, Division of Ophthalmology
Director, Low Vision Rehabilitation
   Program
Pediatric Ophthalmology & Adult
   Strabismus
Cincinnati Children's Hospital
   Medical Center
Cincinnati, OH
36: Hydrocephalus

Jean Shein, MD, FAAO
Director of Pediatric Ophthalmology
Eye Care Center of Kauai
Lihue, HI
49: Thermal Injury

Carol L. Shields, MD
Codirector, Oncology Service
Wills Eye Institute
Professor of Ophthalmology
Thomas Jefferson University Hospital
Philadelphia, PA
24: Retinoblastoma

Jerry A. Shields, MD
Director, Oncology Service
Wills Eye Institute
Professor of Ophthalmology
Thomas Jefferson University
   Hospital
Philadelphia, PA
24: Retinoblastoma

Ryan W. Shultz, MD
Department of Ophthalmology
Mayo Clinic
Rochester, MN
36: Hydrocephalus

Sorath Noorani Siddiqui, FCPS
Consultant Pediatric
   Ophthalmologist
Clinical Fellow, Pediatric
   Ophthalmology and Strabismus
Head of Department, Pediatric
   Ophthalmology and Strabismus
Al Shifa Trust Eye Hospital,
   Rawalpindi
Rawalpindi, Punjab, Pakistan
75: Sickle Cell Retinopathy

Lance M. Siegel, MD, FAAP, FAAO
Director, Children's Eye Institute
Upland, CA
39: Retinopathy of Prematurity
73: Down Syndrome

John W. Simon, MD
Professor and Chairman,
   Department of Ophthalmology
Professor of Pediatrics
Albany Medical College
Albany, NY
78: Juvenile Idiopathic Arthritis

David Stager, Jr, MD, FAAP, FACS
Pediatric Ophthalmology and
 Adult Strabismus
Plano, TX
Assistant Clinical Professor of
 Ophthalmology
University of Texas Southwestern
 Medical Center
Dallas, TX
87: Myasthenia Gravis

Sri Thyagarajan, MRCOphth, BSc
74: Pigmentary Retinopathy

Benjamin H. Ticho, MD
Associate Professor
University of Illinois at Chicago
 Eye and Ear Infirmary
Chicago, IL
60: Sixth Cranial Nerve Palsy

Elias I. Traboulsi, MD
Professor of Ophthalmology
Cleveland Clinic Lerner
  College of Medicine of Case
  Western Reserve University
Director, Department of Pediatric
 Ophthalmology
Director, Center for Genetic
 Eye Diseases
Cleveland Clinic Cole Eye Institute
Cleveland, OH
40: Leber Congenital Amaurosis

Anya A. Trumler, MD
Assistant Professor
Wilmer Eye Institute, The Johns
 Hopkins Hospital
Baltimore, MD
15: Congenital Glaucoma

Deborah K. VanderVeen, MD, FAAP
Associate in Ophthalmology,
 Associate Professor of Ophthal-
 mology, Harvard Medical School
Boston Children's Hospital
Boston, MA
27: Heterochromia Iridis
29: Conjunctival Nevus

Federico G. Velez, MD
Assistant Clinical Professor of
 Ophthalmology
David Geffen School of Medicine
 at University of California
 Los Angeles
Department of Ophthalmology
Jules Stein Eye Institute, University
 of California Los Angeles
Los Angeles, CA
Physician Specialist, Olive View–
 University of California Los
 Angeles Medical Center
Sylmar, CA
63: Duane Syndrome

**Anthony J. Vivian, FRCS,
 FRCOphth**
Consultant Paediatric
 Ophthalmologist
Cambridge University Hospitals
Cambridge, United Kingdom
70: Neurofibromatosis
74: Pigmentary Retinopathy
77: Sturge-Weber Syndrome

Xiaolei Wang, MD
University of California San Diego
La Jolla, CA
68: Non-proliferative Diabetic
 Retinopathy

David R. Weakley, MD
Professor of Ophthalmology
University of Texas Southwestern
  Medical Center
Director of Pediatric Ophthalmology
Children's Medical Center
Dallas, TX
13: Acute Dacryocystitis
46: Orbital Floor Fracture
48: Hyphema

Oren L. Weisberg, MD, MA
Pediatric Ophthalmology and
  Strabismus
D'Ambrosio Eye Care
Courtesy Staff, Boston Children's
  Hospital
Lancaster, MA
8: Subconjunctival Hemorrhage

Avery H. Weiss, MD
Chief, Division of Ophthalmology
Seattle Children's Hospital
Professor of Ophthalmology
Affiliate Professor, Department
  of Pediatrics
University of Washington School
  of Medicine
Seattle, WA
35: Optic Neuritis
66: Visual Inattention

David T. Wheeler, MD, MCR, FAAP
Affiliate Associate Professor of
  Ophthalmology and Pediatrics
Oregon Health and Science University
Portland, OR
Pediatric Ophthalmology, Child Eye
  Care Associates
Lake Oswego, OR
32: Peters Anomaly

Katherine M. Whipple, MD
Clinical Instructor
Division of Oculofacial Plastic and
  Reconstructive Surgery
University of California San Diego
  Department of Ophthalmology
La Jolla, CA
51: Canalicular Laceration

M. Edward Wilson, MD
Professor of Ophthalmology and
  Pediatrics
N. Edgar Miles Endowed Chair
Department of Ophthalmology
Albert Florens Storm Eye Institute,
  Medical University of South
  Carolina
Charleston, SC
79: Cerebral Palsy

Kenneth W. Wright, MD, FAAP
Medical Director
Wright Foundation for Pediatric
  Ophthalmology and Strabismus
Los Angeles, CA
18: Ptotis

Sara Yoon, MD
Ophthalmologist
Roseville, CA
10: Herpes Simplex Virus Keratitis

Kang Zhang, MD, PhD
Professor of Ophthalmology
University of California San Diego
La Jolla, CA
68: Non-proliferative Diabetic
  Retinopathy

†Deceased

To Leslie Julia "Julie" Baber (1971–2009),

our fellow and more importantly, our friend. Julie inspired

and initiated this text; its completion is a tangible manifestation

of her commitment to making a difference in the lives of

children, despite a career and life cut much too short.

For Julie, her memory, and her husband and family—

you will be thought of often and remembered always.

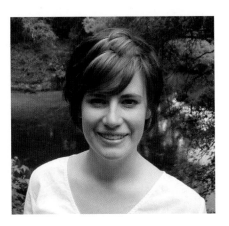

Table of Contents by Symptom*

*Table of Contents by Condition included as Appendix A (page 609).

Acknowledgments

We are deeply grateful to our colleagues who took on the chapters in this text, as well as the instructors, referring pediatricians, and students who have affected our understanding of how best to teach over the years. It is impossible to acknowledge all of these persons individually, but each should know that we are deeply aware of the value of their contributions.

The children who are represented in this book enable readers to learn and therefore help other children. We thank these children and their families for participating in this project.

Jo Adamcik and Terri Spano, administrative assistants extraordinaire from the University of California, San Diego, along with Eileen Glasstetter and Martha Cook from the American Academy of Pediatrics editorial office, deserve special mention for being the midwives attending the birth of this text.

Personal Acknowledgments

David B. Granet, MD: To my amazing wife Lisa: I have not enough words to adequately express the depth of my feelings; only because of the love and understanding you unselfishly give has our family been strong enough to allow me to edit a text that helps other people's children. To my children, Elijah, Isaiah, and Ezra: Grandpa once wrote, "I hope one day you'll understand why the time Dad took to write this book was not spent with you," and I'll say the same. Dad, I do understand, and I have passed along your love to my boys. To my parents, Arlene and Irving Granet: thanks for the greatest childhood a son could hope for; Mom, I have never forgotten any of it.

Shira L. Robbins, MD: To my beloved husband Peter, who makes everything possible: you are my rock. To my daughters Johana and Lily, whose love and ridiculous cuteness bring me joy every day: when you grow up I hope you find a profession that is as fulfilling to you as being a pediatric ophthalmologist is to me. Finally, to my parents, Saundra and Robby, and my sister Marlie: you said I could do anything, and I believed you.

Preface

Why this book? Why now? Why by these writers?

Learning via case studies is a classic and important part of the ongoing education of physicians. The American Academy of Pediatrics (AAP) has embarked on creating a series of subspecialty-based texts just for this purpose. But pediatric ophthalmology is different. This specialty is reached via ophthalmology training followed by a fellowship, not traditional pediatric training. That leaves pediatricians as the physicians expected to identify and coordinate care in a field where the referral goes to an MD who did not "grow up" as a pediatrician.

Every pediatrician office faces ocular problems regularly. How can you tell when decreased vision is because of the need for glasses or uveitis? How does one distinguish an inflamed eye from an allergy or Kawasaki disease? What do you do when there is ocular trauma or an abnormal red reflex? When to refer, treat, or observe are questions that pediatricians ask routinely.

To bridge this gap, we have asked many of the top pediatric ophthalmologists to contribute short, easily readable cases representative of the types of problems that will face pediatricians each week. While not a photographic atlas, the included representative images will be invaluable for the pediatrician. More detail has been included in discussion sections to augment the learning process. Via editing, we have taken many dissimilar voices and put them into a standard, easy-to-read format without losing the individuality of each writer. After review by the physician editors, AAP medical editors combed through the copy to ensure synergy with current medical knowledge and AAP guidelines. What you hold in your hand is unique.

As members of the AAP Section on Ophthalmology, the editors are passionate about physicians sharing information with one another. To better care for our precious patients, the generalist and the specialist need to learn more from each other. Had this book been about croup, we'd be the ones reading!

The story of this text goes deeper and is even more personal. It was begun by our beloved fellow Leslie Julia "Julie" Baber, MD, and finished by us after her passing; you will find a little bit of love in every chapter. No one could meet Julie and not be touched by her honest voice and caring heart. The chapter authors all were originally contacted by her and committed to this project while she headed it—none complained during the delays incurred while she underwent treatments. Julie's husband Ronan, a model of graciousness and loving dedication, has chosen to donate royalty proceeds to The Julie Baber Educational Fund stewarded by the University of California, San Diego (UCSD) Abraham Ratner Children's Eye Center. He ensures that the knowledge in this book helps in multiple ways. For more information about this fund, contact Karen Anisko Ryan, UCSD Shiley Eye Center, 9415 Campus Point Dr, Room 241B, La Jolla, CA 92093-0946; 858/534-8017; kanisko@ucsd.edu.

David B. Granet, MD, FAAP, FACS, FAAO

Shira L. Robbins, MD, FAAP, FAAO

Diagram of the Eye

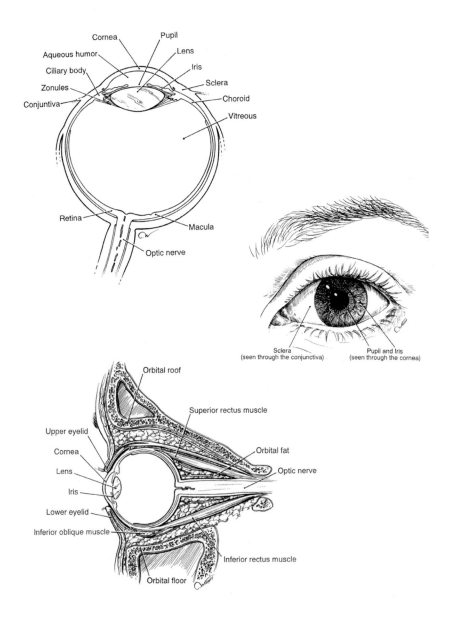

Reproduced with permission from Simon JW, Calhoun JH, eds. *A Child's Eyes: A Guide to Pediatric Primary Care.* Gainesville, FL: Triad Publishing Company; 1998.

Section 1

Red Eye

Chapter 1

Newborn With Ocular Discharge

Leslie Julia Baber, MD
Shira L. Robbins, MD

Presentation

A 6-day-old boy is seen in his pediatrician's office because he has discharge from both eyes. The newborn's mother reports that the problem began 1 day earlier, 2 days after his first well-baby visit.

On examination, the newborn has thick, purulent discharge from both eyes. There is moderate swelling of the eyelids but no lesions on the eyelids. The conjunctiva is moderately injected. Despite the thick discharge (Figure 1-1), the corneas appear clear. The newborn is afebrile and otherwise appears well. Remaining findings of the physical examination are normal.

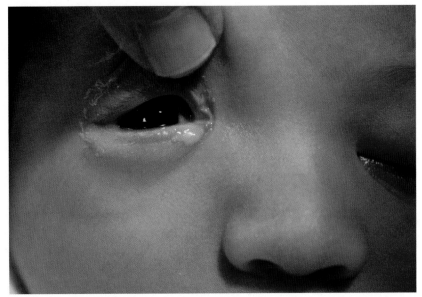

Figure 1-1. Newborn with thick, yellow discharge and eyelid swelling. Courtesy of Shira L. Robbins, MD.

History shows that the patient was born full term via vaginal delivery and there were no known complications during pregnancy or delivery. However, the mother received prenatal care on an irregular basis.

The newborn is sent to the emergency department for evaluation by a pediatric ophthalmologist because of his age and concern regarding the offending pathogen involving the cornea or other organ systems. The same physical findings noted by the pediatrician are present. No preauricular lymphadenopathy is present. After staining the corneas with fluorescein for slit-lamp examination, the pediatric ophthalmologist finds no epithelial defects. Also with the portable slit lamp, the ophthalmologist sees no follicles on the conjunctiva. Cultures of conjunctival scrapings, specimens for Gram and Giemsa stains, and a rapid *Chlamydia* test are ordered.

Diagnosis

The newborn has ophthalmia neonatorum (neonatal conjunctivitis). The differential diagnosis of discharge from one or both eyes of a newborn also includes nasolacrimal duct obstruction and dacryocystitis.

Ophthalmia neonatorum refers to conjunctivitis that develops in the first month of life. It may be infectious or noninfectious. The noninfectious form of conjunctivitis usually manifests within the first 24 hours of life and resolves spontaneously within a day or so. Classically, noninfectious cases were caused by chemical prophylaxis with silver nitrate. However, in the United States this regimen has been replaced, typically with topical erythromycin or tetracycline, therefore reducing the incidence of chemically induced neonatal conjunctivitis. Infectious causes include *Neisseria gonorrhoeae, Chlamydia trachomatis,* other bacteria, and herpes simplex virus (HSV). Onset of *Neisseria* neonatal conjunctivitis typically occurs within several days of birth. Eyelid swelling is marked, and generally there is copious purulent discharge. This type of conjunctivitis may involve the cornea and may progress rapidly to corneal perforation. Chlamydial conjunctivitis generally presents slightly later (usually within 5 to 14 days of birth) and has a milder clinical course. The conjunctivitis itself is self-limited, but a substantial percentage of affected newborns will experience chlamydial pneumonia within 3 months of age.

Nongonococcal bacterial conjunctivitis has a variable presentation. Management depends on severity at presentation. Herpetic neonatal conjunctivitis typically presents within the first 2 weeks of life. Vesicular skin lesions may or may not be present. Disseminated neonatal HSV has a mortality rate of up to 85%, and ocular involvement may precede or follow dermal and systemic manifestations.

Differential Diagnosis

Diagnoses besides neonatal conjunctivitis that should be considered include the following:

Nasolacrimal Duct Obstruction

The discharge is typically more mucoid than in neonatal conjunctivitis, and the conjunctiva and eyelids are minimally affected, if at all (Figure 1-2).

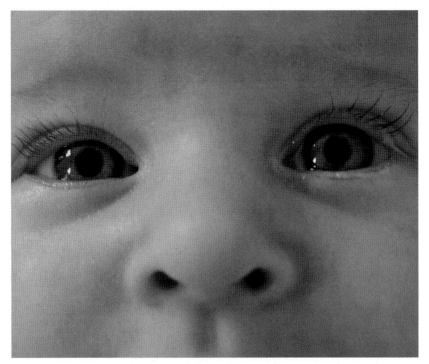

Figure 1-2. Nasolacrimal duct obstruction, left eye, with tearing and mucoid discharge. Courtesy of Shira L. Robbins, MD.

Dacryocystitis

The swelling and erythema are located over the medial canthal area, and discharge often is expressed from the punctum by rolling a finger over the swelling toward the eyeball.

Congenital Glaucoma

Discharge and eyelid involvement are rarely seen. The clinical triad of tearing, photophobia, and blepharospasm are typical with enlargement of the globe and high intraocular pressures.

When to Refer

Referral for testing to determine the causative agent is needed when symptoms persist more than 24 hours or in cases of copious discharge. In this case, the gram-negative intracellular diplococci strongly suggest *N gonorrhoeae* as the infective agent. The Giemsa stain did not show intracytoplasmic inclusion bodies in the cells from the conjunctival scrapings, which, if they had been present, would be consistent with *C trachomatis*. Cultures were negative.

Treatment

Prompt treatment of gonococcal conjunctivitis is essential to avoid the complication of a corneal ulcer and rapid progression to corneal perforation, which can result in blindness. Treatment of *N gonorrhoeae* conjunctivitis is on an inpatient basis, with intravenous (IV) or intra-muscular ceftriaxone sodium as the antibiotic of choice. Irrigation of the cornea and topical antibiotics also are used.

If the causative agent was *Chlamydia,* treatment would involve erythro-mycin orally for 2 to 3 weeks in addition to topical therapy. Treatment of nongonococcal and non-chlamydial bacterial conjunctivitis without corneal involvement is performed in an outpatient facility and is topical; the patient should be admitted to the hospital only if there is corneal involvement. Treatment of herpetic conjunctivitis is admission for administration of IV acyclovir and ocular topical antiviral agents.

No treatment is needed for chemical conjunctivitis, as it resolves spontaneously within days.

Discussion

Without prompt diagnosis and treatment of neonatal conjunctivitis, serious complications can occur. Neonatal conjunctivitis caused by an infectious agent can result in blindness. *N gonorrhoeae*, for example, can penetrate an intact cornea. The underlying infection also can lead to severe systemic sequelae and even death.

In most cases, neonatal conjunctivitis responds to appropriate treatment and prognosis is good. Newborns should be monitored for the development of a secondary infection, such as pneumonia, in the case of chlamydial conjunctivitis.

When the causative agent is a sexually transmitted infection, the newborn's mother and partners should be referred for treatment as well.

Key Points

- Prompt diagnosis and treatment of neonatal conjunctivitis are necessary to prevent serious complications due to the underlying infection, such as blindness, systemic sequelae, and even death.
- For gonorrheal and chlamydial infections, mothers and their partners also need treatment.

Suggested Reading

Gomi CF, Robbins SL, Heichel CW, Gross RD, Granet DB. Conjunctival diseases. In: Nelson LB, Olitsky SE, eds. *Harley's Pediatric Ophthalmology.* Philadelphia, PA: Lippincott Williams and Wilkins; 2005:201–216

Chapter 2

Red, Watery Eye

Leslie Julia Baber, MD
Shira L. Robbins, MD

Presentation

A 10-year-old girl presents to the pediatrician's office because she has been sent home from school by the school nurse due to "pinkeye." She has had an itchy, burning left eye since yesterday. Her mother states that she had a sore throat last week. Several other children in her class have also had "a pinkeye."

On examination, a well-appearing child has an injected (red) left eye, with mild swelling of the upper and lower eyelids (Figure 2-1). There is a watery, nonpurulent discharge from the eye, with crusting in the eyelashes. There is no staining of the cornea with instillation of fluorescein. The right eye appears normal. An enlarged left preauricular lymph node can be palpated. The remaining findings of the physical examination are normal.

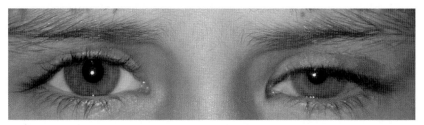

Figure 2-1. Injected left eye with mild eyelid swelling. Courtesy of Shira L. Robbins, MD.

Diagnosis

The pediatrician diagnoses the child with likely adenoviral conjunctivitis and explains to the parent that antibiotics are not indicated to treat this kind of infection. Artificial tears and cool compresses to the eyes are recommended for comfort. After counseling them about the importance of good hygiene to prevent spread to other members of the household, the pediatrician recommends that the girl stay home from school until the symptoms subside.

Her mother calls 2 weeks later. Her symptoms spread to the right eye several days after her last visit, and she is now complaining of a sandy feeling in the eyes, blurred vision, and light sensitivity. An appointment is scheduled for her to see a pediatric ophthalmologist.

The ophthalmologist sees the patient the next day. Her visual acuity is 20/30 in the right eye and 20/40 in the left. Both eyes are moderately injected, but there is no eyelid swelling at this time. On slit-lamp microscopic examination, the ophthalmologist sees small white spots (subepithelial corneal infiltrates), more in the left eye than the right, with punctate epithelial defects overlying the infiltrates. The eye examination yields otherwise normal results.

Differential diagnosis of a red eye is extensive. When the red eye is accompanied by itching, burning, and discharge, the differential is more limited and includes allergic, bacterial, and viral conjunctivitis; trauma (especially in a child unable or unwilling to give an accurate history); and foreign body. In this case, the history of recent pharyngitis and other similarly affected children in the girl's class and the finding of the preauricular lymph node make the diagnosis of adenoviral conjunctivitis the most likely. Adenovirus can also present as a hemorrhagic conjunctivitis.

Other viruses that can cause conjunctivitis include measles, mumps, Epstein-Barr virus, molluscum contagiosum, herpes simplex virus, and rarely in children, herpes zoster virus.

When seeing a patient with an injected eye, the pediatrician always needs to examine the cornea well. It should be stained with fluorescein to rule out the possibility of herpetic infection, corneal abrasion, and corneal ulcer. The eyelids should also be examined well for any lesions indicating trauma or herpes and should be everted to look for a hidden foreign body.

Cultures are generally not indicated unless there is substantial discharge or symptoms do not resolve as expected. Despite all of this, a narrowed differential diagnosis can be difficult to create because in actual presentation, there is much overlap among the diseases.

Symptoms often worsen in the affected eye over the first several days. It is also common for the infection to spread to the second eye. With adenoviral conjunctivitis it is also not uncommon to develop an immunologic response that leads to infiltration of white blood cells under the corneal epithelium. This condition causes increased discomfort and light sensitivity.

Differential Diagnosis

Diagnoses besides adenoviral conjunctivitis that should be considered for a red eye include the following:

Allergic Conjunctivitis

Itching, burning, and watery or mucous discharge accompany eye redness, and symptoms are usually bilateral. One would not find an enlarged preauricular lymph node. One would also expect "hay fever" symptoms, rather than an antecedent upper respiratory tract infection.

Bacterial Conjunctivitis

If the discharge were purulent, bacterial conjunctivitis would be higher in the differential diagnosis.

Trauma or Foreign Body

Itching, burning, and discharge may accompany a red eye. This diagnosis should be considered, especially in a child unable or unwilling to give an accurate history.

When to Refer

If patients with suspected adenoviral conjunctivitis complain of pain and light sensitivity, or if the condition does not resolve within 1 or 2 weeks, referral to an ophthalmologist is indicated.

Treatment

In this case, the ophthalmologist begins treatment with topical steroids in both eyes and schedules a follow-up appointment in 1 week.

Initial treatment of viral conjunctivitis is supportive. Cool compresses to the eyes and artificial teardrops, as needed, will help with discomfort. Because adenoviral conjunctivitis is highly contagious, hygiene is crucial to prevent spreading. Pediatricians should counsel patients to wash their hands frequently, avoid touching the eyes, avoid sharing of towels, and so on. Patients also should be warned that their symptoms may worsen over the first several days or that the infection may spread to the other eye.

The 2012 American Academy of Pediatrics *Red Book* advises a policy of school attendance as follows: "Except when viral or bacterial conjunctivitis is accompanied by systemic signs of illness, infected children should be allowed to remain in school once any indicated therapy is implemented, unless their behavior is such that close contact with other students cannot be avoided."

If patients complain of pain and light sensitivity, referral to an ophthalmologist is indicated. If subepithelial infiltrates have developed and symptoms are severe, they will be treated with topical corticosteroids, assuming there are no contraindications. Topical steroids have, however, been shown to prolong the period of viral shedding. Because topical steroids have potential devastating visual side effects, they should be prescribed only by an ophthalmologist who can monitor for the development of these side effects.

Discussion

Adenovirus infection is the most common cause of viral conjunctivitis but not the most common cause of routine pinkeye that makes it to the pediatrician's office—bacterial conjunctivitis is. Separating those entities can often be challenging.

> ## Key Points
> - Many conditions may present like viral conjunctivitis, including allergic and bacterial conjunctivitis.
> - If the condition is not resolving, referral to an ophthalmologist is indicated.
> - Topical corticosteroids should be prescribed only by an ophthalmologist. Failure to monitor for vision-threatening side effects is malpractice.

Suggested Reading

American Academy of Pediatrics. Infections spread by direct contact. In: Pickering LK, Baker CJ, Kimberlin DW, Long SS, eds. *Red Book: 2012 Report of the Committee on Infectious Diseases.* 29th ed. Elk Grove Village, IL: American Academy of Pediatrics; 2012:156

O'Brien TP, Jeng BH, McDonald M, Raizman MB. Acute conjunctivitis: truth and misconceptions. *Curr Med Res Opin.* 2009;25(8):1953–1961

Wagner RS, Aquino M. Pediatric ocular inflammation. *Immunol Allergy Clin North Am.* 2008;28(1):169–188

Chapter 3

Red Eye With Mucopurulent Discharge

Leslie Julia Baber, MD

Presentation

A father brings his 3-year-old daughter to the office urgently on a Monday morning after she was sent home from child care because of a "red, goopy eye" (Figure 3-1). The father states that the eye was crusted shut this morning and he had to use a damp washcloth to clean it off before she could open it. It was a little crusty Sunday morning but has definitely worsened. She has not been otherwise ill, and the father is unaware of any contact she has had with other people with red eyes.

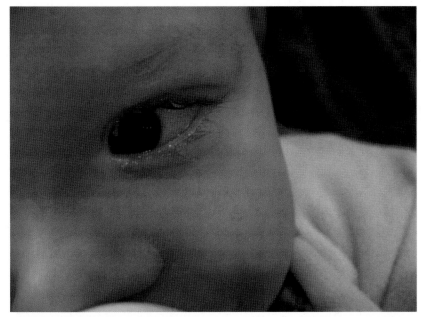

Figure 3-1. Mild conjunctival injection and mucopurulent discharge. Representative photo courtesy of David B. Granet, MD.

On examination, she has moderate injection (redness) and chemosis (excessive edema of the ocular conjunctiva) of the right eye with a mucopurulent discharge on the ocular surface and in the eyelashes. Her right upper and lower eyelids are mildly swollen, but there are no lesions. After instillation of fluorescein, it appears as if there may be an epithelial defect, but after the child blinks, the stained area moves to a different spot, showing that it is just mucus. The covering pediatrician is confident that the cornea is unaffected. A preauricular lymph node cannot be palpated. The ears and throat are normal. The remaining findings of the physical examination are normal as well.

Diagnosis

Purulent discharge is indicative of bacterial conjunctivitis, which this child has. One study found that the most predictive physical findings for bacterial conjunctivitis are matted sticky eyelids and mucoid or purulent discharge.

If there is acute onset of copious discharge, one must consider gonococcal disease. Preauricular lymphadenopathy is generally found with gonococcal or viral conjunctivitis. Gonococcus may infect the cornea and is one of the few infections that can cause corneal perforation rapidly, so it is crucial to examine the cornea well. If *Neisseria gonorrhoeae* is suspected, one should perform a Gram stain immediately, looking for the organism. Cultures and sensitivity analyses should also be performed. However, this child's cornea appears normal, so there is no need.

When gonococcal infection is not suspected, Gram stain, culture, and sensitivity analyses should be performed in severe cases but are generally otherwise omitted. Bacterial conjunctivitis is the most common cause of conjunctivitis in children who come to medical attention. In a 2007 study, 78% of the children with an emergency department diagnosis of conjunctivitis had culture-positive bacterial conjunctivitis. *Haemophilus influenzae* accounted for 82% of these bacterial infections, and 32% of these children had conjunctivitis-otitis syndrome. Most studies evaluating bacterial conjunctivitis in the pediatrician's office confirm it is a gram-positive disease, especially including *Streptococcus pneumoniae*.

Unilateral conjunctivitis is a red flag in the differential diagnosis. Uveitis and herpes ocular infections are more likely to occur in one eye, whereas viral, bacterial, and allergic conjunctivitis are generally bilateral.

Differential Diagnosis

Diagnoses besides bacterial conjunctivitis that should be considered include the following:

Viral Conjunctivitis

Generally bilateral, viral conjunctivitis typically presents with a watery, nonpurulent discharge in addition to eye redness; preauricular lymphadenopathy; and no itching. There may be a history of an upper respiratory tract infection.

Allergic Conjunctivitis

Itching, burning, and watery or mucous discharge accompany eye redness, and symptoms are usually bilateral. There is no preauricular lymphadenopathy. Symptoms of "hay fever" are present.

Uveitis

In this deep eye inflammation, a red eye typically is accompanied by pain, blurred vision, and light sensitivity, features that are rarely part of conjunctivitis.

Ocular Herpes

The most common ocular manifestation of herpes simplex virus is a blepharoconjunctivitis. However, instillation of fluorescein dye under cobalt-blue light shows a bright-green staining pattern that corresponds to a branching corneal lesion.

When to Refer

If patients do not respond to appropriate antibiotic treatment as quickly as expected (preferably within 2 to 3 days), they should be referred to an ophthalmologist for evaluation of a more severe infection, such as herpetic infection, or uveitis. The sooner this is identified, the better. A child suspected of having gonococcal conjunctivitis should be referred to an ophthalmologist.

Treatment

For nongonococcal bacterial conjunctivitis, as in this case, empiric therapy with topical broad-spectrum antibiotics is indicated to shorten the course of this self-limited disease. Cultures are not needed for the routine presenting disease because the offending bacteria are well known. Morbidity to the child, limitation of contagion, more rapid diagnosis of masquerade diseases, and economic benefit to the family, parents, and school system all strongly warrant the shortest treatment. A recent report indicated that with fourth-generation fluoroquinolones, the infection can usually be cured within 2 days. Fortunately, there has been no evidence that the use of these medications causes resistance or safety issues. The *Sanford Guide to Antimicrobial Therapy* agrees and recommends use of fourth-generation antimicrobials as first-line treatment.

From a practical standpoint, return to school or out-of-home child care can occur after 24 hours of treatment with a rapid-acting, broad-spectrum bacteriocidal antibiotic. Local school rules may require additional time off regardless of the antibiotic chosen. Recommendations from the 2012 American Academy of Pediatrics *Red Book* are as follows: "Except when viral or bacterial conjunctivitis is accompanied by systemic signs of illness, infected children should be allowed to remain in school once any indicated therapy is implemented, unless their behavior is such that close contact with other students cannot be avoided." The *Red Book* also states that "Most minor illnesses do not constitute a reason for excluding a child from child care." It goes on to list conjunctivitis without fever and without behavioral change as one of the minor illnesses not requiring exclusion from out-of-home child care. It adds, however, "...if 2 or more children in a group care setting develop conjunctivitis in the same period, seek advice from the program's health consultant or public health authority." For this reason, limitation of contagion is important.

If the conjunctivitis appears atypical, modification of treatment may be needed based on cultures and sensitivity analyses. Patients should be seen again in several days if there has been no improvement while receiving treatment.

Gonococcal conjunctivitis requires systemic and topical antibiotics and may require hospitalization. Ophthalmologic consultation should be obtained to thoroughly examine and monitor the cornea if this organism is suspected. Patients with gonococcal conjunctivitis should be followed up daily until resolution.

Additionally, *H influenzae* may also require systemic and topical antibiotics if conjunctivitis-otitis syndrome is suspected.

Discussion

Bacterial conjunctivitis is the most common cause of conjunctivitis in children. It generally will resolve even without treatment over a period of about 2 weeks. Treatment is to limit morbidity to the child, speed return to school and work (for the parent), prevent contagion, and identify masquerade disease. As such, the purpose of treatment is to shorten the course of disease, which is thus cost-effective at the same time.

Key Points

- Gonococcal conjunctivitis past the neonatal period is suggestive of sexual activity or abuse.
- Empiric therapy with a rapid-acting, bacteriocidal, broad-spectrum antibiotic can begin without obtaining cultures.
- Conjunctivitis that does not respond to empiric therapy must be reevaluated.

Suggested Reading

American Academy of Pediatrics. Infections spread by direct contact. In: Pickering LK, Baker CJ, Kimberlin DW, Long SS, eds. *Red Book: 2012 Report of the Committee on Infectious Diseases.* 29th ed. Elk Grove Village, IL: American Academy of Pediatrics; 2012:156

American Academy of Pediatrics. Recommendations for inclusion or exclusion. In: Pickering LK, Baker CJ, Kimberlin DW, Long SS, eds. *Red Book: 2012 Report of the Committee on Infectious Diseases.* 29th ed. Elk Grove Village, IL: American Academy of Pediatrics; 2012:137

Gilbert DN. *Sanford Guide to Antimicrobial Therapy 2011.* Sperryville, VA: Antimicrobial Therapy, Inc; 2011

Granet DB, Dorfman M, Stroman D, Cockrum P. A multicenter comparison of polymyxin B sulfate/trimethoprim ophthalmic solution and moxifloxacin in the speed of clinical efficacy for the treatment of bacterial conjunctivitis. *J Pediatr Ophthalmol Strabismus.* 2008;45(6):340–349

Patel PB, Diaz MC, Bennett JE, Attia MW. Clinical features of bacterial conjunctivitis in children. *Acad Emerg Med.* 2007; 14(1):1–5

Chapter 4

Itchy, Irritated Eyes

David B. Granet, MD

Presentation

On Cinco de Mayo, May 5, a family brings their 6-year-old girl to the pediatrician for evaluation of ocular irritation. From across the room the pediatrician notices that she has irritated eyes. On close observation, her conjunctiva and eyelids appear red and mildly swollen. She also has dark circles under her eyes, and the skin there is dry and flaky. She rubs her eyes and sniffles.

The patient's family history includes her father's asthma but is otherwise unremarkable. The family recently moved from San Diego. The patient's signs and symptoms began about the same time as the move. In addition, the family recently adopted a cat, and the animal and girl have been inseparable. She plays with the cat mostly in her bedroom, which has shag carpeting. She has experienced no trauma, chemical exposure, or recent upper respiratory tract infection. When she began rolling and blinking her eyes, the parents decided she needed medical attention.

On examination, mild wheezing is auscultated. Her visual acuity is 20/20 in both eyes. When the pediatrician pulls down her lower eyelids, small bumps are evident on the inner surface (Figure 4-1). On direct ophthalmoscopy, the conjunctiva and eyelids are swollen, the conjunctival vessels are enlarged, and there is increased tearing. After instillation of fluorescein dye in the eyes, a smooth green sheen is observed using a blue light called a Wood light (normal result indicating no breakdown of the epithelium). She is mildly photophobic (sensitive to light) but not out of the realm of ordinary for her age. She has no obvious "cold sores."

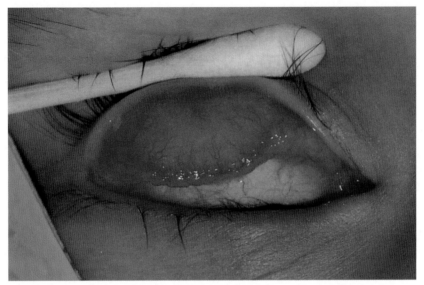

Figure 4-1. Conjunctival papillary inflammation seen most clearly at border of palpebral conjunctiva (pink) and bulbar conjunctiva (white) in photo. Courtesy of Shira L. Robbins, MD.

Diagnosis

The differential diagnosis for an irritated eye under the rubric of *conjunctivitis* is quite broad. Interestingly, the more concerning causes, such as herpes, iritis, and trauma, typically occur in only one eye. This child has both eyes involved, which do not stain on fluorescein testing; she has no substantial ocular discharge and no preauricular lymph node or antecedent upper respiratory tract infection; the pupils are normal; and she is not greatly photophobic.

The constellation of symptoms and signs indicate the patient almost certainly has allergic conjunctivitis. Itching is a cardinal symptom of allergies. A rule of thumb can be thought of as, "If it doesn't itch, it's not an allergy." Any irritated eye will tear and become injected because the eye has a limited number of responses to irritation. The infraorbital dark circles, called *allergic shiners,* are exceedingly common in allergic patients.

The environmental changes are another compelling risk factor for allergic conjunctivitis. Regions such as southern California have less seasonal plant growth and less incidence of seasonal allergic conjunctivitis. The patient's symptoms are occurring in early May, when plants begin to bloom. Also, she obtained a new cat and plays with it on shag carpeting. These represent the major environmental allergens—pollen, animal dander, and dust mites.

Differential Diagnosis

Diagnoses besides allergic conjunctivitis that should be considered include the following:

Herpes Simplex Virus

This is typically a dendritic lesion and occurs more often monocularly.

Other Viral Conjunctivitis

Features of viral conjunctivitis include an acute follicular conjunctival reaction and preauricular lymphadenopathy.

Iritis

This can occur in a quiet eye but often with photophobia and is usually monocular.

Trauma

This is typically monocular. Foreign bodies particularly can present with acute or chronic conjunctival reaction.

Bacterial Conjunctivitis

Generally bilateral with green or yellow discharge and matting of lashes. Streptococcal pneumococcus may be very contagious.

When to Refer

A referral to a specialist is not needed at this time. Should the child not improve with treatment, referral is needed to an allergist or ophthalmologist to confirm the diagnosis.

Treatment

The hallmark of treatment of allergic conjunctivitis is avoidance of the allergen. Environmental factors for this child will include not sleeping with the cat. If her symptoms persist or worsen and she has a positive skin test result for cat dander, the family may need to remove the cat from the household or not allow the cat to enter the girl's bedroom. Dust mite control includes sealing pillowcases, washing all bedding in hot water, and eliminating carpeting. Other environmental control measures include washing the girl's hair before she goes to sleep to eliminate the transfer of allergens from her hair to her bedding. Unfortunately, not all allergens can be avoided.

Other nonmedical interventions include avoidance of eye rubbing. Mechanical irritation activates the mast cell to release histamine and also causes autoinoculation of the eyes.

Medical treatment includes the use of over-the-counter antihistamine eyedrops and nonprescription oral medications. These tend, however, to be less effective than available prescription treatment. Currently available prescription topical therapies include a combination mast cell stabilizer and antihistamine. To increase patient compliance, the pediatrician should prescribe medications with the least dosing frequency possible that have good efficacy and patient tolerance data compared with alternatives. Currently, topical olopatadine hydrochloride is the most commonly prescribed treatment of allergic conjunctivitis.

Discussion

Allergic conjunctivitis is one of the most common causes of red eye. Allergies typically begin to present at around age 3 years. Elimination of the offending allergen, if possible, is the core of treatment. If that is not possible or is ineffective, topical treatment with a once-a-day combined mast cell stabilizer and antihistamine is generally the next step. If allergic disease is persisting, a pulsed treatment of topical steroids may be needed. Treatment with steroids should be instituted by an ophthalmic specialist.

Key Points

- The more worrisome causes of ocular disease typically occur in only one eye.
- A thorough history and examination can separate out the many forms of conjunctivitis.
- Allergies almost always cause itching.
- Avoidance of the allergen and elimination of eye rubbing are the first steps in management.
- Treatment is with a combination mast cell stabilizer and antihistamine, dosed as infrequently as possible.
- If the child does not improve, referral to an ophthalmologist or allergist is advised.

Suggested Reading

Granet D. Allergic rhinoconjunctivitis and differential diagnosis of the red eye. *Allergy Asthma Proc.* 2008;29(6):565–574

Relief from springtime allergies. *Consumer Reports.* March 2010. http://www.consumerreports.org/health/conditions-and-treatments/allergy/allergy-treatment/overview/allergy-treatment.htm. Accessed March 13, 2012

Chapter 5

Red Eye With Periocular Pearly Rash

Erick D. Bothun, MD

Presentation

A 9-year-old boy is seen in the clinic for evaluation of a red eye. He reports good vision in that eye, but he has had mild redness and tearing for a number of weeks. The mother comments on the many bumps on his face and neck. The boy is well known to the pediatrician's practice and is healthy. He has a history of strabismus with normal growth and development. Immunizations are current. He is active in school and is learning tae kwon do.

Examination reveals multiple 1- to 3-mm dry, pearly lesions on the skin of the right upper and lower eyelids (Figure 5-1). The right eye is mildly injected. Similar skin lesions are present on the boy's neck and periocular area. They are skin colored and range in size from pinpoint

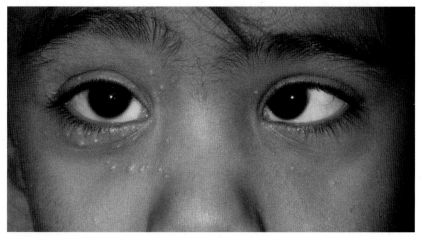

Figure 5-1. Erythematous and thickened right upper eyelid with multiple periocular skin lesions. Courtesy of Ken K. Nischal, FRCOphth.

to that of a pencil eraser. The larger lesions have rolled edges with a central depression (Figure 5-2). A closer inspection of the child's body reveals 2 smaller yet identical lesions on the right side of his waist.

Diagnosis

None of the skin lesions appear inflammatory. Their distribution and color are wartlike in nature. However, the smooth, firm shape of the larger lesions, with rolled, pearly edges and a depressed center, leads to the diagnosis. The child has molluscum contagiosum with an associated conjunctivitis.

If the child were cooperative enough for the pediatrician to prick open one of the large lesions and squeeze or use a curette to remove the central material, it would be pale and cheesy. A Gram stain of this material shows brick-shaped inclusion bodies.

The pediatrician advises the family that this rash is typically a self-limited infection of the epidermis. Molluscum is spread from direct skin contact. The rash will typically appear weeks to months after exposure and spreads to normal skin through self-inoculation.

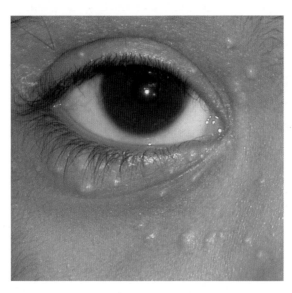

Figure 5-2. Multiple flesh-colored periocular lesions of varying size with pearly edges and occasional umbilicated centers. Courtesy of Ken K. Nischal, FRCOphth.

Differential Diagnosis

Diagnoses besides molluscum contagiosum that should be considered include the following:

Warts

Painless, rough skin growth resembling a solid blister

Chalazia

Tender, erythematous, and deep swelling of the eyelid margin with occasional drainage and crusting of overlying skin

Granulomata

Small, bright red nodule typically located at sight of previous trauma

Phthiriasis

Eyelid lice appearing as crusting at the eyelid margin and occasionally associated with lid and ocular injection

When to Refer

Although a conservative watch-and-wait approach is recommended, the redness on the patient's right eye may be a related complication. When molluscum is present on or around the eye, the infection may cause a chronic conjunctivitis. A referral to the pediatric ophthalmologist is made, and the pediatrician's diagnosis is confirmed. Treatment of the conjunctivitis is initiated.

Treatment

Because most molluscum infections are self-limited, treatment is not typically initiated in an immunocompetent patient. Children should not be restricted from school or child care attendance. Although there is no consensus on management, intervention may be chosen when a child's picking and scratching at lesions cause scarring, if conjunctivitis is diagnosed, or if lesions remain longer than 1 to 2 years.

Rapid treatments include cryotherapy, enucleation, and curettage with local or general anesthesia and coating with fingernail polish or duct tape. Pulse dye laser is also effective but is cost prohibitive in most cases. Systemic cimetidine has been found effective in children who will not cooperate with a local regimen. Various topical medications, with varying risk levels, have been shown effective, including podofilox, iodine and salicylic acid, potassium hydroxide, cantharidin, tretinoin, and imiquimod.

Treatment also may include recommendations to limit transmission of the virus to close contacts.

Discussion

The cause of molluscum contagiosum is a poxvirus *(Molluscipoxvirus)* that affects the skin and mucous membranes. The incubation period is usually 2 to 7 weeks but can be longer.

Molluscum contagiosum is spread from direct skin contact or by fomites such as bath towels or swimming pool equipment. The rash may not appear until weeks or months after exposure and spreads to healthy skin through self-inoculation. Usually, lesions are found on the face, trunk, and extremities in children between 1 and 10 years of age. Molluscum may be localized on or around the genitalia and may spread as a sexually transmitted infection. In the setting of immunosuppression, this infection may be more severe and resistant to treatment.

Because most molluscum infections are self-limited, treatment is not typically initiated in an immunocompetent patient unless there is conjunctivitis. Generally, resolution of the molluscum contagiosum rash takes 6 to 12 months without treatment.

Key Points

- Advise families about practices at child care or school that might transmit the molluscum poxvirus to other children.
- Affected areas should be kept clean and covered by clothing or bandage.
- Objects such as towels and swimming toys should not be shared until the lesions have resolved.
- Molluscum contagiosum lesions on or around the eyelids can lead to chronic conjunctivitis, which should be evaluated by a pediatric ophthalmologist.

Suggested Reading

Centers for Disease Control and Prevention. Molluscum (molluscum contagiosum). http://www.cdc.gov/ncidod/dvrd/molluscum/index. htm. Accessed March 13, 2012

Hanson D, Diven DG. Molluscum contagiosum. *Dermatol Online J.* 2003;9(2):2. http://dermatology.cdlib.org/92/reviews/molluscum/ diven.html. Accessed March 13, 2012

Shapiro W. Molluscum contagiosum. Stöppler MC, ed. eMedicineHealth. http://www.emedicinehealth.com/molluscum_contagiosum/article_ em.htm. Accessed March 13, 2012

Chapter 6

Eyelid Crusting and Redness

Jena Mills, BA
Shira L. Robbins, MD

Presentation

A 4-year-old girl is brought to the pediatrician's office presenting with bilateral ocular redness and irritation as well as eyelid crusting. Her mother has noticed frequent eye rubbing, and the child often complains of a "burning" sensation in her eyes. Her mother has also noted some mild photophobia (light sensitivity) within the past few weeks. Although no other children in her preschool class have had pinkeye this year, her mother claims that this has been a recurrent problem and is concerned that it has not disappeared. A review of the patient's history confirms the absence of any generalized skin conditions or other systemic problems.

A close examination of the child's eyelid area reveals swollen eyelid margins, dandruff-like scales on the lids, collarettes surrounding eyelash follicles, and inflammation of the conjunctival tissue (Figure 6-1).

Diagnosis

This child has chronic blepharitis (eyelid inflammation) with associated conjunctivitis (also known as blepharoconjunctivitis). Diagnosis of blepharitis is often made solely based on patient history and, when possible, physical examination of signs. Because of the collarettes surrounding the girl's eyelash follicles, the pediatrician suspects a staphylococcal anterior blepharitis and performs a swab of the discharge on the eyelid margin for bacterial culture testing. This test will help to confirm diagnosis and ensure that treatment with antibiotic drops or ointment will resolve the problem.

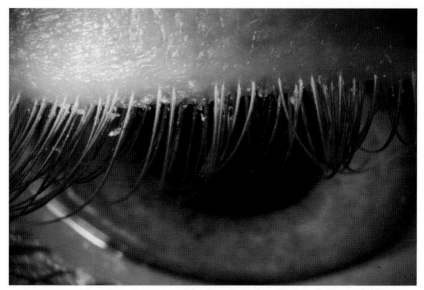

Figure 6-1. Dandruff-like scales on eyelashes. Courtesy of Shira L. Robbins, MD.

Blepharitis is often mistaken for simple recurrent conjunctivitis or dry eye, although both are commonly seen as secondary developments. When inflammation does not resolve with time or artificial tears, blepharitis should be considered as a cause of ocular discomfort.

Classification of blepharitis may be difficult because there can be a wide variety of causes and a large overlap in signs and symptoms. The disease can be divided into anterior and posterior blepharitis, with anterior being primarily staphylococcal or seborrheic in origin, and posterior being directly related to meibomian gland dysfunction. Anterior blepharitis is much more common in children and is most often staphylococcal. However, other causes may include allergies, arthropods (mites), viruses, fungi, generalized skin conditions, systemic medical disorders, or a combination of these factors. This can be problematic when constructing a treatment plan and can sometimes lead to difficult management.

Posterior blepharitis is less common and is often asymptomatic in children, aside from development of an occasional chalazion that will usually resolve within 3 or 4 weeks.

Angular blepharitis is a less common variation that principally affects the outer corners of the eyelids typically making the lids red, dry, and scaly. It may involve blockage of lacrimal ducts caused by bacterial infection.

Blepharitis may occasionally be secondary to a systemic disorder (eg, lupus) or a wide variety of generalized skin conditions. Although most of these conditions are far less common in children, they should be considered depending on the patient's history. Molluscum contagiosum is a viral infection of the skin or mucous membranes that occurs with higher frequency in children and can lead to the development of blepharitis.

Differential Diagnosis

Diagnoses besides blepharitis that should be considered include the following:

Recurrent Conjunctivitis

If there is no eyelid involvement, conjunctivitis should be considered and treated, as it is often contagious and may cause vision damage if left untreated.

Keratitis

This involves inflammation of the cornea and is often accompanied by significant ocular pain and blurred vision. Keratitis may have a variety of causes and associated treatments, all of which should be promptly pursued to prevent permanent corneal damage and vision changes.

Orbital Cellulitis

This acute infection of tissues surrounding the eye (eg, eyelids, eyebrow, cheek) is usually accompanied by fever, discolored eyelid, and decreased vision.

Dacryocystitis

This infection and inflammation of the tear drainage system is characterized by pain, erythema, and edema.

Trichiasis

Children may have abnormally positioned eyelashes, congenitally or as a result of an infection or other trauma. This abnormality can be detected on careful examination and should be treated if it is affecting corneal or conjunctival tissues.

When to Refer

An ophthalmologic evaluation is needed if blepharitis symptoms persist or worsen despite treatment. A patient with chronic blepharitis and symptoms of allergies should be referred to an allergist for allergy testing.

Treatment

After prescribing antibiotic drops, the pediatrician instructs the patient's mother to begin a twice daily face-washing regimen, followed by application of warm compresses to the girl's eyelids. You explain that compresses should be a clean, moderately warm washcloth or other object that can retain heat. In addition, using a washcloth or cotton-tipped applicator, she should perform very gentle eyelid scrubs using a mild, tearless baby shampoo diluted with warm water (1:100) or a nonprescription eyelid soap to help clean eyelid scaling. The pediatrician asks that the patient be brought in again if symptoms persist or worsen, which would require an ophthalmologic evaluation.

Topical steroids may be prescribed by a pediatric ophthalmologist in conjunction with antibiotic drops in severe cases of inflammation or if other complications, such as phlyctenules (small white bumps or blisters on the corneal surface of the eye) or marginal keratitis (peripheral corneal lesions), arise.

If there is an underlying condition, it must be addressed for blepharitis to subside.

Discussion

Blepharitis is a common cause of chronic eye irritation in children older than 3 years. There is no cure and treatment is ongoing to manage the symptoms. This patient showed improvement within days of initiating treatment. However, she suffers from recurrences when her family is lax with eyelid hygiene recommendations.

> ## Key Points
>
> - Blepharitis is the most common cause of chronic eye irritation in children, but unlike conjunctivitis, it is not contagious.
> - Chronic blepharitis is characterized by intermittent exacerbations and remissions, although blepharitis may also occur acutely.
> - Blepharitis may be asymmetrical, especially in children.
> - Children with Down syndrome are at higher risk of blepharitis.

Suggested Reading

Kanski JJ, Pavésio CE, Tuft T. *Ocular Inflammatory Disease.* Philadelphia, PA: Elsevier Mosby; 2006

Seal DV, Pleyer U. *Ocular Infection.* 2nd ed. New York, NY: Informa Healthcare; 2007

Taylor D, Hoyt CS, eds. *Pediatric Ophthalmology and Strabismus.* 3rd ed. Philadelphia, PA: Elsevier Saunders; 2005

Wright KW, Spiegel PH. *Pediatric Ophthalmology and Strabismus.* 2nd ed. New York, NY: Springer; 2003

Chapter 7

Unilateral Eye Redness Without Discharge

Monte Dean Mills, MD

Presentation

A 4-year-old girl presents to the pediatrician's office with a 1-week history of unilateral eye redness. She was initially diagnosed over the phone with acute infectious conjunctivitis based on her symptoms. Topical antibiotic drops were prescribed and have been used for the past 4 days without improvement.

The patient has been healthy, but on the pediatrician's review of systems, the girl's mother reports that she has complained of leg pain with occasional limping during the past 3 months. The leg pain and limping resolved spontaneously.

Examination of the eyes shows bilateral redness of the sclera, most prominent close to the cornea (at the limbus, as shown in figures 7-1 and 7-2). The redness is not associated with mucous or purulent discharge but is associated with light sensitivity (photophobia). The redness does not extend to the inner eyelid surface (tarsal conjunctiva). There is also no preauricular adenopathy.

Examination of the knees demonstrates mild tenderness and swelling bilaterally.

Diagnosis

The findings of scleral redness without other evidence of conjunctivitis, as well as sparing of redness on tarsal conjunctiva, are characteristic of acute anterior uveitis or iritis. As shown in figures 7-1 and 7-2, the redness is usually most intense near the cornea, at the corneal limbus.

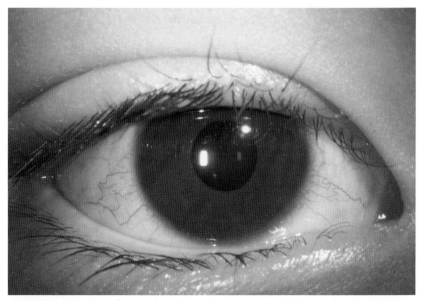

Figure 7-1. Injection of conjunctival blood vessels is more pronounced at the limbus. Courtesy of Shira L. Robbins, MD.

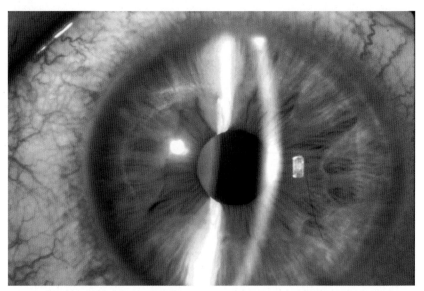

Figure 7-2. Slit-lamp photograph of anterior uveitis with conjunctival redness, most prominent at the corneal limbus, without signs of conjunctivitis. Courtesy of Monte D. Mills, MD.

Acute anterior uveitis is frequently misdiagnosed as conjunctivitis, but it will not respond to topical antibiotics and generally will persist longer than acute infectious conjunctivitis. Acute anterior uveitis is frequently associated with photophobia and pain but may also be asymptomatic.

In children, the most common systemic disease associated with acute anterior uveitis is juvenile idiopathic arthritis (JIA), which is found in 40% to 80% of patients. The most common type of JIA seen with uveitis is oligoarticular, with positive serology for antinuclear antibodies (ANA).

Differential Diagnosis

Diagnoses besides anterior uveitis or iritis that should be considered include the following:

Infectious Conjunctivitis

In children, infectious conjunctivitis is usually bilateral, with redness extending onto the tarsal conjunctival surfaces. It is usually associated with mucopurulent discharge. Frequently, preauricular adenopathy is present with viral conjunctivitis, and it may also be associated with rhinitis and pharyngitis. Viral conjunctivitis is often epidemic in children; there may be a history of other affected family members or school or child care contacts.

Trauma, Corneal Abrasion

Eye trauma with or without corneal abrasion may cause acute redness, pain, and photophobia but may usually be distinguished by the history of trauma and abrupt onset, and with examination using fluorescein staining of the cornea, which will stain and identify epithelial defects of the cornea and conjunctiva. There is usually rapid improvement in symptoms over 24 to 48 hours with spontaneous healing.

Exposure Keratitis

Exposure keratitis occurs primarily in children with abnormal eyelid closure, as with facial palsy and facial deformity or with sedated or anesthetized patients. Exposure and drying of the cornea leads to redness, pain, and photophobia. Treatment by correcting the underlying eyelid abnormality and providing ocular surface lubrication reverses the abnormality, with usually rapid improvement.

Infectious Keratitis

Herpesvirus, varicella, or bacterial infections of the cornea cause redness, pain, and photophobia. Additional signs of keratitis may include associated adjacent dermatitis (eg, herpes, varicella), corneal fluorescein staining with dendritic patterns (herpes), or associated eyelid margin blepharitis. Detailed clinical examination with slit-lamp microscope by an ophthalmologist is usually sufficient to make a clinical diagnosis, although culture or polymerase chain reaction detection of pathogens may also be useful. Specific antimicrobial treatment is based on the clinical diagnosis.

When to Refer

Any patient with a red, painful eye not responding to treatment (in this case, for infectious conjunctivitis) should be referred for ophthalmic examination. The diagnosis of anterior uveitis is very difficult without detailed examination of the anterior segment of the eye with a slit-lamp microscope.

The girl is referred to a pediatric ophthalmologist. Examination of the eyes with a slit lamp is essential for the diagnosis. Acute anterior uveitis is defined by the presence of inflammatory cells in the anterior chamber of the eye, seen only with slit-lamp microscopy. Other signs of acute anterior uveitis may include keratic precipitates (aggregations of inflammatory cells on the inside of the cornea), band keratopathy (calcium deposition in the superficial aspect of the cornea), glaucoma (elevated intraocular pressure), and cataract. The eye examination will include dilation of the pupils to observe for posterior synechiae (adhesions of iris to the lens, which cause the pupil to dilate irregularly) and to examine the retina, optic disc, and vitreous for additional signs of posterior uveitis.

The consulting pediatric ophthalmologist may send the patient back to the pediatrician for further workup. Rheumatologic consultation is indicated in any cases of uveitis associated with arthritis symptoms, as in this case, because of the strong association between JIA and anterior uveitis. Other systemic associations may include psoriatic arthritis, ankylosing spondylitis, Lyme disease, acute interstitial nephritis, sarcoidosis, congenital or acquired syphilis, Reiter syndrome, and toxoplasmosis.

The pediatrician or rheumatologist should direct laboratory evaluation toward the most likely systemic diagnoses based on the history and physical examination. Laboratory studies may include ANA, rheumatoid factor, toxoplasmosis antibodies, Lyme disease antibodies, and other studies related to potential systemic-associated abnormalities.

Treatment

The pediatric ophthalmologist prescribes topical steroids. Topical prednisolone or dexamethasone drops or ointments are usually adequate to control acute anterior uveitis. Depending on the severity of the inflammation and initial response to treatment, initial treatment with prednisolone 1% 4 to 6 times daily, with gradually tapering of frequency over several weeks, is generally prescribed. Topical steroid treatment avoids many of the potential side effects of systemic steroids, including systemic immunosuppression, adrenal suppression, and growth retardation. However, local complications, including steroid-induced glaucoma and cataract, are possible. Patients using topical steroids require monitoring by an ophthalmologist for assessment of treatment response and potential complications, including measurement of intraocular pressure and visual acuity.

Long-term immunosuppression, systemic steroids, or other agents may be necessary to supplement topical steroids, if anterior uveitis becomes recurrent or chronic. Systemic treatment may also reduce the risks of local complications of topical steroids if recurrent or longer-term treatment is necessary.

Discussion

Anterior uveitis can lead to corneal and pupillary scarring. Ocular complications tend to occur after extended or recurrent anterior uveitis lasting more than a few weeks. Because of the risk of vision-threatening complications and the need for slit-lamp examination to monitor response to treatment, all patients should be monitored by an ophthal-mologist once the diagnosis of anterior uveitis has been made.

Most children with acute anterior uveitis who are diagnosed and treated early in the course of the condition, and who have appropriate treatment of any underlying systemic condition, will respond to treat-ment without permanent vision loss. Ocular complications causing loss of vision are uncommon and are often associated with delayed diagnosis, unsupervised use of topical steroids, or inadequate diagnosis and treatment of underlying medical conditions. Cataracts, synechiae, amblyopia, and glaucoma occurring as complications of anterior uveitis or steroid treatment are treatable if detected promptly.

Anterior uveitis occurs frequently in patients with JIA; therefore, these patients should all have periodic slit-lamp examination, even if they have not had anterior uveitis in the past. The frequency of these exami-nations can be based on age and JIA classification, as recommended by the American Academy of Pediatrics (Table 7-1). Generally, patients with newly diagnosed JIA should have an initial ophthalmic examination including slit-lamp microscopy, followed by periodic reexaminations every 3 to 12 months depending on age and risk for anterior uveitis.

Table 7-1. Frequency of Ophthalmologic Examination in Patients With Juvenile Idiopathic Arthritis

Type of JIA	ANA Status	Age at Onset, y	Duration of Disease, y	Risk Category	Eye Examination Frequency, mo
Oligoarthritis or polyarthritis	Positive	≤6	≤4	High	3
		≤6	>4	Moderate	6
		≤6	>7	Low	12
		>6	≤4	Moderate	6
		>6	>4	Low	12
	Negative	≤6	≤4	Moderate	6
		≤6	>4	Low	12
		>6	N/A	Low	12
Systemic onset (rash, fever)	N/A	N/A	N/A	Low	12

Abbreviations: ANA, antinuclear antibodies; JIA, juvenile idiopathic arthritis; N/A, not applicable.

Adapted from Cassidy J, Kivlin J, Lindsley C, Nocton J; American Academy of Pediatrics Section on Rheumatology, Section on Ophthalmology. Ophthalmologic examinations in children with juvenile rheumatoid arthritis. *Pediatrics*. 2006;117(5):1843–1845. http://pediatrics.aappublications.org/content/117/5/1843. Accessed March 13, 2012

Key Points

- Redness of the conjunctiva at the corneal limbus without discharge or eyelid involvement is highly associated with an anterior uveitis.
- Children with the clinical diagnosis of infectious conjunctivitis, without resolution or response to treatment, should be referred for ophthalmic examination to exclude anterior uveitis.
- Confirmation of this condition requires a slit-lamp examination by an ophthalmologist.
- Juvenile idiopathic arthritis (JIA) is the most common underlying systemic condition leading to anterior uveitis. Children with JIA should be screened for anterior uveitis, even if asymptomatic.
- Anterior uveitis can lead to glaucoma, cataract, corneal scarring, and pupillary scarring, which can all compromise vision. Early detection is important to prevent vision-threatening complications.
- Treatment is usually topical steroids, with severe cases requiring systemic anti-inflammatory agents. Treatment must be monitored with frequent ophthalmic examinations.

Suggested Reading

Cassidy J, Kivlin J, Lindsley C, Nocton J; American Academy of Pediatrics Section on Rheumatology, Section on Ophthalmology. Ophthalmologic examinations in children with juvenile rheumatoid arthritis. *Pediatrics.* 2006;117(5):1843–1845. http://pediatrics. aappublications.org/content/117/5/1843. Accessed March 13, 2012

Kump LI, Cervantes-Castañeda RA, Androudi SN, Foster CS. Analysis of pediatric uveitis cases at a tertiary referral center. *Ophthalmology.* 2005;112(7):1287–1292

Päivönsalo-Hietanen T, Tuominen J, Saari KM. Uveitis in children: population-based study in Finland. *Acta Ophthalmol Scand.* 2000;78(1):84–88

Chapter 8

Acute Well-Circumscribed Red Eye

Oren L. Weisberg, MD, MA

Presentation

A 5-year-old girl is brought to the pediatrician's office by her parents, who noticed that "the white part of her right eye is all bloody." It was first observed when she awoke that morning. The parents have not seen any tearing or discharge from the eye and have not noticed sensitivity to light (photophobia) or problems with the child's vision. The patient has not had any concurrent illness and has had no contact with others who are ill. She is not complaining of pain or foreign body sensation. She has no significant past medical history and does not take any medications on a daily basis.

The previous day the child played outside with her 2 older brothers, and although no specific trauma was noted, it cannot be ruled out. The children often play roughly together, and several times they were out of view of the parents.

On examination, the child appears healthy and comfortable without any signs of distress. She is afebrile. Her blood pressure is normal. Her visual acuity in each eye is 20/20 when measured with the Snellen wall eye chart. Her extraocular motility is full. There is no evidence of strabismus. The pupils are round and reactive to light, and there is no evidence of an afferent pupillary defect. The eyelids appear healthy, and there are no areas of ecchymosis, edema, or lacerations. An accumulation of bright red blood is seen under the conjunctiva infero-nasally in her right eye (Figure 8-1). The underlying sclera is not visible. There is no dilation of the surrounding conjunctival vessels. The cornea is clear, and after instillation of fluorescein dye, no epithelial defects are seen. A red reflex is appreciated and is symmetric between the eyes.

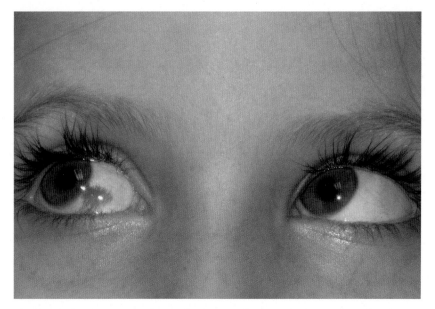

Figure 8-1. Representative photo of right eye infero-nasal subconjunctival hemorrhage. Courtesy of Shira L. Robbins, MD.

Diagnosis

The diagnosis is unilateral subconjunctival hemorrhage, defined as blood between the conjunctiva and sclera. Although this first episode of subconjunctival hemorrhage may be isolated and benign, the possibility of subtle trauma should be considered. In this case, because no trauma has been reported, the examination is crucial in identifying any signs of possible trauma.

Findings that might indicate trauma include: (1) a decrease in vision in either eye; (2) lack of full extraocular motility, in which both eyes move in all directions and in unison (restricted ocular motility can sometimes be seen with accumulation of large amounts of subconjunctival blood); (3) strabismus (misalignment of one or both eyes); (4) asymmetry of the pupil size or shape (ie, oval or teardrop instead of round), which might be a result of trauma with the possibility of a ruptured globe; (5) lacerations of the eyelids, eyelash margins, or conjunctiva; or (6) presence of a foreign body in the eye.

By pulling down the lower eyelid and flipping up the upper eyelid, the clinician can perform an examination of the inferior and superior conjunctival fornices to look for lacerations and foreign bodies. If a ruptured globe is suspected, this examination would be deferred because such a maneuver could extrude the contents of the eye. However, this patient has none of these findings suggesting trauma. In addition, direct ophthalmoscopy does not reveal any signs of optic nerve edema or retinal hemorrhages and decreases the already low likelihood of nonaccidental trauma.

The other causes of subconjunctival hemorrhage include infection, drugs, systemic illness, Valsalva maneuver, and blood abnormalities. Infectious causes include viruses (eg, adenovirus, coxsackievirus) and bacteria (eg, pneumococcus). The lack of contact with sick people, the absence of concurrent illnesses, and a lack of an increase in tear film or discharge on the lashes all make an infectious cause unlikely.

A review of the patient's chart and discussion with the parents confirm that the child has no medical problems and is not taking any medications on a regular basis. Patients with systemic illnesses, including diabetes mellitus, hypertension, Ehlers-Danlos syndrome, hemochromatosis, and vitamin C deficiency, may experience recurrent subconjunctival hemorrhages. Consideration also needs to be given to anemias (eg, aplastic anemia), thrombocytopenia purpura, leukemia, and splenic disorders. Numerous drugs (including blood thinners) can also lead to subconjunctival hemorrhages.

Finally, a Valsalva maneuver, including prolonged coughing, vomiting, or seizure activity, can cause subconjunctival hemorrhages. No such history was described by the parents.

Differential Diagnosis

Differential diagnoses for this type of ocular appearance include a subconjunctival hemorrhage, infective conjunctivitis, and episcleritis.

When to Refer

A high suspicion for accidental and inflicted trauma is necessary in cases of subconjunctival hemorrhage, and if suspected, an examination by a pediatric ophthalmologist is recommended. A pediatric ophthalmologist is able to measure intraocular pressures and perform a dilated retinal examination to assess the health of the retina and optic nerve. Other findings besides trauma that should prompt referral to an ophthalmologist include pain, decrease in vision, double vision, bilateral subconjunctival hemorrhages, or total (360°) subconjunctival hemorrhage (which can indicate a ruptured globe).

Treatment

No treatment is needed for an isolated unilateral subconjunctival hemorrhage. The blood will be reabsorbed over several weeks, likely progressing through the typical color changes seen in other parts of the body (from dark red or purplish to green, then yellow).

Discussion

Subconjunctival hemorrhages are self-limiting. If recurrent subconjunctival hemorrhages are noted without a history of trauma or infections, an additional workup seeking systemic causes can be performed.

Key Points

- Subconjunctival hemorrhage without apparent cause is common and requires no intervention.
- A high suspicion for accidental or inflicted trauma is necessary.
- Findings that should prompt referral to an ophthalmologist include trauma, pain, decrease in vision, double vision, bilateral subconjunctival hemorrhages, or total (360°) subconjunctival hemorrhage.
- Underlying systemic conditions should be considered in cases of recurrent subconjunctival hemorrhages.

Suggested Reading

Liebowitz HM. The red eye. *N Engl J Med.* 2000;343(5):345–351

Roy FH. *Ocular Differential Diagnosis.* 9th ed. New Delhi, India: Jaypee Brothers Medical Publishers Ltd; 2012

Chapter 9

Fever and Red Eyes

John T. Z. Kanegaye, MD
Jane C. Burns, MD

Presentation

A 14-month-old Hispanic boy comes to his pediatrician's office with the chief complaint of 2 days of fever and red eyes. The child has had no cough, rhinorrhea, vomiting, or diarrhea. Examination reveals an irritable toddler with bilateral, non-exudative conjunctival injection and apart from mild temperature elevation (38.7°C), no other abnormal findings. The physician prescribes an ophthalmic antibiotic solution and reassures the parent that the fever is probably caused by a viral infection that will resolve without specific treatment. The parent is instructed to bring the child back within 2 days if the fever persists.

Two days later (illness day 4) the child returns to the pediatrician's office because of persistence of the fever and red eyes. Additional medical history from the mother includes the appearance today of a non-pruritic rash, red palms and soles, and red, peeling lips. There is a 6-year-old sibling at home, and the sibling and both parents are well. The child attends a child care center but has no known contact with ill people. The child's immunizations are up to date. The mother reports that her son has no respiratory or gastrointestinal tract symptoms. She does state that her son has been very cranky, which is unusual for this normally easygoing child. The mother has noticed no photophobia, tearing, or conjunctival exudate.

Physical examination reveals an irritable child with a diffuse maculo-papular rash over the trunk and extremities. Axillary temperature is 38.4°C. There is bilateral symmetric conjunctival injection without exudate. There is sparing of the limbus, suggesting the absence of edema in the conjunctiva (Figure 9-1). Oropharyngeal examination shows dry, peeling, red lips (Figure 9-2); a red oropharynx without specific lesions; and a strawberry tongue. There is no substantial cervical lymphadenopathy. Cardiac examination reveals a rapid heart rate of 160 beats per minute and an S4 gallop at the apex. Abdominal examination is notable for fullness in the right upper quadrant with involuntary guarding. No spleen is palpable. The hands are swollen and the palms slightly red (Figure 9-3). The child refuses to walk and cries when placed in a standing position.

Given the constellation of fever, bilateral conjunctival injection, rash, and swollen hands with red palms and soles, the pediatrician suspects Kawasaki disease (KD) and sends the patient to the clinical laboratory. Results show a white blood cell count of 16,500 cells/μL with 67% neutrophils, 13% band forms, 12% lymphocytes, and 8% eosinophils.

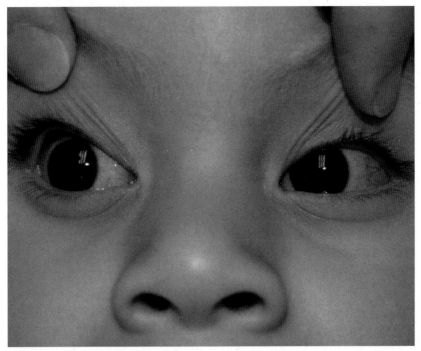

Figure 9-1. Bilateral symmetric conjunctival injection with limbal sparing and no exudate. Courtesy of John T. Z. Kanegaye, MD.

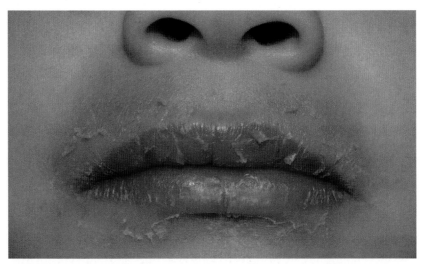

Figure 9-2. Dry, peeling, red lips. Courtesy of John T. Z. Kanegaye, MD.

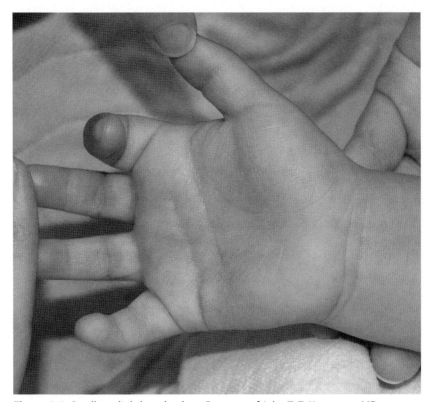

Figure 9-3. Swollen, slightly red palms. Courtesy of John T. Z. Kanegaye, MD.

The hemoglobin level and hematocrit are low for age (9.8 g/dL and 29%, respectively) with normal red blood cell indices. The platelet count is elevated at 475,000 cells/μL. The erythrocyte sedimentation rate (ESR) is elevated (62 mm/h), as is the C-reactive protein level (8.9 mg/dL). Alanine aminotransferase and gammaglutamyltranspeptidase levels are elevated at 115 U/L and 89 U/L, respectively. Urine obtained by bag contains 6 to 8 white blood cells per high-power field. The patient is admitted to the hospital for treatment.

Diagnosis

The conjunctival injection in association with fever and rash suggests a systemic illness with ocular manifestations. The differential diagnosis of the triad of fever, rash, and conjunctival injection in a toddler is broad. The most common cause of this triad is viral infection, with adenovirus and enterovirus at the top of the list. Measles must be considered, but the child's immunizations are up to date and there have been no known ill contacts and no history of foreign travel. The absence of exudate or conjunctival edema on examination of the eyes also argues against viral infection. The rapid heart rate with gallop rhythm suggests myocardial involvement. The fullness in the right upper abdominal quadrant and guarding suggest hepatitis or hydrops of the gallbladder.

The physical findings in combination with leukocytosis, anemia, thrombocytosis, and elevated levels of acute phase reactants and hepatobiliary enzymes suggest the systemic vasculitis of KD, the most common cause of acquired heart disease in childhood. Because there is currently no diagnostic test for KD, the diagnosis is based on a constellation of clinical signs (Table 9-1) and laboratory data suggesting acute systemic inflammation.

Table 9-1. Diagnostic Criteria for Kawasaki Disease

Fever ≥4 days,[a] in association with ≥4 of the following criteria[b]:
Extremity changes

Acute: Palmar, plantar erythema; hand, foot swelling
    Subacute: Desquamation of fingers and toes in a periungual distribution
    (week 2–3 of illness)

Polymorphous rash
Bilateral conjunctival injection without exudates
Oral changes (cracked, red lips; strawberry tongue; mucosal injection)
Cervical adenopathy >1.5 cm
Exclusion of other diseases

[a] By convention, each calendar day is included as a day of illness. Experienced clinicians may make the diagnosis before day 4 when 4 of 5 criteria are present.
[b] In the presence of coronary artery abnormalities by echocardiography, the diagnosis may be made with <4 criteria.

Adapted from Newburger JW, Takahashi M, Gerber MA, et al. Diagnosis, treatment, and long-term management of Kawasaki disease: a statement for health professionals from the Committee on Rheumatic Fever, Endocarditis, and Kawasaki Disease, Council on Cardiovascular Disease in the Young, American Heart Association. *Pediatrics.* 2004;114(6):1708–1733

Differential Diagnosis

Diagnoses besides KD that should be considered include the following:

Viral Infections

- Adenoviral infection
- Enteroviral infection
- Measles
- Rubella
- Mononucleosis

Other Infections

- Lyme disease
- Rocky Mountain spotted fever
- Leptospirosis

Drug Reaction

Staphylococcal or Streptococcal Toxin-Mediated Disease

Scarlet fever is *not* associated with injected conjunctivae.

- Staphylococcal scalded skin syndrome
- Toxic shock syndrome

Stevens-Johnson Syndrome or Toxic Epidermal Necrolysis

When to Refer

With an established or highly suspected diagnosis of acute KD, admit for treatment or further evaluation, eg, echocardiogram, abdominal ultrasound for hydrops of gallbladder.

For uncertain or incomplete presentations of KD, in early illness these patients may be followed closely on an outpatient basis with repeated examinations, laboratory investigations, and consideration of echocardiography. The ophthalmologist may be useful in confirming the KD-type conjunctivitis and also use a slit-lamp biomicroscope to identify fine (small) cells in the anterior chamber. That examination changes and needs to be done by days 8 or 9 of the disease to be useful.

Treatment

The major complications of KD are damage to the myocardium and vascular wall; 25% of untreated patients will experience coronary artery aneurysms. Treatment with high-dose intravenous immunoglobulin (IVIG) (2 g/kg) within the first 10 days after onset of fever reduces the rate of aneurysms to 5%. Intravenous immunoglobulin resistance (persistence or recurrence of temperature ≥38.0°C ≥36 hours follow-ng completion of infusion) warrants repeated administration of IVIG or consideration of additional anti-inflammatory therapy. Aspirin is given in high doses (80–100 mg/kg/day divided in 4 doses) until fever has resolved and is continued at 3 to 5 mg/kg/day until markers of inflammation (eg, ESR, platelet count) have returned to normal, or indefinitely if coronary lesions persist.

Discussion

The etiology of KD remains unknown, although an environmental trigger, possibly a microbial agent, is suspected. Genetic factors clearly play a role in disease susceptibility and outcome. Asian children are affected more frequently than children of northern European or Hispanic descent. Boys are affected more often than girls. Eighty percent of patients are younger than 5 years, and half are younger than 2 years.

Key Points

- Timely recognition and treatment of Kawasaki disease (KD) are essential to prevent or mitigate the damage caused by the acute vasculitis.
- Diagnosis requires a high index of suspicion. Incomplete forms are especially difficult to diagnose unless the clinician specifically considers KD and follows the patient closely for development of additional diagnostic criteria. An algorithm for the diagnosis of incomplete cases is provided in the 2004 American Heart Association guidelines.
- Kawasaki disease should be considered in the differential diagnosis of any infant or child with prolonged fever.
- Cervical lymph node involvement is seen in only one-third of cases and is the least common of the physical signs of KD, as illustrated by this case.
- After treatment, patients should be followed indefinitely by a physician knowledgeable of the cardiovascular sequelae of KD, as late complications in adulthood have been observed. However, the prognosis for most patients without coronary artery complications is excellent. Patients with aneurysms should be followed by a pediatric cardiologist or KD specialist.

Suggested Reading

Burns JC, Mason WH, Glode MP, et al. Clinical and epidemiologic characteristics of patients referred for evaluation of possible Kawasaki disease. United States Multicenter Kawasaki Disease Study Group. *J Pediatr.* 1991;118(5):680–686

Gordon JB, Kahn AM, Burns JC. When children with Kawasaki disease grow up: myocardial and vascular complications in adulthood. *J Am Coll Cardiol.* 2009;54(21):1911–1920

Newburger JW, Takahashi M, Gerber MA, et al. Diagnosis, treatment, and long-term management of Kawasaki disease: a statement for health professionals from the Committee on Rheumatic Fever, Endocarditis, and Kawasaki Disease, Council on Cardiovascular Disease in the Young, American Heart Association. *Pediatrics.* 2004;114(6):1708–1733

Smith LB, Newburger JW, Burns JC. Kawasaki syndrome and the eye. *Pediatr Infect Dis J.* 1989;8(2):116–118

Chapter 10

Ocular Pain, Redness, Photophobia, and Tearing

Christopher W. Heichel, MD
Sara Yoon, MD

Presentation

A 7-year-old boy presents to the pediatric clinic complaining of right eye pain associated with decreased vision, sensitivity to light, and tearing for the past 5 days. His ocular history is otherwise unremarkable. He is healthy and developing normally, and his immunizations are up to date.

On eye examination, his visual acuity is 20/60 in the right eye and 20/20 in the left eye. A penlight examination of the eye shows a large, white, branching lesion covering 25% of the cornea (figures 10-1 and 10-2). There is conjunctival redness with no discharge.

Instillation of fluorescein dye under cobalt-blue light (Wood lamp) shows a bright-green staining pattern that corresponds to the branching corneal lesion (Figure 10-3). The central portion of the corneal lesion is confluent, whereas the border of the lesion is irregular and stains less intensely.

Because eye pain has lasted for 5 days and the lesion is irregular and involves the visual axis (central cornea), a simple corneal abrasion is unlikely. The pediatrician discusses the case with her local pediatric ophthalmologist, who recommends an immediate referral. The pediatric ophthalmologist confirms the pediatrician's findings and additionally notes a mild uveitis (inflammatory reaction in the anterior chamber).

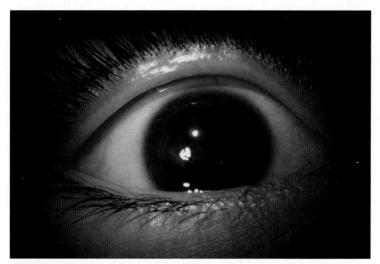

Figure 10-1. Large white branching lesion in the cornea. Courtesy of Shira L. Robbins, MD.

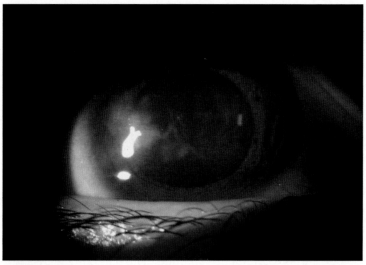

Figure 10-2. Close-up view of white branching corneal lesion. Courtesy of Shira L. Robbins, MD.

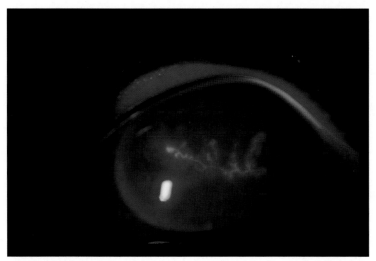

Figure 10-3. Fluorescein staining of branching corneal lesion. Courtesy of Shira L. Robbins, MD.

Diagnosis

Given the patient's main symptoms of pain and photophobia, diagnosis is likely a corneal process with an associated uveitis. The corneal staining pattern is consistent with a dendrite (corneal ulcer with a branch-like pattern) and is likely herpes simplex infection of the cornea. The differential diagnosis is on the next page.

The most common ocular manifestation of herpes simplex virus (HSV) is blepharoconjunctivitis affecting eyelids and conjunctiva. However, HSV keratitis is the most concerning manifestation of primary ocular HSV infection because it can lead to permanent vision loss. Typically HSV keratitis affects the epithelium, the most superficial layer of the cornea. Cysts develop that erode the overlying epithelium and coalesce, forming a dendritic lesion. This lesion stains bright green with fluorescein because of the eroded epithelium. Borders of these lesions consist of raised and swollen epithelial cells, which contain the virus. Underlying corneal stroma can be affected in severe or recurrent disease. This can cause stromal edema and inflammation that can lead to visually debilitating corneal scarring if not treated quickly and appropriately.

Because HSV affects the trigeminal nerve (fifth cranial nerve), decreased corneal sensation is invariably present. It is not uncommon to appreciate concomitant anterior chamber inflammatory reaction, or uveitis, which can cause photophobia.

Differential Diagnosis

Diagnoses besides HSV keratitis that should be considered include the following:

Simple Corneal Abrasion

A simple corneal abrasion would heal within 5 days unless it becomes infected.

Infectious Conjunctivitis

Infectious conjunctivitis is usually marked by itching and copious discharge.

Herpes Zoster

Herpes zoster is extremely uncommon in the pediatric population. If herpes zoster is diagnosed, an underlying immunodeficiency should be strongly considered. Herpes zoster is a reactivation of the same virus that causes chickenpox, varicella-zoster virus. When herpes zoster reactivates along the ophthalmic branch of the trigeminal nerve, it can affect the eye. Presentation and clinical course of herpes zoster can be quite similar to those of HSV. Classically, a dendriform corneal lesion can be appreciated. However, this corneal lesion is a pseudo-dendrite, as it does not cause epithelial erosion and stains less intensely than does a true HSV dendrite.

When to Refer

If HSV keratitis is suspected, prompt evaluation and follow-up care by an ophthalmologist are recommended for multiple reasons. Keratitis caused by HSV can progress rapidly, causing long-term sequelae such as corneal scarring and subsequent amblyopia. Also, the differences between HSV and herpes zoster can be subtle, and making the correct diagnosis without microscopic evaluation with a slit lamp can be difficult. In stromal corneal disease, topical corticosteroids may be indicated to reduce risk of corneal scarring. Management of topical steroids and their potential side effects can be challenging. Finally, HSV recurrences are higher in children than adults (48% vs 18%, respectively).

Treatment

The goal of treatment is to minimize corneal stromal scarring. Physical debridement of the dendrite to remove infectious virus should be performed, and antiviral therapy should be initiated. Traditionally, a topical antiviral such as 1% trifluridine has been used effectively (dose: 1 drop 5 to 9 times daily). However, this medication can cause substantial corneal toxicity; therefore, the dosage must be tapered rapidly. Acyclovir and ganciclovir are available in ophthalmic ointment form, which younger children may tolerate better than drops (dose: thin ribbon 3 times daily).

An oral antiviral agent such as acyclovir is an effective treatment option for children, especially as administration of eyedrops may be an obstacle for some children (dose: 30 mg/kg/day in 3 divided doses). Additionally, acyclovir has the advantage of treating the lesion without causing corneal toxicity. Prolonged antiviral treatment is usually indicated in patients following initial resolution of the disease. Prolonged use of antivirals has been shown to decrease risk of recurrence of herpetic eye infections, especially for patients in the pediatric age group with higher risk of recurrence.

Treatment of herpes zoster can include antivirals and topical corticosteroids as well. However, dosing of the oral antiviral agent can be different from that for HSV, and topical trifluridine has not been shown to be effective in herpes zoster.

Discussion

Herpes simplex virus is spread by direct contact with mucosal membranes. By age 5 years, nearly 60% of the population has been infected with HSV. While the eyes and face are more commonly affected by HSV type 1, it is not uncommon for HSV type 2 to affect these areas as well. Most infected individuals remain as viral carriers, but 6% of those carriers experience clinical manifestations. These manifestations are much more common in the perioral region than the eye.

Children seem to have greater incidence of bilateral ocular involvement, whether simultaneous or sequential, compared with adults. Bilateral involvement has also been associated with atopy.

Prompt diagnosis and treatment are crucial in patients with HSV keratitis.

Key Points

- Pain, light sensitivity, and tearing are the hallmarks of herpes eye infections.
- Herpes should be considered in a case of non-resolving redness of the eye.
- Keratitis due to herpes simplex virus (HSV) is a leading cause of corneal scarring in the United States.
- Transmission of HSV is by direct contact with mucosal membranes.
- Children have greater incidence of HSV recurrence than do adults. Therefore, families of affected children should be alert to future eye redness, pain, tearing, or photophobia and have their children promptly evaluated for herpetic recurrence.
- Children seem to have greater incidence of bilateral involvement (simultaneous or sequential) compared with adults. Bilateral involvement has also been associated with atopy.

Suggested Reading

Chong EM, Wilhelmus KR, Matoba AY, Jones DB, Coats DK, Paysse EA. Herpes simplex virus keratitis in children. *Am J Ophthalmol.* 2004;138(3):474–475

Darougar S, Wishart MS, Viswalingam ND. Epidemiological and clinical features of primary herpes simplex virus ocular infection. *Br J Ophthalmol.* 1985;69(1):2–6

Goodman JL. Infections caused by herpes simplex viruses. In: Hoeprich PD, Jordan C, Ronald AR, eds. *Infectious Diseases.* 5th ed. Philadelphia, PA: JB Lippincott; 1994

Herpetic Eye Disease Study Group. Acyclovir for the prevention of recurrent herpes simplex virus eye disease. *N Engl J Med.* 1998;339(5):300–306

Herpetic Eye Disease Study Group. Predictors of recurrent herpes simplex virus keratitis. *Cornea.* 2001;20(2):123–128

Holland EJ, Brilakis HS, Schwartz GS. Herpes simplex keratitis. In: Krachmer JH, Mannis MJ, Holland EJ, eds. *Cornea: Fundamentals, Diagnosis and Management.* Philadelphia, PA: Elsevier Mosby; 2005

Kielar RA, Cunningham GC, Gerson KL. Occurrence of herpes zoster ophthalmicus in a child with absent immunoglobulin A and deficiency of delayed hypersensitivity. *Am J Ophthalmol.* 1971;72(3):555–557

McMullen WW, D'Amico DJ. AIDS and its ophthalmic manifestations. In: Albert DM, Jakobiec FA, eds. *Principles and Practice of Ophthalmology.* Philadelphia, PA: WB Saunders; 2008

Schwartz GS, Holland EJ. Oral acyclovir for the management of herpes simplex virus keratitis in children. *Ophthalmology.* 2000;107(2):278–282

Chapter 11

Red, Painful Eye

Jennifer Bernabe-Ko, MD
Myoung Joon Kim, MD
David J. Schanzlin, MD

Presentation

A 5-year-old boy comes to the pediatrician's office because of acute ocular pain after his playmate's fingernail accidentally scratched his eye. He is tearing and unable to open his eyes. After instillation of topical proparacaine (anesthetic), his pain is relieved and he is able to open his eyes. The pediatrician then performs an ocular examination.

The visual acuity of the scratched eye is 20/400. The visual acuity of the other eye is 20/20. On penlight examination, a focal rough surface of the cornea is apparent, which might be an area of epithelial defect (Figure 11-1). The pediatrician confirms this with fluorescein dye staining (Figure 11-2). There was mild conjunctival hyperemia. No other injuries are observed.

Diagnosis

This patient has a corneal abrasion. The injury in corneal abrasion is superficial, without involvement of the deeper corneal stroma. Corneal abrasions are indicated by the loss of corneal epithelium. Tangential impact by hard objects can cause this condition. Some common agents of corneal abrasion include fingernails, plants, paper, and toys.

Symptoms of corneal abrasion include pain, light sensitivity (photophobia), foreign body sensation, and tearing. Because symptoms tend to be intense, patients have a difficult time holding their eyes open. Instillation of topical anesthetic can relieve symptoms for the examination but cannot be used long term secondary to corneal toxicity. Visual acuity may be decreased because of an irregular ocular surface caused by the abrasion.

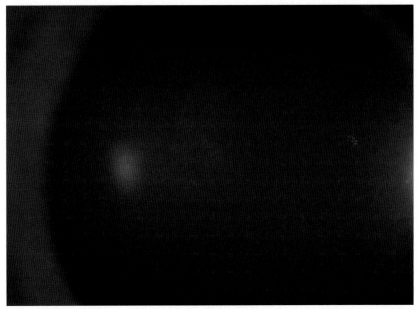

Figure 11-1. Focal area of corneal whitening with linear area centrally. Courtesy of Myoung Joon Kim, MD.

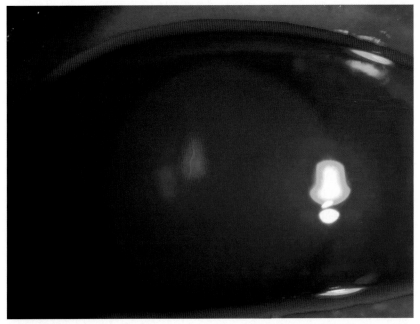

Figure 11-2. Corresponding fluorescein staining denoting denuded epithelium with central linear deeper involvement. Courtesy of Myoung Joon Kim, MD.

Ciliary injection (dilation of vessels around the corneal limbus) can be present in patients with corneal abrasion. A penlight or slit lamp can reveal the area where the epithelium is denuded or loose. The area of epithelial defect can be confirmed by staining with fluorescein dye. The stained area will show as bright green with cobalt blue light illumination.

Differential Diagnosis

Diagnoses besides corneal abrasion that should be considered include the following:

Infectious Keratitis

Infectious keratitis may present with similar symptoms. However, typically, an infectious keratitis will show a demarcated area of stromal suppuration and thinning, whereas an abrasion will present a clear yet de-epithelialized cornea. In addition, infectious keratitis may be accompanied by inflammation in the anterior chamber.

Corneal Foreign Body

The presence of a corneal foreign body is most easily identified under the biomicroscopic slit lamp. It appears as an area of negative and linear staining with fluorescein dye. Patients may indicate the location of the foreign object.

Recurrent Erosion Syndrome

This occurs in patients with a previous history of a sharp, sudden corneal abrading injury. The presentation is sudden, severe pain; however, there may not be any precipitating event. It often happens on waking up, lasting from a few minutes to hours. The cause of the spontaneous de-epithelialization is believed to be from poor epithelial adhesion after healing.

Traumatic Iritis

Traumatic iritis results from a blunt trauma to the eye causing intraocular inflammation. Aside from redness, there is significant photophobia and vague eye discomfort that is often described as heavy and aching. The cornea is absent of any epithelial defect.

When to Refer

If the corneal abrasion is not greatly improved within 24 hours after treatment or if there are signs of infection or whiteness to the cornea, the patient should be seen by a pediatric ophthalmologist. If the lesion is seen soon after the injury, stromal infiltration by inflammatory cells may not be observed immediately. To detect and treat associated infectious keratitis early, it is necessary to carefully document inflammatory signs, such as corneal infiltration (deeper stromal involvement) and anterior chamber reaction, on follow-up examinations by an ophthalmologist. Associated ocular or adnexal injuries and infectious keratitis after corneal abrasion require referral to an ophthalmologist. Furthermore, if corneal abrasion recurs spontaneously or by minor trauma in both eyes, some types of corneal dystrophy should be suspected and evaluated by a pediatric ophthalmologist.

Treatment

The pediatrician is comfortable removing loose corneal epithelium using a cotton-tipped applicator, forceps, or a spatula instrument to prevent imperfect healing and recurrent erosion syndrome. This is not always needed, especially if the pediatrician is not comfortable with the procedure. A broad-spectrum topical antibiotic is prescribed. A short-acting cycloplegic agent (eg, 1% cyclopentolate) is used for the relief of pain from traumatic iritis and ciliary body spasm.

Patching or a bandage contact lens may be considered for the patient's comfort. However, in the case of trauma from plant matter or potentially infectious material, it is best to avoid placing a patch or contact lens. Moreover, the use of a topical corticosteroid is avoided because it retards epithelial healing and potentiates infection. A topical nonsteroidal anti-inflammatory drug can be considered for pain control.

Follow-up depends on the severity of the injury. Patients should return in 24 hours when they have a central or large abrasion or are treated with an eye patch.

Discussion

The patient's epithelial cells normally grow and cover the denuded area within 24 to 48 hours depending on the extent of the injury. This happens by a migrating sheet of cells from the peripheral limbal area. It appears as thin leading edge of epithelium meeting centrally. If the Bowman membrane is not affected, corneal abrasions will heal without scarring. The process of reestablishing the full thickness of the cornea may take up to 6 weeks. Imperfect repair of hemidesmosomes between cells may lead to recurrent erosion syndrome.

If the area of abrasion is not greatly improved within 24 hours or if there are signs of infection or whiteness to the cornea, the patient should be seen by an ophthalmologist.

Key Points

- Most corneal abrasions heal without any problems, even though presenting symptoms can be intense.
- Treatment is targeted at relieving the patient's symptoms and preventing complications.
- A corneal abrasion should not be treated with a topical corticosteroid because it retards epithelial healing and potentiates infection.

Suggested Reading

Krachmer JH, Palay DA. Corneal trauma. In: Krachmer JH, Palay DA, eds. *Cornea Atlas*. 2nd ed. Philadelphia, PA: Elsevier; 2006:263–287

Sutphin JE. External disease and cornea. In: *Basic and Clinical Science Course*. San Francisco, CA: American Academy of Ophthalmology; 2008–2009

Chapter 12

Sudden Eye Redness and Pain

Myoung Joon Kim, MD
Jennifer Bernabe-Ko, MD
David J. Schanzlin, MD

Presentation

A 5-year-old girl comes into the pediatrician's office for an emergency consultation because of sudden sharp pain and a gritty feeling on the surface of her right eye. Her mother tells the pediatrician that the little girl was playing in the backyard and suddenly complained of severe discomfort of the right eye.

During the pediatrician's examination, the little girl is copiously tearing and has light sensitivity (photophobia) and conjunctival redness. On penlight examination the pediatrician sees a small, brown object lodged on the corneal epithelium.

Diagnosis

This child has a corneal foreign body. It is very important to take note of the history of the patient. In cases in which there is a corneal foreign body, often there is a history of a moving projectile toward the eye. In this case, the child was most likely playing in the soil or garden. Common materials encountered that are associated with ocular injury are metallic objects, sand, and soil. When children have an eye injury, it is usually associated with something around their immediate play area—pieces of candy wrapper, parts of their toys, and so on.

To be able to examine patients thoroughly, it is sometimes necessary to apply topical anesthetic eyedrops such as proparacaine. In the ophthalmologist's clinic, a slit-lamp biomicroscopic examination enables the eye care specialist to determine the location and depth of penetration of the foreign body (Figure 12-1). In some cases in which the foreign body is not grossly visible, fluorescein dye can be used to stain the de-epithelialized tissue to localize the foreign body.

Differential Diagnosis

Diagnoses besides a corneal foreign body that should be considered include the following:

Corneal Abrasion

This presents mostly with a foreign body sensation and sharp pain. However, the cornea will present as a clear area of de-epithelialization.

Traumatic Iritis

This presents with the same symptoms of red eye and light sensitivity, but there is a history of blunt trauma to the eye. Examination by slit lamp reveals a specific pattern of ciliary injection and aqueous flare and cells.

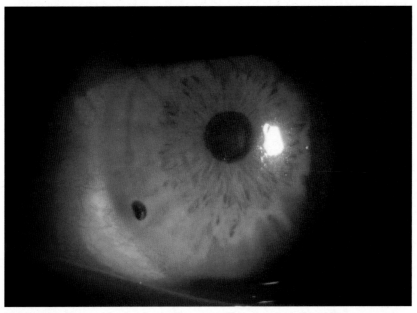

Figure 12-1. Corneal foreign body. Courtesy of Myoung Joon Kim, MD.

Infectious Conjunctivitis

This similarly presents as redness and discomfort. However, very prominent is the purulent discharge, conjunctival swelling, and diffuse pattern of conjunctival hyperemia.

When to Refer

In most cases, the foreign body is best removed by an ophthalmologist. The attempt to remove the object should only be done after assessment of the depth of penetration via slit lamp. Removal in a setting of full-thickness corneal penetration may result in aqueous leak. Referral is best done immediately, most especially if it is an organic material. If this is not possible, coverage with a broad-spectrum topical antibiotic may be initiated until proper referral can be made. The instillation of such eyedrops should be done with care to avoid disrupting the foreign body and further damaging the eye.

Treatment

The definitive treatment is removal of the metallic foreign body using forceps or a hypodermic needle with the use of the slit-lamp microscope. If the child is uncooperative, the pediatric ophthalmologist may need to do the examination and removal procedure while the child is under anesthesia. If the object is metallic, it is important to remove it entirely because it may cause some corneal staining and may even later cause recurrent erosions. A dental burr instrument is sometimes used to remove the iron stain on the cornea.

It is very important not to attempt a removal of a foreign body without first making sure that the globe has not ruptured. If the anterior chamber is compromised, surgical preparation may be required if the wound does not seal.

Inspection of the upper and lower palpebral conjunctiva is performed to ensure no other foreign body is left undetected. Because conjunctival foreign bodies can sometimes be easily missed, the upper and lower palpebral conjunctiva should be examined thoroughly via eyelid eversion. After instillation of proparacaine in the eye, the removal of a conjunctival foreign body can be done gently with a cotton swab (if superficial) or forceps.

Antibiotic drops or ointment is prescribed. Oral analgesia and cycloplegic drops are given depending on the severity of pain and photophobia.

Often, the epithelium will heal quite rapidly—within 24 to 48 hours. For the patient's comfort, the eye may be patched or a bandage contact lens applied.

Discussion

The patient should be seen the following day. If the foreign body is organic, such as soil or plant material, closer follow-up examination is necessary to detect and treat infection. Organic material is very antigenic and can cause significant corneal inflammation. Fungal keratitis is a definite danger and subsequent laboratory tests such as culture and sensitivity tests must be performed if there are signs of infection.

If the foreign body is inorganic and inert, such as glass or plastic, the patient is treated as if it is a corneal abrasion and followed accordingly on removal.

Key Points

- Organic material contains bacteria and fungi. Patching in that setting may potentiate infection.
- When the pupil moves in an inflamed eye, it hurts. Therefore, using a dilating eyedrop will make these patients more comfortable but will blur vision temporarily.
- Small defects in the ocular epithelium heal quickly.

Suggested Reading

Krachmer JH, Palay DA. Corneal trauma. In: Krachmer JH, Palay DA, eds. *Cornea Atlas.* 2nd ed. Philadelphia, PA: Elsevier; 2006:263–287

Sutphin JE. External disease and cornea. In: *Basic and Clinical Science Course.* San Francisco, CA: American Academy of Ophthalmology; 2008–2009

Chapter 13

Periocular Redness and Pain

David R. Weakley, MD

Presentation

A 4-year-old is seen in the pediatrician's office because of a 3-day history of increasing redness and pain around the right eye. The parents, well known to the pediatrician, report that the problem began as a small area adjacent to the nose but in the past 2 days has worsened and spread. The medial area is firm, very tender, and warm to the touch (Figure 13-1). The parents also noted tearing and purulent discharge from the right eye.

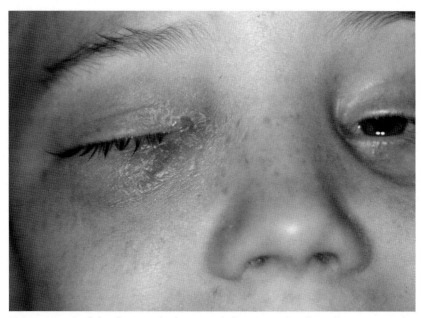

Figure 13-1. Eyelid redness and edema medially greater than laterally. Courtesy of David R. Weakley, MD.

Diagnosis

This child has acute dacryocystitis (inflammation of the lacrimal sac) with an early secondary preseptal cellulitis. Acute dacryocystitis can best be differentiated from primary preseptal cellulitis by the location of the initial infection medially in the area of the lacrimal sac. Additionally, there will generally be localized tenderness and an abscess or discharge in the lacrimal sac. Although this condition can occur spontaneously, it usually occurs when there is obstruction of the nasolacrimal drainage system.

Dacryocystitis most commonly occurs in babies who have nasolacrimal duct obstruction associated with a dacryocystocele (also called dacryocele or amniotocele) that has become secondarily infected. Figure 13-2 demonstrates the typical appearance of a dacryocystocele that has not progressed to dacryocystitis.

Differential Diagnosis

Diagnoses besides acute dacryocystitis that should be considered include primary preseptal cellulitis, encephalocele, and orbital cellulitis.

When to Refer

A patient with dacryocystitis should be referred to a pediatric ophthalmologist for monitoring vision and because relief of the obstruction by probing the nasolacrimal duct is often necessary once infection subsides.

A neonate with a dacryocystocele should be referred to a pediatric ophthalmologist soon after birth. Resolution of the dacryocystocele by manual decompression or probing will greatly decrease the risk of developing dacryocystitis. Some patients with dacryocystocele may have an associated nasal mucocele (Figure 13-3) caused by bulging mucosa at the distal end of the nasolacrimal duct. In some patients this nasal mucocele may result in airway compromise and require intranasal marsupialization by a surgeon. If breathing difficulty occurs with a dacryocele, a pediatric otolaryngologist should be consulted.

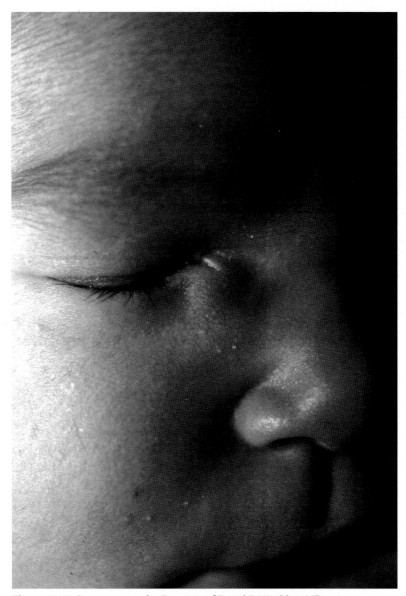

Figure 13-2. Dacryocystocele. Courtesy of David R. Weakley, MD.

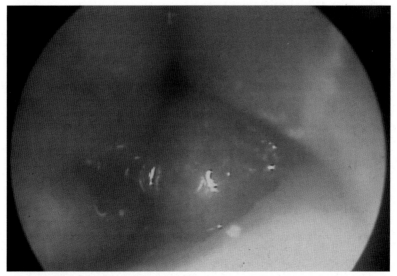

Figure 13-3. Intranasal mucocele (cyst) on endoscopic examination. Courtesy of David R. Weakley, MD.

Treatment

Although great variability exists in choice of treatment, many recommend intravenous antibiotics, especially in babies in whom posterior spread can occur. Orbital computed tomography should be considered if there are any signs of posterior spread.

Manual decompression of the lacrimal sac by digital compression is usually attempted, and any pus expressed should be cultured. This can be performed in a pediatrician's office by applying digital pressure over the distended lacrimal sac if you are comfortable with such a maneuver. Otherwise manual probing by an ophthalmologist may be indicated once acute symptoms reside. In patients for whom manual decompression is successful, it should be repeated as necessary to prevent reaccumulation of pus in the lacrimal sac, which will hasten resolution.

Discussion

Acute dacryocystitis most commonly occurs in babies with nasolacrimal duct obstruction, particularly if a dacryocele is present. If left untreated, it may lead to spread of the cellulitis. Management includes treatment of the secondary infection with antibiotics followed by management of the underlying obstruction.

Key Points

- Acute dacryocystitis is usually caused by an obstruction of the nasolacrimal duct.
- Acute dacryocystitis is most common in babies but may occur in older children, typically with a history of nasolacrimal duct obstruction.
- Acute dacryocystitis can best be differentiated from primary preseptal cellulitis by the location of the initial infection medially in the area of the lacrimal sac.
- Treatment of acute dacryocystitis is often with intravenous antibiotics and subsequent surgical intervention if necessary.
- Referral to a pediatric ophthalmologist is necessary to monitor vision and in most cases, for relief of the nasolacrimal duct obstruction.

Suggested Reading

American Academy of Ophthalmology. Section 6. Pediatric ophthalmology and strabismus. In: *Basic and Clinical Science Course.* San Francisco, CA: American Academy of Ophthalmology; 2006:240–241

MacEwen CJ. The lacrimal system. In: Taylor D, Hoyt CS, eds. *Pediatric Ophthalmology and Strabismus.* 3rd ed. Philadelphia, PA: Elsevier Saunders; 2005:285–294

Section 2

Teary Eye

Chapter 14

Tearing and Mucoid Discharge in an Infant

Bobby S. Korn, MD, PhD
Don O. Kikkawa, MD
Shira L. Robbins, MD

Presentation

A 6-week-old boy comes to his pediatrician's office because his parents have noted persistent tearing and mucoid discharge in both eyes since birth. The parents are concerned that their son has infectious pinkeye. A review of the birth history reveals no history of intrauterine infections; the patient received prophylactic erythromycin ophthalmic ointment at birth. He has otherwise been healthy on prior examinations.

On examination, the child has tears running down both cheeks, and a cloudy white discharge is expressed with palpation over the lacrimal sac (Figure 14-1).

Diagnosis

This child has congenital nasolacrimal duct obstruction (NLDO). The site of obstruction in the nasolacrimal system affects the type of discharge noted. High obstructions, at the level of puncta or canaliculi, typically have the presenting symptom of clear tearing. Low obstructions, distal to the lacrimal sac, can present with mucoid or mucopurulent discharge secondary to infection of pooled tears within the lacrimal sac. Such lower obstructions are the most common cause of congenital NLDO and result from a membranous lining at the valve of Hasner caused by delayed maturation of the lacrimal system (Figure 14-2). This patient's presentation is most consistent with a lower obstruction because of his cloudy discharge.

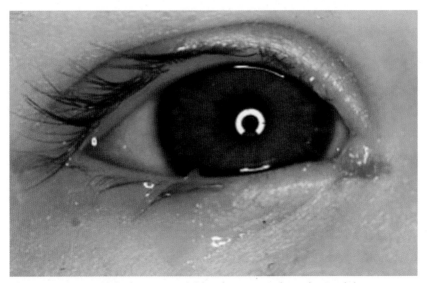

Figure 14-1. Mucoid discharge in a child with congenital nasolacrimal duct obstruction. Courtesy of Bobby S. Korn, MD, PhD.

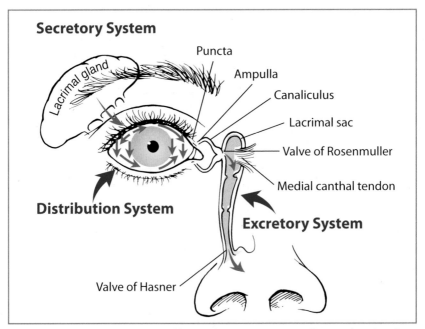

Figure 14-2. Schematic diagram of lacrimal system. Courtesy of Kenneth W. Wright, MD. From Wright KW. *Pediatric Ophthalmology for Primary Care*. 3rd ed. Elk Grove Village, IL: American Academy of Pediatrics; 2008:146.

For confirmation of NLDO diagnosis, a fluorescein dye disappearance test may be performed by the pediatrician or ophthalmologist. In this test a drop of fluorescein dye is instilled into the inferior conjunctival cul-de-sac of both eyes. Normally, fluorescein is cleared through the lacrimal system by 5 minutes. Therefore, a substantial amount of fluorescein in the eye at 5 minutes, seen with a Wood lamp (blue light), is diagnostic for NLDO. Overflow of fluorescein onto the cheek also confirms the diagnosis of NLDO. Frequently, in a patent lacrimal duct system, fluorescein can be visualized in the nares. Presence of fluorescein in the nose with overflow onto the cheek indicates a partially obstructed lacrimal system. This patient has overflow tearing and substantial fluorescein in the eyes at 5 minutes, which confirms the presence of NLDO.

Differential Diagnosis

Diagnoses besides nasolacrimal duct obstruction that should be considered include the following:

Punctal or Canalicular Atresia

This congenital anomaly results from failure of the lacrimal system to canalize during development. Atresia is evident (by near absence of puncta) on clinical inspection of the lacrimal punctum.

Conjunctivitis

Ophthalmia neonatorum describes the spectrum of conjunctivitis occurring in the first month of life (see Chapter 1). These range from gonococcal infection to *Chlamydia trachomatis* infection, herpes viral conjunctivitis, and chemical conjunctivitis. The advent of widespread antibiotic prophylaxis has greatly reduced incidence of gonococcal conjunctivitis. Incidence of late conjunctivitis with possible pneumonitis raises concern for *Chlamydia conjunctivitis,* whereas presence on fluorescein staining of corneal dendrites favors herpes infection. Conjunctivitis is commonly associated with discharge and a red eye, in contrast with NLDO, which typically presents with discharge and *no* red eye. Occasionally the lower eyelid will be red and excoriated in conjunctivitis.

Congenital Glaucoma

Tearing, photophobia, and blepharospasm can be presenting signs of congenital glaucoma. There may be associated corneal enlargement (appearance of big eyes) or corneal clouding. Suspicion of this diagnosis requires prompt ophthalmic referral to preserve vision.

When to Refer

Spontaneous remission is the rule in congenital NLDO. The pediatrician should recommend an ophthalmologic evaluation if the patient with NLDO is still symptomatic at 1 year of age.

In some patients with distal NLDO, acute dacryocystitis (infection of the lacrimal sac) can develop (see Chapter 13). These patients should be referred to a pediatric ophthalmologist after resolution of acute infection so that the site of obstruction can be relieved with surgical intervention.

Treatment

Initial management of NLDO is massage over the area of the lacrimal sac (Figure 14-3). In many instances, membranous obstruction of the valve of Hasner is relieved by increased hydrostatic pressure afforded by lacrimal massage. Parents should be instructed on how to perform this massage at home. Nasolacrimal duct massage is performed by pressing with a finger on the sac below the medial canthus in a downward fashion, approximately 5 strokes 2 times a day. It is important to apply pressure to the sac and not the nasal bone.

In this case, the pediatrician should ask the parents to return to the office if the infant's ocular discharge changes color from white to yellow or green.

Antibiotics should not be used for a quiet, tearing eye. If there is an element of mucoid (clear or white) or purulent discharge (usually yellow or green), topical antibiotics (eg, polymyxin B/trimethoprim or, for faster resolution, fluoroquinolone eyedrops, alternatively erythromycin or bacitracin ointment) generally reduce the discharge. However, it is important to let parents know that unless the obstruction is relieved,

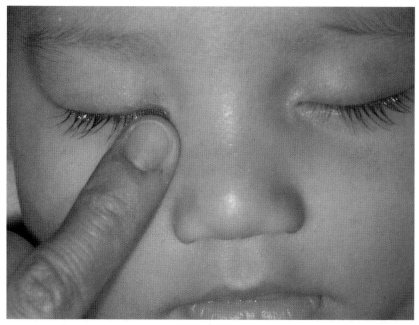

Figure 14-3. Nasolacrimal duct obstruction massage technique. Courtesy of Shira L. Robbins, MD.

mucoid discharge tends to recur after cessation of antibiotics because antibiotics do *not* open a blocked drainage system.

If acute dacryocystitis develops, systemic antibiotics are indicated, followed by surgical intervention.

Timing of initial surgical treatment of NLDO is bimodal. Some surgeons advocate early (younger than 6 months) in-office lacrimal duct probing, whereas most recommend waiting until the infant is 1 year old to perform a surgical procedure using anesthesia. Both approaches have high success rates. Early in-office intervention avoids the need for anesthesia but results in many more children undergoing probing of the lacrimal duct. Later intervention allows NLDO to resolve on its own without a procedure in many cases. However, later intervention mandates an operating room setting. Each ophthalmologist will have an individual approach to this condition. Most ophthalmologists in the United States opt to perform surgery after the infant reaches 1 year of age, by which time most cases spontaneously resolve. Ophthalmologists will operate earlier in the face of recurrent infections or symptomatic tearing, which can blur vision and affect the child's daily activities.

The usual treatment algorithm is to perform lacrimal duct probing and lacrimal irrigation in the operating room if tearing persists beyond 1 year. Various authors have reported success rates greater than 90% for lacrimal duct probing. If probing fails, next line of treatment is intubation of the nasolacrimal system with silicone tubing that is often combined with infracture of the inferior nasal turbinate. An alternative line of treatment is balloon catheter dilation (dacryoplasty). Finally, if all other measures have been exhausted, dacryocystorhinostomy (opening a new passageway through bone to the nasal cavity) is performed to create a new outflow channel for tears.

Some parents apply human milk to a newborn's eye as a treatment of neonatal conjunctivitis. Topical human milk has not been shown to relieve NLDO, which is a structural condition. Whether it is safe and effective for treating an infectious conjunctivitis associated with NLDO has not been conclusively demonstrated.

Discussion

Congenital NLDO is common, seen in up to 20% of all infants. In 95% of these cases, onset of tearing or discharge is recognized within the first month of life. Another 3% of these cases present in the second month of life, and the remaining cases present in the third and fourth months. If onset of tearing occurs after the fourth month, an acquired cause of tearing should be sought.

Approximately 95% of congenital NLDO cases spontaneously resolve by 1 year. The pediatrician should recommend an ophthalmologic evaluation if the patient is still symptomatic at 1 year of age or earlier if the diagnosis is not conclusive.

Key Points

- Nasolacrimal duct obstruction (NLDO) is very common.
- Antibiotics need to be used only if there is associated purulent ocular discharge.
- Glaucoma and acute dacryocystitis should be considered because they are associated with ocular morbidity.
- Most NLDOs resolve within the first year of life, which lends itself to a watch-and-wait approach. If tearing persists beyond 1 year, surgical intervention may be needed.

Suggested Reading

American Academy of Ophthalmology. Pediatric ophthalmology and strabismus. In: *Basic and Clinical Science Course.* San Francisco, CA: American Academy of Ophthalmology; 2005–2006

Kushner BJ. The management of nasolacrimal duct obstruction in children between 18 months and 4 years old. *J AAPOS.* 1998;2(1):57–60

Nelson LB, Calhoun JH, Menduke H. Medical management of congenital nasolacrimal duct obstruction. *Pediatrics.* 1985;76(2): 172–175

Robb RM. *Nasolacrimal Duct Obstruction in Children.* In: Focal Points, Clinical Modules for Ophthalmologists. San Francisco, CA: American Academy of Ophthalmology. Module 8, 2004

Chapter 15

Infant With Tearing and Light Sensitivity

Anya A. Trumler, MD
Shira L. Robbins, MD
Carl B. Camras, MD, PhD

Presentation

A 9-month-old girl is brought to the pediatric clinic because her parents have noticed that her eyes have been watery and more light-sensitive than usual over the past few weeks. In the sunlight she has been squeezing her eyes closed. They have not noticed any discharge or crossing of the eyes. There is no history of trauma. She was born at 38 weeks by normal vaginal delivery. She has otherwise been reaching normal developmental milestones and has no known health problems. The patient has no family history of ocular disease.

On examination, the infant appears to fix and follow objects with each eye when tested individually. When shining a direct ophthalmoscope into the eye, she closes her eyes and turns away. In a dimly lit room, there is an obvious difference in the size of the eyes. There is also a slight haziness or blue hue to the right eye, which causes iris details to appear less distinct (Figure 15-1). Red (Brückner) reflex is asymmetric. By holding each eye open, the pediatrician is able to view the central retina with the direct ophthalmoscope. The right optic nerve appears to have a larger central depression than the left optic nerve (Figure 15-2).

Diagnosis

This patient has congenital glaucoma. This disease leads to progressive damage to the optic nerve in patients related to elevated intraocular pressure.

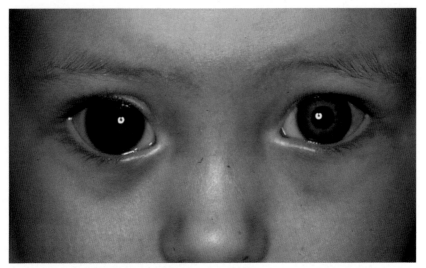

Figure 15-1. External photograph of patient showing enlarged right cornea with decreased iris details of right eye caused by corneal clouding. Note that right eye pupil is smaller. Courtesy of Anya A. Trumler, MD.

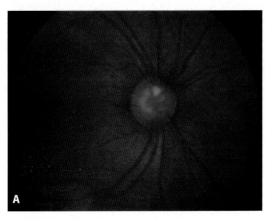

Figure 15-2. A, Right eye optic nerve with enlarged central depression, known as the optic cup. In glaucoma there is increased size of the optic cup relative to the optic nerve. Courtesy of Anya A. Trumler, MD.

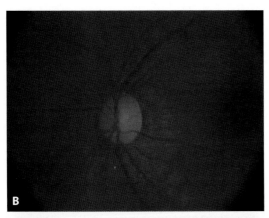

B, Left eye with normal-appearing optic nerve and optic cup. Courtesy of Anya A. Trumler, MD.

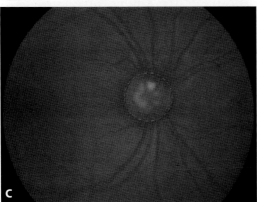

C, Black-and-white image of right eye optic nerve outlined with a red dotted line; optic cup is outlined with a blue dotted line. Courtesy of Anya A. Trumler, MD.

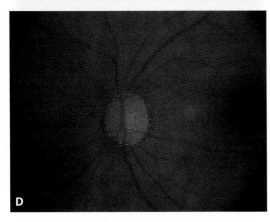

D, Black-and-white image of left eye optic nerve outlined with a red dotted line; optic cup is outlined with a blue dotted line. Comparison of the right and left eyes shows asymmetry in optic cup size, with the right optic cup larger than the left. Courtesy of Anya A. Trumler, MD.

The classic symptom triad for congenital glaucoma is epiphora (excessive watering), blepharospasm (uncontrolled closure of eyelids), and photophobia (light sensitivity). Elevated intraocular pressure in these younger eyes is thought to cause gradual stretching of the tissues, resulting in enlarged corneas, enlarged eye size, corneal cloudiness, tears in the inner corneal layers, and increased optic nerve cupping. Excessive tearing caused by congenital glaucoma can lead to a false diagnosis of nasolacrimal duct obstruction (see "Differential Diagnosis"). If intraocular pressure is not controlled, the eye can develop buphthalmos (sometimes called ox eye). There also can be stretching of all the tissues, resulting in high myopia, scleral thinning, lens dislocation, and microscopic tears in the inner corneal layers causing corneal swelling and cloudiness. Without treatment, complete blindness can result.

If disease presentation occurs in children after age 4 years, it is termed *juvenile glaucoma.* In these patients, because of age, tissues are less elastic, so the eye does not enlarge from high eye pressure. Clinical examination and subjective complaints in juvenile glaucoma are fairly unremarkable other than elevated intraocular pressure and optic nerve head cupping. Juvenile glaucoma usually has autosomal-dominant inheritance and is treated more like adult-onset glaucoma.

Differential Diagnosis

Diagnoses besides congenital glaucoma that should be considered include the following:
- Nasolacrimal duct obstruction
- Trauma to cornea during birth
- Corneal abrasion
- Uveitis
- Conjunctivitis
- Corneal infection
- Corneal disorders

When to Refer

Patients suspected of having glaucoma require urgent referral to an ophthalmologist for further examination and diagnostic testing. Examination includes visual acuity, refraction, corneal examination, intraocular pressure measurement, and dilated eye examination. Pediatric patients may have difficulty cooperating with the detailed eye examination required to make the diagnosis of congenital glaucoma; therefore, most infants require general anesthesia for the examination. Examination using anesthesia is done not only to confirm diagnosis but also to evaluate for other associated ocular abnormalities, such as other embryologic dysgenesis.

Treatment

Treatment of primary congenital glaucoma is surgical. Medical treatment with eyedrops or oral glaucoma medications are used as temporizing agents until a specialist can perform the surgical procedure. Surgery entails creating a surgical opening connecting the aqueous drainage system to the anterior chamber. Approximately 80% of congenital glaucoma patients younger than 1 year achieve adequate intraocular pressure control with 1 or 2 surgical procedures.

After surgery, some patients may also require treatment with antiglaucoma drops. Topical medications used in the treatment of glaucoma are beta-blockers, carbonic anhydrase inhibitors, prostaglandin analogues, miotic therapy, and adrenergic agonists. The alpha-2-adrenergic agonist brimonidine is an effective treatment to lower intraocular pressure, but in children younger than 2 years, this ophthalmic solution is contraindicated because of its severe side effects of lethargy, hypothermia, apnea, and central nervous system depression. The oral carbonic anhydrase inhibitors acetazolamide and methazolamide, prescribed by ophthalmologists, are also effective intraocular pressure–lowering therapies, but children should be monitored for weight loss, lethargy, and metabolic acidosis.

Discussion

The precise pathologic defect in congenital glaucoma is not known, but it is thought to be caused by abnormal development in the aqueous fluid drainage pathway from the eye.

Incidence of congenital glaucoma is 1 in every 10,000 births and results in blindness if not treated. Congenital glaucoma can occur in utero and manifest at birth in 25% of patients, with 80% of all cases developing before 1 year of age. Ninety percent of cases occur sporadically, with others having an autosomal-recessive or autosomal-dominant inheritance. Incidence of congenital glaucoma is higher in males (70% males to 30% females). Two-thirds of cases are bilateral.

There are also pediatric glaucomas associated with other ocular developmental abnormalities which can be elucidated on ophthalmic examination (Box 15-1). Secondary glaucoma may arise in pediatric patients due to ocular diseases that affect the aqueous fluid drainage mechanism (Box 15-2). A third category are those pediatric glaucomas associated with other systemic and ocular developmental abnormalities (Box 15-3).

If congenital glaucoma presents at birth, prognosis is poor, with at least 50% of patients becoming legally blind, often having visual acuity of 20/400 or worse, despite adequate intraocular pressure treatment. Congenital glaucoma that initially presents within the first year after birth has a better prognosis, with 53% to 79% having visual acuity of 20/50 or better, and only 2% to 15% becoming legally blind. Patients with a diagnosis of congenital glaucoma require lifelong frequent follow-up to monitor and treat further disease progression.

Box 15-1. Developmental Glaucomas With Associated Ocular Abnormalities

Aniridia (congenital and acquired glaucoma)

Axenfeld-Rieger anomaly

Congenital ectropion uvea

Congenital iris hypoplasia

Mutations in *CYP1B1* gene

Mutations in *FOX4* gene

Anterior segment dysgenesis

Box 15-2. Secondary Glaucomas

Aphakic glaucoma

Traumatic glaucoma

Secondary to intraocular neoplasm

Secondary to chronic uveitis

Lens-related glaucoma

Steroid-induced glaucoma

Secondary to rubeosis or neovascularization of anterior segment of eye

Angle closure

Box 15-3. Primary Glaucoma Associated With Systemic/Ocular Abnormalities

- Sturge-Weber syndrome: facial port-wine stain with cerebral calcifications
- Neurofibromatosis type 1: café au lait spots and neurofibromas
- Stickler syndrome: collagen disorder affecting joints, auditory system, and eyes
- Lowe syndrome: bilateral cataracts, mental delay, and kidney disease
- Rieger syndrome: craniofacial, ocular, and dental abnormalities
- SHORT syndrome: short stature, hyperextensible joints, and Rieger syndrome
- Zellweger syndrome: enlarged liver, facial deformities, and mental delay
- Marfan syndrome: connective tissue disorder with tall height and organ abnormalities
- Aniridia: abnormal iris with other ocular abnormalities; can be associated with Wilms tumor and WAGR (Wilms tumor, aniridia, genitourinary anomalies, mental retardation) syndrome in sporadic cases
- Multiple craniofacial syndromes

> ## Key Points
>
> - Pediatric glaucoma is the abnormal elevation of eye pressure, with resultant ocular and optic nerve injury causing loss of vision.
> - Congenital glaucoma classically presents with cloudy enlarged corneas, light sensitivity, and excessive tearing.
> - Excessive tearing caused by congenital glaucoma can lead to a false diagnosis of nasolacrimal duct obstruction.
> - Suspicion of pediatric glaucoma requires immediate referral to a pediatric ophthalmologist or glaucoma specialist.
> - Treatment of congenital glaucoma is most successful if initiated early and consists of surgery and antiglaucoma eyedrops.
> - Pediatric glaucoma can be associated with underlying genetic syndromes.

Suggested Reading

Bowman RJ, Cope J, Nischal KK. Ocular and systemic side effects of brimonidine 0.2% eye drops (Alphagan) in children. *Eye (Lond).* 2004;18(1):24–26

Gencik A, Gencikova A, Ferák V. Population genetical aspects of primary congenital glaucoma. I. Incidence, prevalence, gene frequency, and age of onset. *Hum Genet.* 1982;61(3):193–197

Ho CL, Walton DS. Primary congenital glaucoma: 2004 update. *J Pediatr Ophthalmol Strabismus.* 2004;41(5):271–288

Hoskins HD Jr, Shaffer RN, Hetherington J. Anatomical classification of the developmental glaucomas. *Arch Ophthalmol.* 1984;102(9): 1331–1336

Mendicino ME, Lynch MG, Drack A, et al. Long-term surgical and visual outcomes in primary congenital glaucoma: 360 degrees trabeculotomy versus goniotomy. *J AAPOS.* 2000;4(4):205–210

Rhee DJ. *Glaucoma: Color Atlas and Synopsis of Clinical Ophthalmology.* New York, NY: McGraw-Hill; 2003:182–187

Eyelid and Orbit

Chapter 16

Swollen Eyelids

Christina M. Ohnsman, MD

Presentation

A 10-year-old boy presents to the pediatrician's office with a 2-day history of increasing redness and swelling of the right upper and lower eyelids. He complains of pain in his eye and when asked, also reports nasal congestion. He has had sinusitis in the past but is otherwise healthy.

On physical examination, he has a temperature of 38.3°C (101°F). His right upper and lower eyelids are red and tensely swollen shut, and his skin is tender and warm to palpation. His visual acuity (with his eyelids held open) is 20/20 in both eyes. His pupils react normally and equally, but he cannot fully move the eye up and reports that it hurts to try. His conjunctiva appears to have fluid beneath it nasally and is raised.

Suspecting orbital cellulitis, the pediatrician refers the patient to a pediatric ophthalmologist.

Diagnosis

The pediatric ophthalmologist confirms the diagnosis of orbital cellulitis. The patient is admitted to the hospital, where axial and coronal computed tomography (CT) views of the orbits and sinuses confirm the orbital infection as well as pansinusitis (figures 16-1 and 16-2). A complete blood cell count with differential shows elevated white blood cells. Blood cultures also are obtained.

It is critical to differentiate between preseptal cellulitis (in which the infection is anterior to the orbital septum) and orbital cellulitis (in which the infection is posterior to the orbital septum) because orbital cellulitis requires urgent hospitalization. The skin appears red and edematous in either situation, so other clinical features should be used to differentiate between them (Table 16-1).

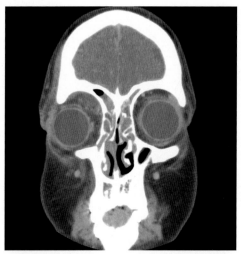

Figure 16-1. Coronal computed tomography reveals bilateral ethmoid sinusitis and inflammatory changes within the right superior and medial orbit, with displacement of the globe inferolaterally. Courtesy of Christina M. Ohnsman, MD.

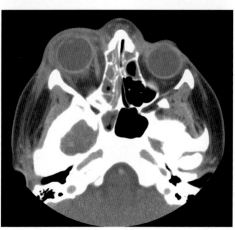

Figure 16-2. Axial computed tomography reveals proptosis of the right globe with inflammatory changes posterior to the orbital septum. Note the ethmoid sinusitis, particularly on the right side. Courtesy of Christina M. Ohnsman, MD.

Table 16-1. Comparison of Symptoms and Signs of Preseptal Versus Orbital Cellulitis

Signs and Symptoms	Preseptal Cellulitis	Orbital Cellulitis
Pain	+	+
Eyelid redness	+	+
Eyelid swelling	+	+
Warmth	+	+
Tenderness	+	+
Fever	+/-	+/-
Conjunctival redness		+
Conjunctival chemosis		+
Proptosis		+
Double vision		+/-
Limited ocular motility		+/-
Afferent pupillary defect		+/-

Conjunctival redness and chemosis (or edema), as well as limitation of extraocular movements, are often present in orbital cellulitis. Proptosis may be present in orbital cellulitis, as may an afferent pupillary defect, indicating optic neuropathy and imminent visual loss. Orbital cellulitis is most often caused by sinusitis, with extension from the ethmoid sinus via the lamina papyracea. Furthermore, it may be associated with a subperiosteal abscess. For these reasons, a CT scan of the orbits and sinuses should be obtained when orbital cellulitis is suspected. It is not necessary to obtain imaging in preseptal cellulitis, although it is imperative to observe the patient closely to be sure that the infection does not progress to an orbital process.

The most common organisms in preseptal and orbital cellulitis are *Staphylococcus* species, including an increasing incidence of methicillin-resistant *S aureus* (MRSA); *Streptococcus* species; and *Haemophilus* species other than *H influenzae*. *H influenzae*–related preseptal or orbital cellulitis has become rare because of the widespread use of the *H influenzae* type b vaccine.

Differential Diagnosis

Diagnoses that should be considered besides orbital cellulitis include the following:

Preseptal Cellulitis

Infection is of the eyelid area anterior to the orbital septum (Figure 16-3). Conjunctival redness and chemosis (or edema) are absent, and there is little or no limitation of extraocular movements.

Idiopathic Orbital Inflammatory Pseudotumor

Rapid onset of a painful, proptotic red eye is caused by inflammation of the extraocular muscles or other orbital structures. Imaging shows thickening of the involved structures without involvement of the sinuses.

Acute Dacryoadenitis

The lacrimal gland is inflamed or infected, causing pain, redness, and swelling of only the lateral eyelid. Extraocular movements are generally unimpaired, and imaging shows lack of sinus involvement.

Chalazion

An early chalazion may present with a red, mildly painful, swollen eyelid prior to formation of a discrete nodule. However, signs and

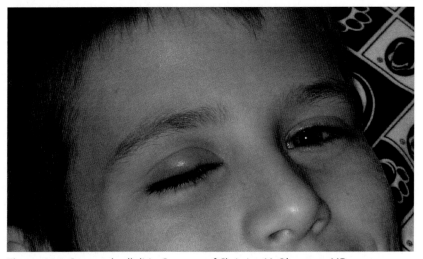

Figure 16-3. Preseptal cellulitis. Courtesy of Christina M. Ohnsman, MD.

symptoms are mild compared with orbital cellulitis, eye movements are uninvolved, and the patient is afebrile.

Insect Bite

An insect bite or sting to the eyelid may result in a similar presentation to that of orbital cellulitis. Careful examination may reveal the puncture wound(s). However, while an insect bite may or may not lead to preseptal cellulitis, the infection typically will not extend posterior to the orbital septum.

Allergic Dermatitis or Angioedema

Eyelid swelling—with or without conjunctival chemosis—is of sudden onset and associated with itching rather than pain. Deeper orbital structures are not involved; therefore, eye movements are full and painless.

Viral Conjunctivitis With Associated Eyelid Edema

Eyelid swelling is associated with diffuse conjunctival redness, watery discharge, and eyelids sticking together on awakening. This is often associated with an upper respiratory infection or pharyngitis. Unlike orbital cellulitis, pain is absent or mild, and extraocular movements are full.

Trauma

Blunt trauma may lead to swollen eyelids, conjunctival redness, and limitation of extraocular movements. If a history is not available, trauma may be differentiated from orbital cellulitis by absence of fever and by the presence of ecchymosis or other signs of injury. Imaging may be necessary for further evaluation.

When to Refer

A pediatric ophthalmologist should always be involved in cases of orbital cellulitis, or whenever the differentiation between this entity and preseptal cellulitis is in doubt.

Treatment

In the hospital the patient is treated with ampicillin-sulbactam (Unasyn) 3 g intravenous (IV) every 6 hours (300 mg/kg/day divided by 4 doses) and vancomycin 800 mg IV every 12 hours (40 mg/kg/day divided by 2 doses). He also receives saline lavage and oxymetazoline spray (Afrin) twice a day.

As opposed to oral antibiotics for patients with preseptal cellulitis, broad-spectrum IV antibiotics are indicated for treatment of orbital cellulitis. These medications may be adjusted according to results of any positive cultures. It is wise to consider the likelihood of MRSA as an etiologic agent when choosing the antibiotic(s).

When sinusitis is also present, a nasal decongestant and saline lavage may be used. Small, medial subperiosteal abscesses may be treated with antibiotics in patients younger than 9 years who do not have visual compromise or intracranial or frontal sinus involvement. However, patients who do not meet these criteria for conservative treatment will require surgery.

After discharge from the hospital, patients will need oral antibiotics for 7 to 10 days.

Discussion

The most common cause of orbital cellulitis is bacterial sinusitis, which may occur as a result of upper respiratory infection in cold weather or as a result of allergic sinusitis during pollen season. Therefore, it may be seen year-round. In addition to sinusitis, other causes of orbital cellulitis include direct infection from local trauma or contiguous spread from sites of infection.

Accurate diagnosis and prompt treatment are essential for patients with orbital cellulitis. Delayed treatment may lead to permanent loss of vision due to optic nerve damage or result in meningitis from intracranial extension. With prompt and accurate treatment, the prognosis is generally good.

Key Points

- Preseptal cellulitis clinical signs are limited to the eyelid area, with no or little involvement of the eyeball or extraocular muscles.
- Orbital cellulitis may be characterized by edematous eyelids, injected or chemotic conjunctiva, limited ocular motility, and possible afferent pupillary defect.
- Delayed treatment of orbital cellulitis may lead to permanent loss of vision due to optic nerve damage or meningitis from intracranial extension.
- A pediatric ophthalmologist should always be involved in cases of orbital cellulitis, or whenever the differentiation between this entity and preseptal cellulitis is in doubt.

Suggested Reading

Donahue SP, Schwartz G. Preseptal and orbital cellulitis in childhood. A changing microbiologic spectrum. *Ophthalmology.* 1998;105(10): 1902–1906

Garcia GH, Harris GJ. Criteria for nonsurgical management of subperiosteal abscess of the orbit: analysis of outcomes 1988–1998. *Ophthalmology.* 2000;107(8):1454–1458

Holzmann D, Willi U, Nadal D. Allergic rhinitis as a risk factor for orbital complication of acute rhinosinusitis in children. *Am J Rhinol.* 2001;15(6):387–390

McKinley SH, Yen MT, Miller AM, Yen KG. Microbiology of pediatric orbital cellulitis. *Am J Ophthalmol.* 2007;144(4):497–501

Yen KG, Chilakapati MC, Coats DK, Miller AM, Paysse EA, Steinkuller PG. Ocular infectious diseases. In: Feigin RD, Cherry JD, Demmler-Harrison GJ, Kaplan SL, eds. *Textbook of Pediatric Infectious Diseases.* 5th ed. Philadelphia, PA: Saunders; 2009:811–835

Chapter 17

Strawberry-Colored Lesion on the Eyelid

Lynnelle Smith Newell, MD
Bobby S. Korn, MD, PhD
Don O. Kikkawa, MD

Presentation

An 18-month-old girl is brought into the pediatrician's office by her mother. Her parents first noted a strawberry-colored lesion involving the right eyelid (Figure 17-1). Initially a red macule at birth, it has continued to grow, now partially obscuring the visual axis. The mother is obviously concerned and wants a suggestion on what to do.

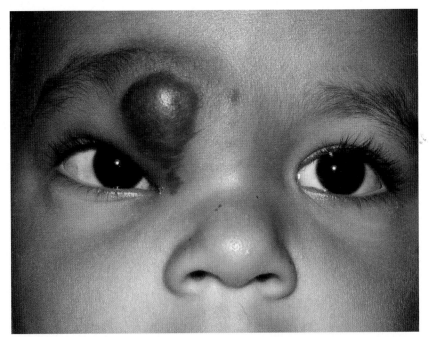

Figure 17-1. An 18-month-old girl presents with a discolored soft tissue mass of the right upper eyelid and eyebrow. Courtesy of Don O. Kikkawa, MD.

The pediatrician knows these lesions usually improve with age but is worried that this lesion might affect the development of vision. Realizing most of such lesions eventually involute (regress) but that more than 50% of patients experience residual skin changes including scarring, atrophy, discoloration, and telangiectasias, the pediatrician warns the parent. Interventions for lesions in the periorbital region are targeted at minimizing visual impairment and optimizing cosmetic results of the eyelid and orbit.

The pediatrician realizes this patient requires ophthalmic examination and refers her to a pediatric ophthalmologist.

Diagnosis

Periocular capillary hemangioma, the diagnosis in this case, is a hamartoma arising from immature, proliferating capillaries and endothelial cells. Capillary hemangiomas are usually absent or barely noticeable at birth, with a premonitory cutaneous mark such as a telangiectasia or macule just like in this patient. Although seemingly predisposed to the head and neck, they can develop anywhere on the skin, mucous membranes, or internal organs. Initial presentation is followed by a phase of rapid growth within the first year of life, followed by a period of stability and then varying degrees of involution by the age of 9 years.

A large spectrum of malformations can affect the eyelid and orbit.

Differential Diagnosis

Diagnoses besides capillary hemangioma that should be considered include the following:

Nevus Flammeus

Nevus flammeus, or port-wine stain, is composed of dilated cavernous vascular channels present and unchanged from birth. These do not blanch with external pressure. Lesions in the ophthalmic division of the trigeminal nerve are associated with Sturge-Weber syndrome.

Arteriovenous Malformation

Arteriovenous malformations are abnormal connections between arteries and veins that do not regress but enlarge with trauma and hormonal states. They may have a palpable thrill on examination.

Cavernous Hemangioma

Cavernous hemangiomas are venous malformations characterized by a soft, compressible mass with a bluish coloration that engorges when dependent. These malformations do not regress.

Lymphangioma

Lymphangiomas are hemodynamically isolated lesions that can show rapid growth that typically manifests after the first decade of life. Recurrent hemorrhage and worsening during upper respiratory tract infections are quite common with lymphangioma.

Tumor

Deep, subcutaneous lesions with an atypical appearance or unusual behavior in the absence of overlying skin changes may warrant a tissue biopsy to rule out atypical benign or malignant tumors. These include neurofibromas, optic nerve gliomas, histiocytosis, rhabdomyosarcoma, lymphoma, or lacrimal gland tumors.

When to Refer

Collaboration is crucial between the pediatrician and ophthalmologist in treating 2 phenomena associated with capillary hemangiomas. Patients with any capillary hemangiomas near the eye should be referred to a pediatric ophthalmologist for examination and testing. The pediatric ophthalmologist will serially measure the size and location, determine the stage of evolution, and create photographic documentation of this lesion. A careful assessment is also necessary to evaluate any effect on the visual and structural development of the eye and orbit. Deep lesions may present with only proptosis or other structural defects. Lesions will blanch with pressure and often increase in size with Valsalva maneuvers.

Small, superficial lesions are more likely to involute with minimal sequelae, and most can be observed without further intervention. Larger, deeper lesions can cause mechanical eyelid problems, eye misalignment, and glaucoma and can compromise visual development by inducing amblyopia. Such lesions require intervention.

Up to 20% of infants will have multiple hemangiomas. Patients with 5 or more cutaneous or segmental lesions with linear or geographic arrangement warrant further workup for visceral involvement and potentially PHACE (posterior fossa anomalies, hemangiomas, arterial, cardiac, and eye abnormalities) syndrome.

The growth and location of the lesion(s) can also create severe systemic complications. While rare, Kasabach-Merritt syndrome develops when rapidly proliferating, large visceral hemangiomas are associated with platelet sequestration and severe thrombocytopenia. Disseminated intravascular coagulopathy can also occur. Second, large hemangiomas of the nasopharynx and oropharynx can obstruct respiratory passages.

The ophthalmologist may use magnetic resonance imaging (MRI) and computed tomography to assess bony involvement, spatial arrangement, and soft-tissue details for large lesions with a diameter larger than 2 cm. The use of MRI is helpful to determine the caliber of feeder vessels and the extent of deeper orbital involvement, both of which contribute to determining prognosis (Figure 17-2). The presence of larger caliber arterial feeders suggests that lesions are unlikely to completely regress.

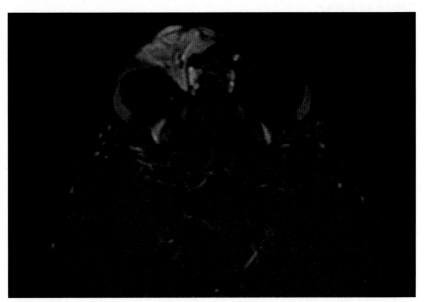

Figure 17-2. Magnetic resonance imaging of brain and orbits of same patient as in Figure 17-1, showing soft tissue mass in right upper lid and glabellar region. Note extension into anterior orbit. Courtesy of Don O. Kikkawa, MD.

Treatment

The goal of treatment often involves interventions made to minimize complications and disfigurement. Growth can cause proptosis, ptosis, eyelid malposition such as entropion and ectropion, and glaucoma and may compromise visual development by inducing strabismus, astigmatism, or amblyopia.

The first line of medical therapy is corticosteroids, with the route of administration decided by the ophthalmologist. Some controversy exists as to the route of administration. Oral and locally administered (eg, injected, topical) steroids have been employed with success. Each has advantages and disadvantages. With local periocular administration, the most feared complication is embolic phenomenon to the retinal arteries with intravascular administration. Interferon-alpha can be considered for visually threatening lesions unresponsive to corticosteroids, but its use is limited because of the more serious potential side effects of this drug, including neurotoxicity. Recently, several individual studies have reported successful results with topical, intralesional, and systemic beta-blocker therapies. Reported side effects of beta-blocker therapies include hypotension, bradycardia, bronchospasm, hypoglycemia, gastrointestinal symptoms, sleep disturbances, and electrolyte abnormalities. Fewer systemic side effects are reported with topical and intralesional treatments because of less systemic absorption. Further examination is currently underway in several randomized controlled trials.

Surgical intervention is considered for lesions unresponsive to medical therapy. It is aimed at debulking the mass and interrupting larger blood vessel feeders to assist with the natural process of involution. With larger lesions, sclerosing agents (ie, alcohol or sodium morrhuate) have been used adjunctively to reduce bleeding and mass effect prior to surgery. Laser treatment can reduce the residual skin pigmentation. Treatment of associated amblyopia and strabismus often improves with patching, atropine, corrective lenses, and strabismus surgery.

Discussion

Periocular capillary hemangioma is one of the most common developmental vascular anomalies of childhood.

One should not underestimate the psychosocial implications that many of these lesions have on patients and their families. Realistic expectations must be established by educating the family on the natural course, potential complications, and treatment options.

Key Points

- Capillary hemangiomas are the most common periocular vascular malformation.
- Most small lesions can be observed and will involute without further intervention.
- Larger lesions causing visual impairment or structural compromise to the orbit require treatment.
- Steroids currently remain the mainstay of medical treatment and surgical intervention being reserved for those that do not respond. Adjunctive treatment includes lasers and sclerosing agents.
- Several studies have demonstrated successful treatment of hemangiomas with beta-blocker therapy. Randomized controlled studies are underway that will determine if this type of therapy becomes a standard of care for future therapies.

Suggested Reading

Ceisler E, Blei F. Ophthalmic issues in hemangiomas of infancy. *Lymphat Res Biol.* 2003;1(4):321–330

Ceisler EJ, Santos L, Blei F. Periocular hemangiomas: what every physician should know. *Pediatr Dermatol.* 2004;21(1):1–9

Drolet BA, Esterly NB, Frieden IJ. Hemangiomas in children. *N Engl J Med.* 1999;341(3):173–181

Ni N, Guo S, Langer P. Current concepts in the management of periocular infantile (capillary) hemangioma. *Curr Opin Ophthalmol.* 2011;22(5):419–425

Ranchod TM, Frieden IJ, Fredrick DR. Corticosteroid treatment of periorbital haemangioma of infancy: a review of the evidence. *Br J Ophthalmol.* 2005;89(9):1134–1138

Chapter 18

Droopy Eyelid

Kenneth W. Wright, MD
Tinny T. Dinh, MD, MS

Presentation

A 6-month-old boy is brought to the pediatrician's office because the mother is concerned about his left eyelid, which she reports has been drooping since birth. She had hoped the eyelid would open fully with age, but it has not changed. She says her son is able to open his left eye only about halfway. Other than the eyelid, she states that he has been doing well.

Physical examination reveals a healthy baby who is reaching his milestones appropriately. During the ocular examination, the pediatrician observes that the infant's left eyelid is much lower than his right eyelid; however, it does not appear to be covering his pupil (Figure 18-1). The pediatrician shines a light at the infant's eyes and measures his upper

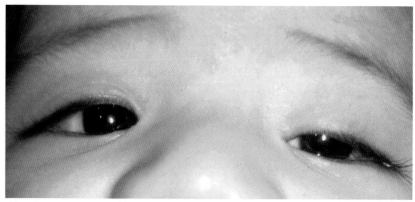

Figure 18-1. Droopy left eyelid. Note the poorly formed lid crease and asymmetric corneal light reflex. Courtesy of Shira L. Robbins, MD.

eyelid margin to pupillary light reflex distance to be 4 mm in the right eye and 2 mm in the left eye. The pediatrician realizes the infant has wrinkles on 1 side of his forehead. The baby is lifting his eyebrow to pull the lid up, and he maintains a slight chin-up head position.

Further ocular examination reveals that the patient is able to fix and follow objects with either eye. His eyes appear properly aligned, and his corneal light reflex appears symmetric. The Brückner test reveals a good and equal red reflex in both eyes, and his pupils are equal, round, and reactive to light without a relative afferent pupillary defect. The pediatrician examines the infant's eye movements and sees that he has full range of motion in both eyes. When the baby looks up, however, his left eyelid does not fully open, and when he looks down, his left eyelid does not fully close.

The pediatrician refers the patient to an ophthalmologist for further ocular examination.

Diagnosis

The child has ptosis of his left eyelid. Because of the normal ocular movements, the pediatrician knows it is most likely not a third cranial nerve palsy. The patient also has a normal pupillary response, which rules out Horner syndrome. A key finding noted by the pediatrician is that the patient's left eyelid does not fully open or close. This suggests that he most likely has congenital blepharoptosis (congenital eyelid ptosis).

Congenital blepharoptosis is a unilateral or bilateral primary dysgenesis of the levator muscle of the upper eyelid. Instead of normal musculature, there is fibrosis of the levator muscle. This results in poor levator muscle function and a minimal or absent upper lid crease. In addition, the fibrotic muscle results in a restriction of the eyelid from closing. A hallmark of congenital ptosis is that the affected eyelid appears higher than the unaffected eyelid on downgaze.

Differential Diagnosis

Diagnoses besides congenital blepharoptosis that should be considered include the following:

Myasthenia Gravis

A rare neo-muscular condition that results in muscle weakness.

Third Cranial Nerve Palsy

Patients with third cranial nerve palsies have abnormal eye movement in addition to blepharoptosis.

Horner Syndrome

Patients with Horner syndrome have an ipsilateral mild ptosis, mild miosis (small pupil), anhidrosis, and in some congenital cases, hetero-chromia (difference in iris color).

When to Refer

Because of the vision-threatening nature of this condition, patients with congenital ptosis should be referred for ophthalmologic evaluation. Severe ptosis in which the eyelid covers the visual axis will result in dense amblyopia. Even a mild ptosis that does not occlude the visual axis can still cause amblyopia by induced astigmatism from the pressure of the eyelid on the cornea.

Treatment

A cycloplegic refraction by the ophthalmologist shows no signs of astigmatism. The patient's vision is appropriate for his age without any signs of amblyopia. His levator muscle function is found to be moderate to good by the movement the eyelid makes. The recommendation from the ophthalmologist is close monitoring until the patient is older, around 3 to 5 years of age, when he will undergo surgical repair of the blepha-roptosis. Delaying the surgery until the child is older allows for a more accurate preoperative examination and more stable long-term results. However, if the examination or any subsequent examinations reveal any signs of amblyopia, more urgent intervention would be warranted.

There are different surgical options for repair of congenital blepharoptosis depending on the levator muscle function of the ptotic eyelid. Patients with moderate to good levator muscle function can be treated with a levator muscle tightening procedure (by plication or resection). Patients with poor levator muscle function may undergo a frontalis suspension procedure. However, ptosis repair surgeries, especially for congenital ptosis, are challenging procedures, and it is not uncommon to require more than one operation.

Ptosis surgery does not improve the function of the dysgenic muscle. As a result, in unilateral cases of congenital ptosis, there will still be asymmetry between the eyelids, especially with upgaze or downgaze. Some surgeons advocate bilateral eyelid surgery, even in unilateral cases, to try to improve symmetry.

Because ptosis surgery elevates the eyelid, after surgery the eyelids may not fully close. This can lead to exposure of the eye while sleeping. The majority of the population has a Bell phenomenon (the eye rolls up when the eyelids are closed) that helps protect the eyes. It is important to note those patients who do not have a Bell phenomenon, as they are at higher risk of corneal injury (exposure keratopathy) and require prophylactic eye lubrication.

Discussion

Ptosis surgery is challenging and children frequently require more than one surgery. Surgery is usually performed at age 4 to 6 years. If there is amblyopia secondary to ptosis, early surgery is done even as young as 6 months.

Key Points

- In all cases of pediatric eyelid ptosis, third cranial nerve palsy and Horner syndrome should be considered.
- Amblyopia can be a resultant condition of eyelid ptosis requiring early medical treatment and is sometimes an indication for early surgical intervention.
- The goal of surgical repair is to elevate the eyelid while providing the best possible cosmesis.
- Ptosis repair surgery does not improve the function of the dysgenic muscle. In unilateral cases of congenital ptosis, there will still be asymmetry between the eyelids, especially with upgaze or downgaze.
- Some surgeons advocate bilateral eyelid surgery, even in unilateral cases of congenital blepharoptosis, to try to improve symmetry.
- It is important to note patients who do not have a Bell phenomenon after ptosis surgery, as they are at higher risk for exposure keratopathy and require prophylactic eye lubrication.

Suggested Reading

American Academy of Ophthalmology. Preferred practice pattern guidelines. http://www.aao.org/ppp. Accessed March 13, 2012

Callahan A. Correction of unilateral blepharoptosis with bilateral eyelid suspension. *Am J Ophthalmol.* 1972;74(2):321–326

Carter SR, Meecham WJ, Seiff SR. Silicone frontalis slings for the correction of blepharoptosis: indications and efficacy. *Ophthalmology.* 1996;103(4):623–630

Hornblass A, Kass LG, Ziffer AJ. Amblyopia in congenital ptosis. *Ophthalmic Surg.* 1995;26(4):334–337

Wright KW. *Pediatric Ophthalmology for Primary Care.* 3rd ed. Elk Grove Village, IL: American Academy of Pediatrics; 2008

Wright KW, Spiegel PH. *Pediatric Ophthalmology and Strabismus.* 2nd ed. New York, NY: Springer; 2003

Chapter 19

Painful Lump on the Eyelid

Daniel J. Karr, MD

Presentation

A 13-year-old girl who has been receiving treatment for acne returns to the pediatrician's office with a new complaint. Over the last week a small, slightly tender bump on her left upper eyelid developed and progressed to a larger, painful lump. Her acne vulgaris is responding to the topical treatments plus oral antibiotics that the pediatrician prescribed.

The new finding, on examination, is a swollen red mass on the left upper eyelid. It is mildly tender and is starting to point through the skin. The entire left upper lid has swelling, but the main inflammatory focus looks like a localized cellulitis or abscess collection (Figure 19-1).

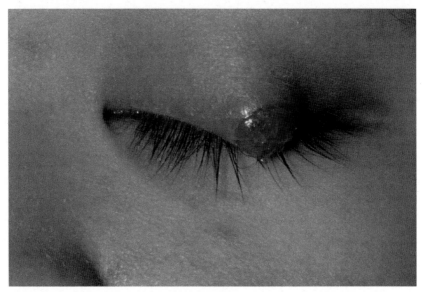

Figure 19-1. Focal inflammation of upper eyelid. Courtesy of Daniel J. Karr, MD.

She gives no history of injury, exposure, or other associations related to her eyelid condition. She reports feeling embarrassed by the lump, wants it treated immediately, and does not want to return to school until it is gone.

Diagnosis

The experienced pediatrician has seen similar lesions in many children of different ages. This lump is obviously a stye (hordeolum externum) or chalazion (Figure 19-2). The distinction between these entities is not always clear, which may have some effect on selecting the best therapy. This teenaged patient has a lesion most consistent with a hordeolum externum, or common stye. This lesion has grown to the point where it is trying to drain through the thinned epithelium.

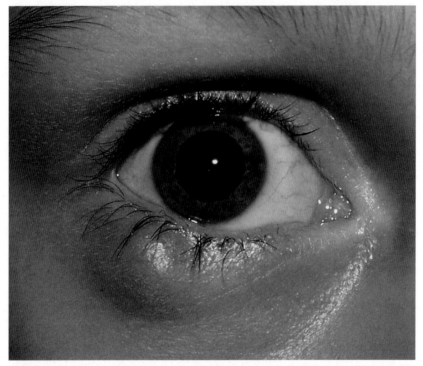

Figure 19-2. Typical chalazion. Courtesy of Shira L. Robbins, MD.

Hordeolum externum is a pyogenic infection, often staphylococcal in nature, localized to the eyelash follicles and their associated glands of Zeis along the eyelid margins (Figure 19-3). The stye begins as a well-localized, painful swelling near the eyelid margin. It typically increases in size and tenderness until it reaches suppuration.

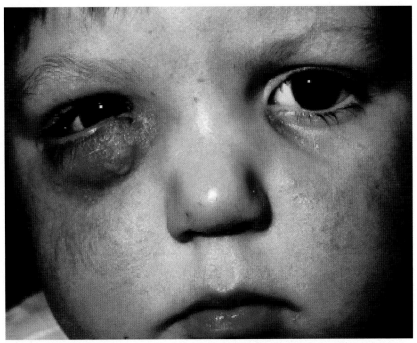

Figure 19-3. Hordeolum externum showing eyelid inflammation with associated gland blockage. From Kanski JJ. Bacterial infections. In: *Clinical Diagnosis in Ophthalmology*. Philadelphia, PA: Mosby; 2006:19, with permission from Elsevier.

Differential Diagnosis

Diagnoses besides hordeolum externum that should be considered include the following:

Chalazion

A chalazion (Greek for "small hailstone") is a chronic inflammatory granuloma of the meibomian gland. It is frequently associated with staphylococcal blepharitis and clinically presents as a slow-growing, firm tarsal mass. It is usually painless unless there is a secondary infection. The natural history of chalazion ranges from spontaneous involution (regression) over weeks to months versus persistence of the mass for many months or development of pain and tenderness secondary to acute infection and abscess formation. Histopathologic analysis reveals a lipogranulomatous inflammatory process (Figure 19-4).

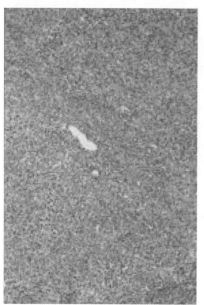

Figure 19-4. Histopathologic specimen of chalazion shows granulomatous inflammation surrounding vacuoles previously containing lipid. Courtesy of Bessie Floyd, MD.

Hordeolum Internum

A hordeolum (Latin for "barley") internum is an acute infection of the meibomian gland, usually caused by staphylococci. This suppurative inflammation of the meibomian gland is analogous to acne (Figure 19-5). Because meibomian glands are larger and more securely encased in dense fibrous tissue, hordeolum interna presents more with pain and edema and localized tenderness over the abscessed gland. The symptoms of pain, swelling, and tenderness tend to increase and frequently lead to spontaneous drainage.

When to Refer

If a chalazion or hordeolum is large and lasts longer than 3 to 4 weeks with appropriate medical therapy, the patient should be referred to an ophthalmologist for surgical incision and drainage of the lesion. Signs of spreading cellulitis, precentral cellulitis, demand immediate evaluation and systemic antibiotic therapy.

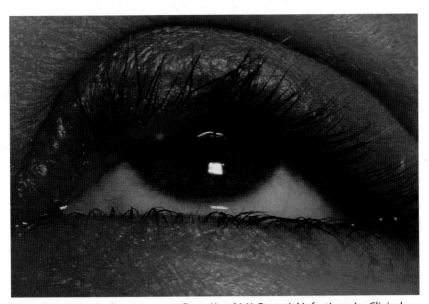

Figure 19-5. Hordeolum internum. From Kanski JJ. Bacterial infections. In: *Clinical Diagnosis in Ophthalmology*. Philadelphia, PA: Mosby; 2006:19, with permission from Elsevier.

Treatment

This patient would benefit from warm, moist compresses applied to the closed eyelid multiple times a day. This will help the stye continue pointing toward and through the skin surface. Then, if local treatment measures do not succeed, surgical incision and drainage by an ophthalmologist are indicated. Most children would need sedation or general anesthesia to incise and drain these lesions.

However, because the patient is most anxious to have this problem resolved quickly, the pediatrician could lance the area pointing under the skin with a hypodermic needle or small scalpel blade. It is very likely the patient would have immediate relief from the drainage. Continuation of warm, moist compresses to encourage further drainage, along with a topical antibiotic such as erythromycin ointment, would be the recommended course of action.

If this lesion were a hordeolum internum, treatment also would consist initially of moist, warm compresses. Incision and drainage could be considered after 3 to 4 weeks of conservative treatment or once the pointing of pus is localized on the conjunctival surface. Likewise, the most frequent treatment of a chalazion consists of warm, moist compresses and massage. If the lesion does not resolve within a reasonable time (3 to 4 weeks), incision and drainage—usually from the conjunctival surface—can be performed. Intralesional injections of steroids or antibiotics can be used to speed healing and treat infection if suspected.

Discussion

A persistent, large lesion on the eyelid can alter the corneal contour, leading to astigmatism and blurred vision. Astigmatism induced by a chalazion or hordeolum increases the risk of developing amblyopia, which can lead to permanent vision loss. Therefore, patients and their families should be instructed to return for follow-up if the lesion grows larger or causes blurred vision.

Chalazia and styes typically respond well to treatment. However, some patients are prone to recurrences. There is a growing body of literature that suggests that recurrences are decreased when children are using omega-3 fatty acids (dietary or supplemental).

Key Points

- Initial treatment of chalazion, stye, and hordeolum internum consists of application of warm, moist compresses to encourage resolution and drainage.
- The clinical course directs the use of topical antibiotic ointment, consideration for adding oral antibiotics for enlarging cellulitis, and possibility of incision and drainage.
- Young patients need sedation or general anesthesia during incision and drainage of these lesions.
- A persistent, large lesion on the eyelid can alter the corneal contour. This can cause astigmatism and blurred vision and increase the risk of developing amblyopia, which can lead to permanent vision loss.

Suggested Reading

Duke-Elder S. Diseases of the eyelids. In: Duke-Elder S, MacFaul PA, eds. *System of Ophthalmology.* Vol VIII. London, England: Henry Kimpton; 1974

Ehlers JP, Shah CP, eds. *The Wills Eye Manual.* 5th ed. Philadelphia, PA: Lippincott Williams and Wilkins; 2008

Chapter 20

Tearing, Eye Rubbing, and Blinking

K. David Epley, MD

Presentation

A 3-year-old Asian boy presents to the pediatrician's office with daily tearing in both eyes. He rubs his eyes frequently throughout the day, and when not rubbing is often forcibly blinking both eyes. The child is otherwise healthy with no systemic illnesses. His symptoms have been present as long as the parents can remember.

On initial examination, the child appears healthy. Eyes are without redness, but the lower eyelid lashes are rotated inward toward the eyes (Figure 20-1). A Wood lamp (blue light) with fluorescein dye shows changes (punctate staining) in the inferior corneas.

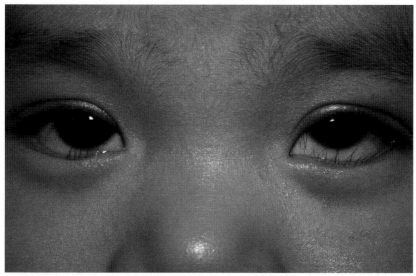

Figure 20-1. Lower eyelid eyelashes are rotated inward toward the eyes. Courtesy of K. David Epley, MD.

Diagnosis

The key to diagnosis is examination of the eyelids. The lower eyelids are turned inward (entropion), causing the eyelashes to touch the corneal surface and creating punctate staining of the lower cornea. Lower eyelid skin and underlying orbicularis muscle appear to be overriding the eyelid margin, forcing it to turn inward. Given the appearance and the child's ethnicity, the condition most likely is epiblepharon, which is similar to congenital entropion.

The lower eyelid is more commonly involved in epiblepharon. This condition is common in Asian children but may also be seen in other races. Children with epicanthal folds (skin covering the nasal aspect of the eyelid conjunctival junction) are more likely to have epiblepharon.

Typical presentation of epiblepharon involves tearing of the affected eye or eyes and may also involve punctate staining of the cornea and mild limbal conjunctival injection. If the conjunctiva is white, there are not likely to be substantial corneal defects. A clear, solid-red reflex and a sharp Hirschberg light reflex with a direct ophthalmoscope suggest that the corneal surface is intact. In more severe cases, it is possible for corneal ulceration with or without infection, corneal neovascularization, or cicatricial conjunctival changes or scarring to occur. If lashes are touching the cornea even in upgaze, the epiblepharon is considered more severe (Figure 20-2).

Differential Diagnosis

Diagnoses besides epiblepharon that should be considered include the following:

For Tearing

- Glaucoma
- Nasolacrimal duct obstruction

Both tend to occur more frequently in infancy, whereas epiblepharon becomes more symptomatic as a toddler and young child. Glaucoma can be distinguished by cloudiness or a glassy appearance to the cornea. In addition, the corneal diameter progressively enlarges with glaucoma, and glaucoma is more likely to be unilateral.

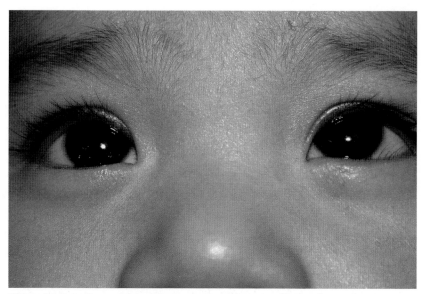

Figure 20-2. Lashes touching the cornea in upgaze usually signify significant rotation of the eyelid. Courtesy of K. David Epley, MD.

Nasolacrimal duct obstruction can be distinguished by the presence of mucus discharge in frequent bouts in infancy. Cornea will be clear and of normal, symmetric diameter with the fellow eye. The child will have an elevated tear lake in the lower eyelid cul-de-sac that doesn't clear with time.

Presence of epiblepharon can be confirmed by eyelid position and by eyelash touch to the surface of the eye.

For Eye Rubbing
- Refractive error
- Blepharitis
- Allergic conjunctivitis

Only proper equipment can test for refractive errors; an auto-refraction device that some pediatricians use for vision screening can help with this, but otherwise refractive error must be determined by an ophthalmologist.

Blepharitis is inflammation of the eyelids and manifests as hyperemia of eyelid margins, crusting of lashes, and collarettes around the base of the eyelashes.

Allergic conjunctivitis is most often bilateral, and lower eyelids will usually have follicles visible without magnification during the acute phase of conjunctivitis. Most often, conjunctiva will be injected.

Presence of epiblepharon can be confirmed by eyelid position and by eyelash touch to the surface of the eye.

For Blinking
- Refractive error
- Dry eye
- Punctate keratitis

Only proper equipment can test for refractive errors; an auto-refraction device that some pediatricians use for vision screening can help with this, but otherwise refractive error must be determined by an ophthalmologist.

Dry eye is rare in children but manifests as ocular discomfort that can lead to blinking. The ocular surface will have a poor tear film with bumps on the conjunctival surface. The Schirmer tear test may show lack of tear production. On fluorescein staining, many small dots of dye uptake can be seen with magnification on the ocular surface (punctate keratitis). Other causes of punctate keratitis can be viral infection, allergy, dry eye, and epiblepharon.

Presence of epiblepharon can be confirmed by eyelid position and by eyelash touch to the surface of the eye.

When to Refer
Children found to have epiblepharon should be examined by a pediatric ophthalmologist, as subjective symptoms (ie, tearing, eye rubbing, and blinking) do not always correlate with severity of disease. Close ophthalmologic follow-up is indicated in children with corneal disease or conjunctival injection.

Treatment
The child in this case received supportive care including artificial tear ointment for a period of 2 years. At that point, the child's eyes were worsening despite the ointment, and he developed punctate keratitis

and decreasing vision from the poor ocular surface. The decision was made to operate, and surgical repair of the epiblepharon was performed without complication. The boy's eyelids healed well, and the subciliary incision was no longer visible 4 months following surgery. His eyelid continues to be in good position without eyelash touch to his ocular surface more than 6 years following surgery.

Treatment of epiblepharon is initially directed at normalizing the corneal surface. In mild cases, artificial tears in a drop or ointment formulation may be used to maintain a healthy corneal and conjunctival surface. In moderate cases, topical antibiotic-corticosteroid combinations may be used to quiet surface inflammation and promote corneal healing.

In severe cases, when symptomatic children do not outgrow the condition or have substantial keratitis, patients require surgery to realign the eyelid margin and prevent lashes from touching the ocular surface. There are several surgical approaches that can be used in treatment of epiblepharon. Surgical correction is an outpatient procedure. Currently, a variety of surgical techniques, including full-thickness eyelid sutures, buried sutures, excision of the skin and orbicularis muscle with or without fixation of the skin or subcutaneous tissue to the tarsal plate, and anterior lamellar repositioning, are used as surgical treatment for epiblepharon.

Discussion

Epiblepharon is a congenital in-turning of the eyelids (usually lower lids). It results from preseptal musculus orbicularis oculi (orbicular muscle of the eye) overriding the eyelid margin. The condition is typically bilateral.

Most children with epiblepharon will outgrow the condition by 5 to 7 years of age. Regular monitoring by a pediatric ophthalmologist is indicated to ensure no permanent damage to the ocular surface occurs, which could affect vision later in life.

Key Points

- If the conjunctiva is white, there are not likely to be substantial corneal defects.
- A clear, solid-red reflex and sharp Hirschberg light reflex with direct ophthalmoscope suggest that the corneal surface is intact.
- Severe epiblepharon can lead to astigmatism and amblyopia. Because these conditions have no external symptoms, an accurate visual assessment is imperative.

Suggested Reading

Choo C. Correction of oriental epiblepharon by anterior lamellar reposition. *Eye (Lond).* 1996;10(Pt 5):545–547

Gigantelli JW. Entropion. In: Yanoff M, Duker JS, eds. *Ophthalmology.* 2nd ed. St. Louis, MO: Mosby; 2004:668–675

Guercio JR, Martyn LJ. Congenital malformations of the eye and orbit. *Otolaryngol Clin North Am.* 2007;40(1):113–140

Hayasaka S, Noda S, Setogawa T. Epiblepharon with inverted eyelashes in Japanese children. II. Surgical repairs. *Br J Ophthalmol.* 1989;73(2):128–130

Khwarg SI, Choung HK. Epiblepharon of the lower eyelid: technique of surgical repair and quantification of excision according to the skin fold height. *Ophthalmic Surg Lasers.* 2002;33(4):280–287

Millman AL, Mannor GE, Putterman AM. Lid crease and capsulopalpebral fascia repair in congenital entropion and epiblepharon. *Ophthalmic Surg.* 1994;25(3):162–165

Olitsky SE, Hug D, Plummer LS, Stass-Isern M. Abnormalities of the lids. In: Kliegman RM, Behrman RE, Stanton BF, Schor NF, eds. *Nelson Textbook of Pediatrics.* 19th ed. Philadelphia, PA: Elsevier Saunders; 2011

Preechawai P, Amrith S, Wong I, Sundar G. Refractive changes in epiblepharon. *Am J Ophthalmol.* 2007;143(5):835–839

Quickert MH, Wilkes TD, Dryden RM. Nonincisional correction of epiblepharon and congenital entropion. *Arch Ophthalmol.* 1983;101(5):778–781

Woo KI, Yi K, Kim YD. Surgical correction for lower lid epiblepharon in Asians. *Br J Ophthalmol.* 2000;84(12):1407–1410

Chapter 21

Bruising Around the Eyes

David A. Plager, MD

Presentation

A 2-year-old girl presents to her pediatrician with a 2-month history of eyelid and lower extremity swelling, some decreased appetite, and poor sleeping. There is no history of easy bruising or bleeding elsewhere on her body.

On examination, she is noted to have bilateral eyelid ecchymosis (bruising) and mild swelling (Figure 21-1).

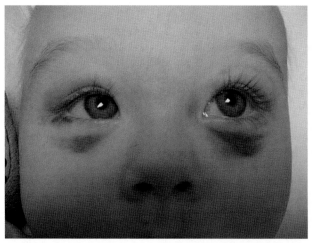

Figure 21-1. Bilateral periorbital ecchymosis and edema. Courtesy of David A. Plager, MD.

Diagnosis

Differential diagnosis is quite short with this classic appearance. In this age group, bilateral eyelid ecchymosis, or so-called raccoon eyes, is highly characteristic of metastatic orbital neuroblastoma. Proptosis or motility disturbance may or may not be present. Other possible ophthalmic findings with neuroblastoma, although not associated specifically with orbital disease, are Horner syndrome (miosis, ptosis, and anhidrosis) and opsoclonus (bizarre, multidirectional nystagmus).

Workup of suspected neuroblastoma includes a thorough physical examination, with particular attention to the abdomen to look for an abdominal mass. Laboratory testing for urine catecholamines is indicated, and 90% to 95% of patients will have elevated homovanillic acid and vanillylmandelic acid. Computed tomography or magnetic resonance imaging of the abdomen, chest, and head will help identify the primary tumor and assess tumor extent (figures 21-2–21-4). Bone scan will help identify skeletal involvement.

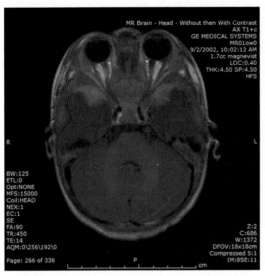

Figure 21-2. Axial magnetic resonance imaging of the head showing metastatic disease. Courtesy of David A. Plager, MD.

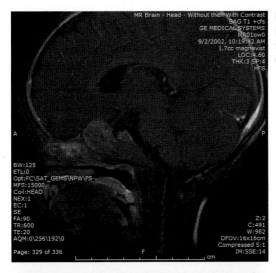

Figure 21-3. Sagittal head magnetic resonance imaging showing metastatic disease. Courtesy of David A. Plager, MD.

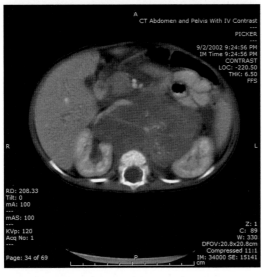

Figure 21-4. Axial body computed tomography showing large primary abdominal tumor. Courtesy of David A. Plager, MD.

Differential Diagnosis

Diagnoses besides metastatic neuroblastoma that should be considered include the following:

Blunt Ocular Trauma

Although bilateral eyelid ecchymosis could be a sequela of direct trauma to the eye, as in a motor vehicle accident, trauma is easy to rule out from history. Non-accidental trauma would more likely include other external signs of trauma, but child abuse should always be a consideration (see Chapter 52).

Bleeding Dyscrasia

Bleeding dyscrasia would typically be associated with other signs of easy bruising or bleeding and can be ruled out by appropriate laboratory testing.

When to Refer

Any child with such ominous signs of ocular pathology—raccoon eyes, proptosis, new onset nystagmus, or Horner syndrome—should be referred promptly to a pediatric ophthalmologist for further evaluation (or a general ophthalmologist if no pediatric ophthalmologist is readily available).

Treatment

Possible treatment regimens are dependent on patient risk factors and may include any combination of surgery, chemotherapy, radiation, stem cell transplantation and immunotherapy.

Discussion

Neuroblastoma is the third most common pediatric cancer and the most common malignancy in infants. It is the most common tumor causing orbital metastasis in children. It is an embryonal tumor arising from anywhere along the peripheral sympathetic nervous system from the pelvis up to the cervical ganglion. It most commonly arises in the abdomen from an adrenal gland or the retroperitoneal area.

Symptoms are frequently related to mass effect of the primary tumor on surrounding tissues and depend on where the primary tumor is located. This may include abdominal pain, bone pain, or symptoms of chest involvement. More general symptoms such as irritability and failure to thrive may also be present.

Prognosis is somewhat complicated and involves assessment of tumor extent, cytogenetic and molecular markers, and age. Neuroblastoma is staged from 1 (disease confined to site of origin) to 4 (distant metastasis). A special stage 4S refers to infants with disseminated disease to skin, bone marrow (not bone), or liver and is associated with a favorable prognosis.

Using this information, patients can be grouped into risk categories— low, intermediate, or high. Approximately 50% of patients will be in the high-risk group; currently, survival rates for this group are less than 50% despite the most aggressive treatment regimes. Survival for low and intermediate risk categories are much higher—approaching 90% and involve less aggressive therapy. A new International Neuroblastoma Risk Group staging system based on clinical criteria and image-defined risk factors has recently been established.

Key Points

- Neuroblastoma is the most common malignancy in infants.
- Symptom presentation is varied based on affected organs. This may include abdominal pain, bone pain, or symptoms of chest involvement. More general symptoms such as irritability and failure to thrive may also be present.
- Metastatic ophthalmologic signs can include any of the following: bilateral periorbital ecchymosis (raccoon eyes), proptosis, eye movement restriction, and Horner syndrome.

Suggested Reading

Brisse HJ, McCarville MB, Granata C, et al. Guidelines for imaging and staging of neuroblastic tumors: consensus report from the International Neuroblastoma Risk Group project. *Radiology.* 2011;261(1):243–257

Maris JM, Matthay KK. Molecular biology of neuroblastoma. *J Clin Oncol.* 1999;17(7):2264–2279

Nickerson HJ, Matthay KK, Seeger RC, et al. Favorable biology and outcome of stage IV-S neuroblastoma with supportive care or minimal therapy: a Children's Cancer Group study. *J Clin Oncol.* 2000;18(3):477–486

Perez CA, Matthay KK, Atkinson JB, et al. Biologic variables in the outcome of stages I and II neuroblastoma treated with surgery as primary therapy: a Children's Cancer Group study. *J Clin Oncol.* 2000;18(1):18–26

Schmidt ML, Lukens JN, Seeger RC, et al. Biologic factors determine prognosis in infants with stage IV neuroblastoma: a prospective Children's Cancer Group study. *J Clin Oncol.* 2000;18(6):1260–1268

Chapter 22

Orbital Mass

Mary O'Hara, MD

Presentation

A 6-year-old girl was noted by her older sister to have a fullness of her left lower eyelid (Figure 22-1). Over the course of 2 weeks, this fullness visibly increased in size. When examined by her pediatrician, the child

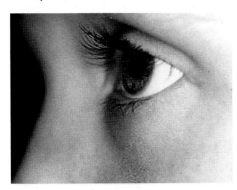

Figure 22-1. Slight fullness evident on left lower lid. Courtesy of Mary O'Hara, MD.

was found to have a discrete, nontender, moveable mass of a rubbery consistency in the lower orbit. The eyelid was not red or painful. The eye moved normally and there was no proptosis. The uncorrected visual acuity in the affected eye was 20/20, and the eye and eyelid were otherwise normal in appearance (Figure 22-2.) There was no prior history of trauma or infections. The child was in good health with no medical problems.

This patient was referred to a tertiary care center with oculoplastic, pediatric ophthalmology, and pediatric oncology services. A computed tomography (CT) scan of the orbit was

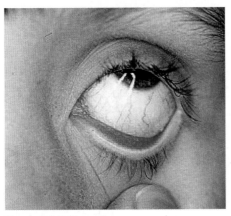

Figure 22-2. Normal eye—no redness. Courtesy of Mary O'Hara, MD.

obtained, which showed a discrete solid mass without bony erosion (Figure 22-3).

Diagnosis

At the tertiary care center the patient underwent orbital exploration, which revealed a discrete solid mass measuring 2 x 1 cm (Figure 22-4). Histopathological evaluation of the tissue was aided by immunohisto-chemical studies that confirmed a diagnosis of embryonal rhabdomyo-sarcoma.

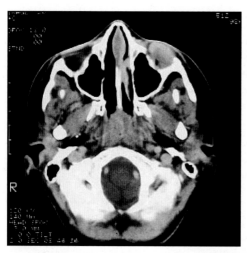

Figure 22-3. Computed tomography scan showing discrete orbital mass in the inferior orbit without bony erosion. Courtesy of Mary O'Hara, MD.

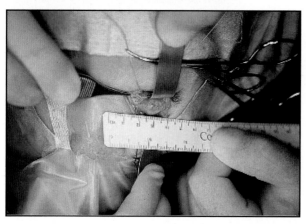

Figure 22-4. Excisional biopsy of mass via subciliary incision. Courtesy of Mary O'Hara, MD.

Lumps in the eyelid are common occurrences in childhood. The differential diagnosis spans the pedestrian chalazion to the uncommon malignant tumors of the orbit. Distinguishing features include pain, limitation of movement, proptosis, redness, eyelid ptosis, and loss of vision. Benign and malignant tumors of the orbit tend to be painless, presenting with gradual or rapid proptosis, ptosis, and globe displacement.

If rhabdomyosarcoma is suspected, imaging studies are essential. Computed tomography and magnetic resonance imaging (MRI) are helpful in the diagnosis of rhabdomyosarcoma. Computed tomography is preferred for evaluation of the extent of bony involvement, whereas MRI is superior for soft-tissue imaging. Orbital imaging can determine the extent and encapsulation of the tumor, intracranial extension, bony erosion, and invasion into the sinuses. Ultrasound of the lesion is a more conservative way to distinguish solid tumor rhabdomyosarcoma.

Although orbital imaging is helpful in the diagnosis of rhabdomyosarcoma, the definitive diagnosis is made by histopathologic examination of tissue obtained via biopsy. Once a rhabdomyosarcoma is suspected, prompt biopsy is recommended because the tumor grows rapidly. Excisional biopsy is preferred if the lesion is discrete. However, if the lesion is diffuse or very posterior in the orbit, incisional biopsy may be more appropriate.

Differential Diagnosis

Diagnoses besides rhabdomyosarcoma that should be considered include the following:

Orbital Pseudotumor or Cellulitis

Inflammatory processes such as orbital pseudotumor and infectious processes such as orbital cellulitis can present with rapid growth and proptosis. However, there is also pain and redness with limitation of movement and systemic signs, such as fever and lethargy.

Chalazion

The common chalazion has a characteristic appearance. The fullness of the eyelid can be explained by eversion of the eyelid to expose the pointing lesion (Figure 22-5).

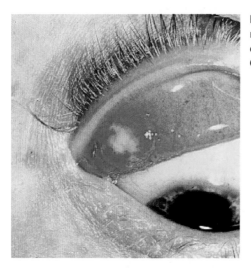

Figure 22-5. Chalazion with redness, pain, and pointing demonstrated on lid eversion. Courtesy of Mary O'Hara, MD.

Capillary Hemangioma

Capillary hemangiomas are benign vascular tumors that usually present in the first few months of life. Initial growth is rapid, with a subsequent quiescent period, followed by slow regression of the tumor over several years. Vascular channels are evident by their high internal reflectivity on ultrasound studies, distinguishing this tumor from a rhabdomyosarcoma.

Lymphangioma

Lymphangiomas are lymphatic malformations that grow slowly but can proliferate rapidly when stimulated by infection. The lymphatic channels of lymphangiomas can be demonstrated by imaging studies. Ultrasound, CT, or MRI can distinguish these masses from the solid tumor of rhabdomyosarcoma. Lymphangiomas demonstrate high internal reflectivity on ultrasound because of the presence of lymphatic channels.

Plexiform Neurofibroma

Plexiform neurofibromas are tumors of the eyelid associated with neurofibromatosis type 1. Although these neurofibromas are rapidly growing, they are distinguished from rhabdomyosarcoma by their characteristic "bag of worms" appearance and by the presence of other stigmata of neurofibromatosis in the patient.

When to Refer

When rhabdomyosarcoma is suspected, the patient should be referred to a tertiary care center for biopsy and histopathologic evaluation of the mass.

Treatment

This patient's mass is removed in toto (Figure 22-6). Once the diagnosis of rhabdomyosarcoma is confirmed, a combination of chemotherapy and external-beam irradiation is used to treat the tumor. The child tolerates the treatment well.

She is now 20 years old and tumor-free. A radiation-induced cataract developed when the girl was 13 years old. The cataract was removed and an intraocular lens was placed. Her visual acuity today is 20/20 in the affected eye. There is mild lash and brow alopecia of the left eye.

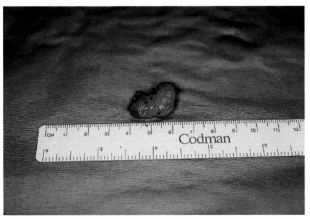

Figure 22-6. Discrete encapsulated tumor. Courtesy of Mary O'Hara, MD.

Discussion

Although the majority of children who develop rhabdomyosarcoma do not have any known risk factors, children with several rare inherited conditions do have an increased risk of rhabdomyosarcoma. Individuals with Li-Fraumeni syndrome, Beckwith-Wiedemann syndrome, neurofibromatosis type 1, Noonan syndrome, and multiple endocrine neoplasia, type 2a syndrome do have an increased incidence of rhabdomyosarcoma as well as other tumors. High birth weight has been linked to an increased risk of embryonal rhabdomyosarcoma, but this may be in association with Costello syndrome.

The treatment of rhabdomyosarcoma with chemotherapy and external-beam irradiation has greatly improved the prognosis for patients with this tumor. Long-term sequelae of radiation therapy can include radiation-induced cataracts, corneal changes, dry eye, and radiation retinopathy. Lash and brow hair loss have also been described.

Factors that affect prognosis for rhabdomyosarcoma are tumor morphology, location of tumor in the orbit, and early diagnosis. Staging of the tumor after biopsy follows the classification systems of the Intergroup Rhabdomyosarcoma Study. Two histopathologic types of rhabdomyosarcoma are seen in the orbit: embryonal and alveolar. A third form of rhabdomyosarcoma, the pleomorphic form, is rarely encountered in the orbit. Embryonal rhabdomyosarcoma is the most common form of rhabdomyosarcoma and also has the most favorable prognosis. The 5-year survival rate is approximately 95%. Alveolar rhabdomyosarcoma has a 5-year survival rate of 75%. Timely recognition and diagnosis of rhabdomyosarcoma can favorably influence the prognosis for this tumor.

Key Points

- Rhabdomyosarcoma is a rare tumor of childhood presenting in the orbit in 10% of cases.
- Diagnostic hallmarks are rapid growth and painless proptosis with globe displacement.
- Orbito-cranial imaging studies are important in the workup of this condition, as they determine the extent of tumor and bony erosion.
- The definitive diagnosis is made by biopsy.
- Prompt referral to an ophthalmologist is necessary.

Suggested Reading

Karcioglu ZA, Hadjistilianou D, Rozans M, DeFrancesco S. Orbital rhabdomyosarcoma. *Cancer Control.* 2004;11(5):328–333

Shields JA, Shields CL. Rhabdomyosarcoma: review for the ophthalmologist. *Surv Ophthalmol.* 2003;48(1):39–57

Chapter 23

Painless Eyelid Bump

Angela N. Buffenn, MD, MPH

Presentation

A 17-month-old boy presents to the pediatrician's office because he has a bump near his left eyebrow, and the boy's mother is convinced that the bump has been enlarging (Figure 23-1). When questioned about recent trauma, the boy's mother denies any such event. The pediatrician has seen this child since birth. He has been growing and developing normally, is healthy, and is fully immunized for his age. The child's medical record contains no mention of a bump or mass on previous examinations.

On examination there is an approximately 1 x 1 cm rounded mass, near the superotemporal margin of the left orbit. The child is comfortable and, in fact, playful throughout the examination. Palpation of the mass does not result in pain. The pediatrician decides to send the child to a pediatric ophthalmologist for further evaluation and treatment.

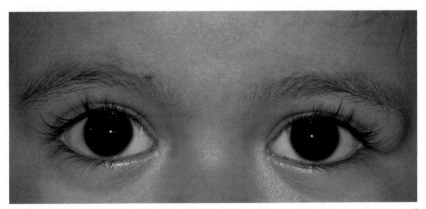

Figure 23-1. Fullness of left lateral eyelid area extending to the eyebrow. Courtesy of Angela N. Buffenn, MD, MPH.

The pediatric ophthalmologist examines the boy and confirms the mass to be painless, nontender, firm, nonfluctuant, and freely mobile. There is no displacement of the eye, and the boy's visual responses are appropriate for his age. The mass can be fully palpated and is not found to extend beyond the superior orbital rim (Figure 23-2).

Diagnosis

Compared with the boy's right orbit, there is increased fullness at the superotemporal margin of his left orbit (Figure 23-1), which could present following trauma. However, there are no other findings on examination consistent with trauma. In addition, the area is painless and nontender, findings not likely to be present following an acute traumatic event. The family also denies any history of trauma.

Although the exact onset of the superotemporal mass is unclear, the major clue in this case is the presence of a painless mass that is smooth, nontender, mobile, and unattached to overlying skin. There are also no visual symptoms and no displacement of the eye itself. This is believed to be a superficial dermoid cyst, which is a type of choristoma.

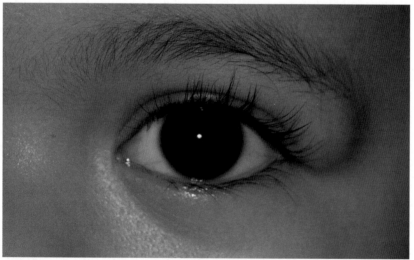

Figure 23-2. Mass in superotemporal orbit. Courtesy of Angela N. Buffenn, MD, MPH.

The term *choristoma* describes growths consisting of normal cells and tissues appearing at an abnormal location. Dermoid cysts are benign choristomas that arise from ectodermal rests trapped at suture lines or within mesenchyme during orbital development. These cysts are present congenitally and enlarge progressively. Histologically, resulting cysts are lined with keratinized, stratified squamous epithelium. Cyst walls contain dermal appendages, including sweat glands, sebaceous glands, and hair follicles (Figure 23-3).

Although dermoid cysts are typically located at the superotemporal margin of the orbit, they can be located in the medial orbit. When diagnosis cannot be confirmed by examination alone, a computed tomography (CT) scan can be used for confirmation. Dermoid cysts have a characteristic appearance on CT scan. They appear as well-circumscribed, discrete masses with low-density lumina. The surrounding bone may also show evidence of remodeling. Imaging may not be necessary when dermoid cysts are small and the entire extent of the cyst can be easily palpated.

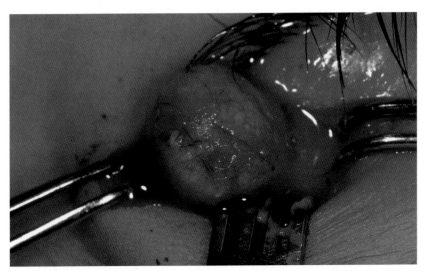

Figure 23-3. Intraoperative photo of orbital dermoid cyst. Courtesy of Angela N. Buffenn, MD, MPH.

Differential Diagnosis

Diagnoses besides dermoid cyst that should be considered include the following:

Trauma

Although increased fullness near the eye may indicate trauma, other characteristic findings of trauma would include abrasions, ecchymosis, or erythema of the skin. The area of fullness also would most likely be painful or tender.

Hemangioma

Capillary hemangiomas are bright red masses that blanch with pressure and may hemorrhage. They may grow rapidly in the first few months of life but, unlike other orbital lesions, tend to spontaneously regress completely by 5 years of age.

Dermolipoma

Dermolipomas are frequently mistaken for orbital dermoids and can occur alone or as part of Goldenhar syndrome. Unlike dermoids, dermolipomas tend to have large amounts of fat and few or no pilo-sebaceous glands. They are pink and skin-like due to keratinization and located laterally on the bulbar surface.

Sinus Mucocele

Ethmoid sinus mucoceles may present early in life. Usual presentation is gradual proptosis with globe displacement, findings not typical of dermoid cysts.

Lacrimal Ductal Cyst

A lacrimal ductal cyst is a smooth, transilluminating, slowly enlarging mass located in the lateral aspect of the upper eyelid. Lacrimal ductal cysts are rare, tending to present in adulthood, but may be seen during the teenage years.

When to Refer

Referral to an ophthalmologist should occur as soon as the cyst is recognized so that treatment can commence before accidental rupture. In addition, early referral allows for removal of the dermoid cyst before it becomes very large. This ultimately gives the ophthalmologist opportunity to consider treatment techniques involving inconspicuous incision sites, which can result in a better overall postoperative appearance.

Treatment

Treatment of dermoid cysts is surgical excision, which was the method of treatment used for this child. Surgery is often delayed until about 1 year of age because it is believed that by age 1 year, risk of general anesthesia is outweighed by risk of accidental cyst rupture from trauma. The entire cyst wall and its contents must be removed to decrease risk of chronic inflammatory reaction with sinus formation and persistent discharge. This is best achieved by removing the cyst intact without rupture (Figure 23-3). When cysts rupture intraoperatively, chronic inflammatory changes can be avoided as long as the cyst wall and its contents are removed completely. All remaining cyst lining should also be removed to help limit possible recurrence.

Discussion

Superficial dermoid cysts are congenital and believed to be one of the most common cystic lesions in childhood. When the entire cyst wall and its contents are removed, risk for recurrence is small, and prognosis is good.

Deep dermoid cysts typically present in adolescence and adulthood. Deep dermoid cysts are more likely to have gradual enlargement and displacement of orbital contents, which makes management of these dermoids complicated.

Epibulbar dermoids are usually found at the corneoscleral junction and can involve the entire thickness of the cornea and sclera. They can be associated with intraocular abnormalities. Management involves surgical excision, but observation is appropriate in cases in which the dermoid is small and without distortion of vision.

Conjunctival dermoids tend to occur in teenagers and adults. They are lined by typical conjunctival epithelium, do not attach to the orbital bones, and are managed by complete excision.

Key Points

- Superficial dermoid cysts are benign congenital choristomas believed to be the most common orbital masses in childhood.
- They present as painless, smooth, nontender, mobile masses that are often unattached to overlying skin.
- These cysts do not tend to cause visual symptoms and do not displace the eye itself.
- Although not required in all cases, a computed tomography scan can be used to confirm diagnosis.
- Treatment of dermoid cysts is complete surgical excision.

Suggested Reading

Ahuja R, Azar NF. Orbital dermoids in children. *Semin Ophthalmol.* 2006;21(3):207–211

Yen KG, Yen MT. Current trends in the surgical management of orbital dermoid cysts among pediatric ophthalmologists. *J Pediatr Ophthalmol Strabismus.* 2006;43(6):337–340

Section 4

Abnormal Red Reflex

Chapter 24

Eye With White Pupil

Carol L. Shields, MD
Jerry A. Shields, MD

Presentation

A 6-month-old boy is noted to have a glassy-looking eye by his mother, who brings the infant to the pediatrician. The infant is one of a set of twins conceived by in vitro fertilization. According to the mother, the eye abnormality has been present for 2 months and the infant apparently can see well and has no pain. She denied the occurrence of ocular trauma or infection. There is no family history of eye problems, including congenital cataracts.

On examination, the infant is cooperative and the eyes appear straight, without strabismus. The surrounding conjunctiva, eyelids, and orbital tissue show no signs of inflammation. The anterior segment of the right eye is normal. The left eye shows obvious leukocoria, or white pupil (Figure 24-1). There is no tearing or redness.

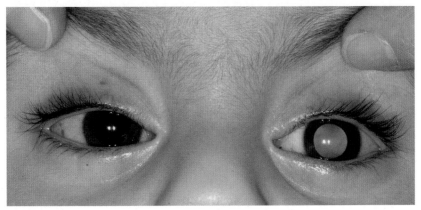

Figure 24-1. Leukocoria (white pupil) is apparent in the left eye. Courtesy of Carol L. Shields, MD.

Ophthalmoscopy reveals that the right fundus and optic disc are normal (Figure 24-2). Evaluation of the left eye discloses a white, elevated retinal mass near the optic disc (Figure 24-3).

The pediatrician refers the patient to an ophthalmologist for dilation of the pupils and fundus examination.

Diagnosis

This infant has retinoblastoma, as found by detailed ophthalmologic examination and imaging studies. Further workup by the ophthalmic consultant, as for any patient with suspected retinoblastoma, includes ophthalmoscopic evaluation for surrounding retinal detachment, vitreous and subretinal seeding, tumor size and exact location, multifocality and bilaterality of tumors, and general assessment of visual potential of the eye. The tumor is intermediate in size (12 mm) and has minimal seeding. Ultrasonography of the eye is performed and reveals a solid intraocular mass with flecks of calcification showing bright echoes. With the patient

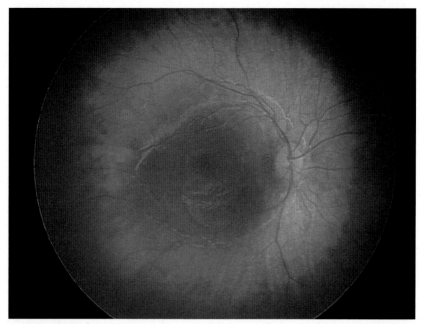

Figure 24-2. Fundus photograph of right eye shows normal optic disc. Courtesy of Carol L. Shields, MD.

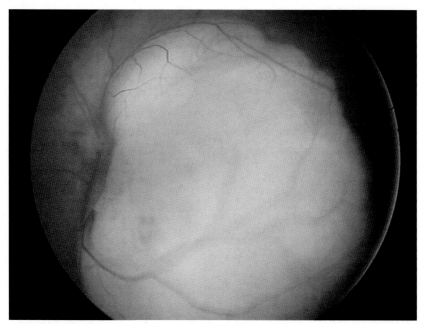

Figure 24-3. Fundus photograph of left eye discloses a white, elevated retinal mass near the optic disc. Courtesy of Carol L. Shields, MD.

under general anesthesia, contrast dye injection with intravenous fluorescein angiography is performed to determine the vascularity in the tumor and feeding the tumor (Figure 24-4). The eye is then classified as group D according to the International Classification of Retinoblastoma (Table 24-1).

There are several causes of a glassy eye, or better stated, an eye with leukocoria (white pupil). Any condition that causes opacity in the ocular media can lead to leukocoria. It is important to understand that even slight whitening in the retina can lead to leukocoria. There are a number of specific ocular disorders in infants and children that can resemble retinoblastoma.

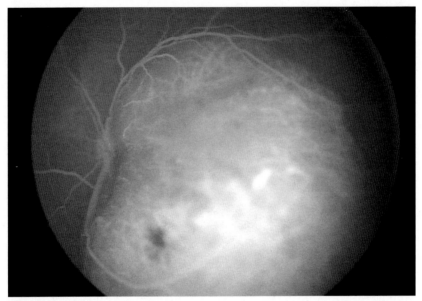

Figure 24-4. Fluorescein angiogram of left eye shows vascularity in the tumor. Courtesy of Carol L. Shields, MD.

Table 24-1. International Classification of Retinoblastoma

Group	Quick Reference	Specific Features
A	Small tumor	Rb ≤3 mm[a]
B	Larger tumor Macula Juxtapapillary Subretinal fluid	Rb >3 mm[a] or • Macular Rb location (≤3 mm to foveola) • Juxtapapillary Rb location (≤1.5 mm to disc) • Additional subretinal fluid ≤3 mm from margin
C	Focal seeds	Rb with • Subretinal seeds ≤3 mm from Rb • Vitreous seeds ≤3 mm from Rb • Subretinal and vitreous seeds ≤3 mm from Rb
D	Diffuse seeds	Rb with • Subretinal seeds >3 mm from Rb • Vitreous seeds >3 mm from Rb • Subretinal and vitreous seeds >3 mm from Rb
E	Extensive Rb	Extensive Rb occupying >50% globe or • Neovascular glaucoma • Opaque media from hemorrhage in anterior chamber, vitreous or subretinal space • Invasion of postlaminar optic nerve, choroid (>2 mm), sclera, orbit, anterior chamber

Abbreviation: Rb, retinoblastoma.
[a]Refers to 3 mm in basal dimension or thickness.

Differential Diagnosis

Diagnoses besides retinoblastoma that should be considered include but are not limited to the following:

Congenital Cataract

Vitreous Hemorrhage

Retinal Detachment

Persistent Hyperplastic Primary Vitreous

Coats Disease

Usually seen unilaterally in young males, Coats disease can resemble retinoblastoma by producing a localized macular lesion or retinal detachment. Unlike retinoblastoma, Coats disease demonstrates irregular, bulb-type telangiectasis in the peripheral aspect of the fundus on fluorescein angiogram.

Ocular Toxocariasis

Retinal Astrocytic Hamartoma of Tuberous Sclerosis

Coloboma

When to Refer

Any infant or child with leukocoria should be referred to an ophthalmologist for full ophthalmic examination including dilated pupil fundus examination. If diagnosis of retinoblastoma is suspected, the patient should be referred to a pediatric ophthalmologist, retina specialist, or preferably, a retinoblastoma specialist (ocular oncologist).

Treatment

Treatment options for patients with retinoblastoma include enucleation (eye removal), external beam radiotherapy, or chemo-reduction plus focal thermotherapy. Given the intermediate tumor size and minimal tumor seeding in this case, chemo-reduction is offered. Following 6 cycles of vincristine, etoposide, and carboplatin, the tumor and related

fluid and seeds would likely show complete regression to a partially cal-
cified remnant scar in the para-macular location. At each examination
by the ocular oncologist, consolidation transpupillary thermotherapy
using an infrared diode laser is applied to the tumor, with good long-
term control (Figure 24-5).

Patching of the right eye to minimize amblyopia of the left eye is suggested for 2 hours daily to maximize visual acuity in the affected eye.
This will be continued until the patient reaches 8 years of age. This boy
will need lifelong evaluation of both eyes on a 6-month basis.

Systemically, this patient will need monitoring for related cancers, including pinealoblastoma and remote second cancers. This will depend
on genetic testing results for germ line versus somatic mutation of
chromosome 13q. Children with a germ-line mutation carry an 8%
risk by age 5 years of pinealoblastoma and a 30% risk by age 30 years
of second cancers. The most common second cancers include bone

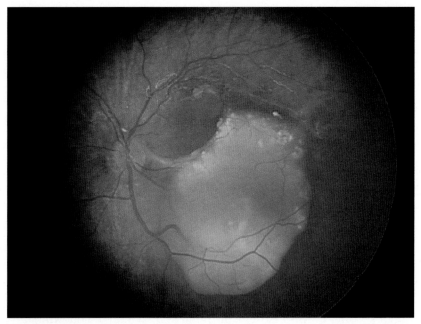

Figure 24-5. Consolidation transpupillary thermotherapy using an infrared diode
laser is applied to the tumor, with good long-term control. Courtesy of Carol L.
Shields, MD.

osteosarcoma, soft-tissue sarcomas, and cutaneous melanoma. If the boy shows somatic mutation, these risks are negligible. All children with bilateral or familial retinoblastoma carry a germ-line mutation. Approximately 10% of children with unilateral sporadic retinoblastoma manifest germ-line mutation. Because this infant has unilateral sporadic retinoblastoma, the chance of having germ-line mutation is about 10%.

Enucleation (eye removal) is an important method of managing retinoblastoma when necessary. Today it is employed less frequently than in the past because of the advent of chemo-reduction and consolidation treatment, as used in this case. Enucleation is mainly reserved for an advanced tumor when there is no hope for useful vision in the affected eye or if there is a concern for invasion of the tumor into the optic nerve, choroid, or orbit. The patient in this case does not need enucleation.

If he did, an orbital implant would be placed after enucleation to provide natural cosmetic appearance of the patient's artificial eye and enable motility of the prosthesis. The patient is fitted with a prosthesis 6 weeks after enucleation. The prosthesis can be enlarged as the child grows. The prosthesis is removed and cleaned twice yearly by the ophthalmologist.

Discussion

After chemo-reduction, children with tumors outside the posterior region of the eye (macula) and who have useful central vision usually achieve visual acuity of 20/20 to 20/40. Those with tumors in the macular region, like this patient, show reduced central vision of approximately 20/200 or worse. Amblyopia patching of the good eye can allow the infant to regain some lost vision.

Retinoblastoma has a 95% cure rate, making it one of the most curable childhood cancers. Siblings of children with retinoblastoma should have an eye examination by an ophthalmologist.

> ## Key Points
>
> - All children with glassy eye or leukocoria should have pupillary dilation and fundus examination by a pediatric ophthalmologist or retina specialist.
> - Chemo-reduction has assumed a major role in the management of retinoblastoma, and enucleation is less often necessary today.
> - Brain imaging (usually magnetic resonance imaging) for pinealo-blastoma in the first 5 years of life is important for patients with germ-line mutation.
> - Lifelong follow-up for second cancers in children with germ-line mutation is important.

Suggested Reading

Shields CL, Mashayekhi A, Au AK, et al. The International Classification of Retinoblastoma predicts chemoreduction success. *Ophthalmology.* 2006;113(12):2276–2280

Shields CL, Shields JA. Basic understanding of current classification and management of retinoblastoma. *Curr Opin Ophthalmol.* 2006;17(3):228–234

Shields JA, Shields CL. Retinoblastoma. In: Shields JA, Shields CL, eds. *Intraocular Tumors: An Atlas and Textbook.* 2nd ed. Philadelphia, PA: Lippincott Williams and Wilkins; 2008:293–365

Chapter 25

White Spots in the Eyes

James B. Ruben, MD

Presentation

A 6-week-old infant new to the pediatrician's practice comes in for a routine well-baby check. The mother thinks the baby is not yet making eye contact with her.

The pediatrician examines the infant with a direct ophthalmoscope and observes normal external ocular adnexa but a diminished red reflex in both eyes. He also notes uninflamed eyes with clear, normal-size cornea; deep anterior chamber; and clear view of the iris. Furthermore, there is a whitish-gray opacity visible through the pupil just behind the iris, and it appears to involve the lens of each eye (Figure 25-1).

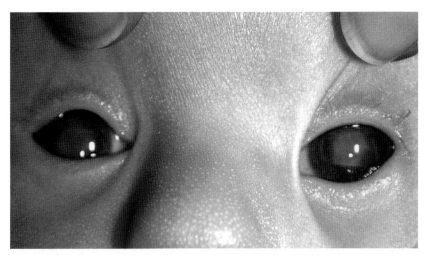

Figure 25-1. A diminished red reflex is apparent in both eyes. Whitish-grey opacities are seen through the pupils just behind the irises involving the lenses. The opacities cover the visual axis. Courtesy of Shira L. Robbins, MD.

The pediatrician is reminded of a similar case he saw the previous week of a 5-year-old with asymmetric red reflex with leukocoria (Figure 25-2).

The pediatrician refers the infant to a pediatric ophthalmologist to obtain a definitive diagnosis. The ophthalmologist performs a complete dilated eye examination.

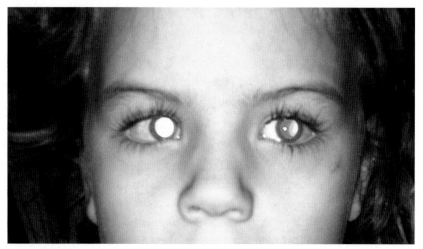

Figure 25-2. Asymmetric red reflex with leukocoria in the right eye. Courtesy of Shira L. Robbins, MD.

Diagnosis

Findings in the pediatrician's office are strongly suggestive of congenital cataracts. On red reflex examination, an infant with normal vision will exhibit a reddish or orange reflex, resulting from reflection off a healthy retina through a clear visual axis, which includes the tear film, cornea, anterior chamber, pupil, lens, and vitreous. The appearance is similar to the red eye common in flash photography. An absent or abnormal red reflex suggests an abnormality in the visual axis that may portend a serious ocular or medical emergency, such as cataract, glaucoma, persistent fetal vasculature, uveitis, retinal detachment, or retinoblastoma (Figure 25-3).

All children with suspected congenital cataracts should undergo thorough evaluation to look for manifestations of other possible components of

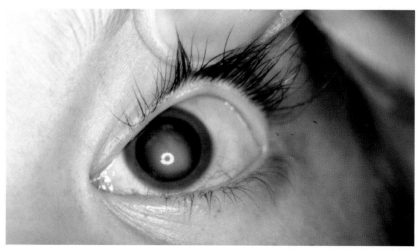

Figure 25-3. Abnormal red reflex with cataract left eye. Courtesy of James B. Ruben, MD.

genetic, infectious, or metabolic association. Family history should be obtained, and particular attention should be paid to ensuring that these babies are meeting growth and developmental milestones. Once a diagnosis of *bilateral* congenital cataracts has been confirmed, directed laboratory studies can also be obtained to rule out disorders that can cause congenital cataracts. Such studies include urinalysis for amino acids to rule out Lowe (oculocerebrorenal) syndrome, urinalysis for reducing substances to rule out galactosemia, and titers for toxoplasmosis, other agents, rubella, cytomegalovirus, and herpes simplex (TORCH).

Differential Diagnosis

Diagnoses besides congenital cataract that should be considered include but are not limited to the following:

Congenital Glaucoma

This generally presents with epiphora and photophobia and is often accompanied by clouding of the cornea and enlargement of the eye.

Persistent Fetal Vasculature

Formerly called persistent hyperplastic primary vitreous, this condition is a congenital malformation that is usually bilateral and sporadic. One eye may appear smaller than the other.

Uveitis

This often presents with photophobia and a red or inflamed eye. Slit-lamp examination is diagnostic with presence of white blood cells in the anterior chamber of the eye.

Retinal Detachment

Leukocoria will emanate from behind the lens with a clear lens visible. Pupil examination will demonstrate a relative afferent papillary defect.

Retinoblastoma

The lens will be clear and there will be leukocoria visible behind the lens.

When to Refer

There often is sufficient information on the pediatrician's physical examination to help determine correct diagnosis. However, definitive diagnosis of the cause of an absent or abnormal red reflex is best made by an ophthalmologist skilled in the care of children. It often requires dilation of the eye and specialized equipment, such as slit-lamp microscope, indirect ophthalmoscope, or ophthalmic ultrasound, which are unavailable in the offices of most primary care practitioners.

It is important for the pediatrician to keep in mind that anything obstructing vision in a young infant or child can result in permanent, severe visual loss or blindness due to deprivation amblyopia—even if the obstructing opacified lens is later removed. Congenital cataracts with sufficient opacity to cause amblyopia should ideally be removed between 4 and 6 weeks of age. Hence, prompt referral is critical.

Treatment

Infants with clinically significant congenital cataracts should undergo early surgical removal of the cataract or cataracts for the best chance of a good visual outcome. After surgery, the patient will need proper refractive correction by eyeglasses, contact lens, or even artificial intraocular lens. Mild cataract that does not affect vision may not need surgical treatment (Figure 25-4).

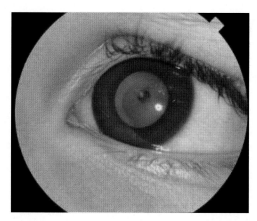

Figure 25-4. Small (<2 mm) anterior polar cataract that was not visually significant because of its size. Courtesy of Shira L. Robbins, MD.

Children with unilateral or asymmetric bilateral cataracts often require intensive visual penalization therapy with patching (occlusion therapy) or cycloplegic eyedrops to treat underlying amblyopia.

In addition, treatment of any underlying disorder may be needed.

Discussion

Congenital cataracts may develop as a result of various conditions. Often there is a genetic component, as part of a systemic syndrome or as an isolated finding, such as with autosomal-dominant congenital cataract. Other causes, such as metabolic conditions, in utero infection, trauma, or congenital eye malformations, may be responsible. Sometimes lens morphology of the cataract can give a clue as to the possible cause, such as the oil-droplet cataract of galactosemia. When cataracts are bilateral, it is more likely that the cause may be genetic or metabolic.

Prognosis after early cataract surgery is usually excellent when compliance with patching therapy is good. However, children with a history of congenital cataracts, particularly those who have undergone early surgery, are at increased lifelong risk of development of glaucoma. Thus, it is important for the pediatrician to reinforce the need for long-term follow-up care with an ophthalmologist.

> ## Key Points
>
> - Red reflex testing should be performed routinely at every infant well-child visit.
> - Congenital cataracts with sufficient opacity to cause amblyopia should ideally be removed between 4 and 6 weeks of age. Delay in diagnosis and treatment generally leads to irreversible amblyopia.
> - Children with unilateral or asymmetric bilateral cataracts often require intensive therapy with patching or cycloplegic eyedrops to treat underlying amblyopia.
> - Children with a history of congenital cataracts, particularly those who have undergone early surgery, are at increased lifelong risk of development of glaucoma. The pediatrician should reinforce to parents the need for long-term follow-up care with an ophthalmologist.

Suggested Reading

American Academy of Pediatrics Section on Ophthalmology, American Association for Pediatric Ophthalmology and Strabismus, American Academy of Ophthalmology, American Association of Certified Orthoptists. Red reflex examination in neonates, infants, and children. *Pediatrics.* 2008;122(6):1401–1404

Chung DC, Traboulsi EI. An overview of the diagnosis and management of childhood cataracts. *Contemp Ophthalmol.* 2004;3(4):1–10

Vishwanath M, Cheong-Leen R, Taylor D, Russell-Eggitt I, Rahi J. Is early surgery for congenital cataract a risk factor for glaucoma? *Br J Ophthalmolol.* 2004;88(7):905–910

Chapter 26

Abnormal Pupillary Light Reflex

Daniel J. Karr, MD

Presentation

The pediatrician meets a 10-week-old patient for the first time. The family had an uneventful planned home delivery attended by a midwife. The immediate postdelivery evaluation by the midwife reportedly showed a healthy, full-term girl. The parents have noted a mild difference in the appearance of the 2 eyes. The mother characterizes this as a smaller left eye.

The infant is active and visually alert. The pediatrician notes that the left eye is smaller than the right (Figure 26-1). Looking more carefully, the pediatrician also is aware of a different color between the pupils, with the left showing white-gray reflex on red reflex test. Despite her excellent visual attention, every time the right eye is covered, the infant becomes agitated and tries to look around the cover. She has no objection to covering her left eye. Her eyes are straight and move well. Pupils have normal reactivity. Remaining findings of general eye examination are completely normal.

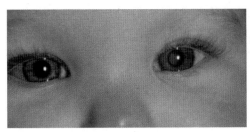

Figure 26-1. Infant with asymmetry of eye appearance. Courtesy of Daniel J. Karr, MD.

Additional history discloses no loss of vision or eye problems in children on either side of the family. The infant has no siblings. One grandparent is being treated for glaucoma, and 2 grandparents have had cataract surgery.

The pediatrician informs the family of the possibility of a serious problem such as congenital cataract or retinoblastoma and recommends a pediatric ophthalmology consultation. Pediatric ophthalmologic evaluation is arranged for later that day. Ultrasonography is performed in the ophthalmology office, which shows no sign of retinoblastoma. Instead, ultrasound reveals a subtle vascular membrane stalk running from the lens anteriorly toward the optic nerve posteriorly (figures 26-2 and 26-3). An axial length is also measured and the involved left eye is found to be atypically short in length.

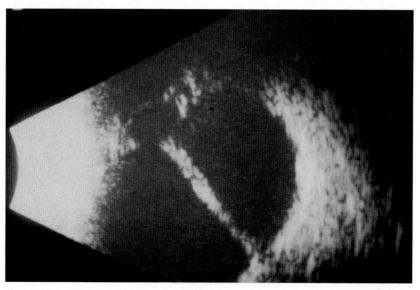

Figure 26-2. Ultrasound image of stalk in vitreous space connecting the lens and optic nerve. Courtesy of Daniel J. Karr, MD.

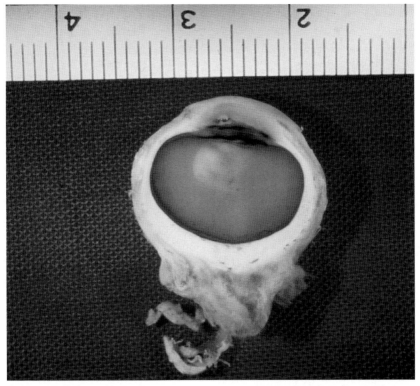

Figure 26-3. Pathology specimen showing stalk relationship (different patient). Courtesy of Daniel J. Karr, MD.

Diagnosis

This patient has a lesion in the left eye that is interfering with vision. It may have been there since birth. The lack of good red light reflex in the left eye and the white-gray membrane seen on eye examination means the child has leukocoria (white pupil). The pediatrician knows that differential diagnoses for leukocoria include retinoblastoma, cataract, and retinopathy of prematurity. Retinopathy of prematurity would not be a consideration, however, because the child was full term.

The pediatric ophthalmologist informs the pediatrician that the left eye is definitely smaller (microphthalmos) and that this finding plus the persistent stalk seen on the ultrasonogram indicate that the diagnosis is persistent fetal vasculature (PFV).

Formerly called persistent hyperplastic primary vitreous, PFV is a con-genital malformation that is usually unilateral, isolated, and sporadic and may be associated with other systemic anomalies.

Untreated PFV usually has progressive cataract formation with the potential of later development of angle-closure glaucoma. When PFV involves primarily the anterior segment of the eye, early surgical inter-vention can result in preservation of the eye and potential for visual development.

Differential Diagnosis

Diagnoses besides PFV that should be considered in the presence of leukocoria in an infant include but are not limited to the following:

Retinopathy of Prematurity

This should be suspected with history of prematurity and normal-sized eyes.

Cataract

Cataract may be difficult to distinguish from PFV because the unilateral congenital cataract eye may be smaller than the fellow eye. Both condi-tions need urgent evaluation.

Ocular Toxocariasis

This presents in an older child, average 7.5 years of age; eye is normal sized and lens is clear.

Uveitis

This can occur in normal-sized eyes. Cataract is a later complication.

Retinoblastoma

Retinoblastoma is the most important and potentially life-threatening leukocoria consideration. The eye is usually normal sized but can be larger from secondary glaucoma. Abnormal reflex can originate from lens region to retina. Every leukocoria patient must have retinoblasto-ma ruled out.

Ultrasonography of the eye reveals a solid intraocular mass with areas of calcifications.

Coloboma of the Retina/Choroid

Here, the eye may be smaller and have diagnostic pupil changes.

Coats Disease

Normal-sized eye with yellow white reflex with characteristic vessel pattern is typical of Coats disease. This is difficult to distinguish from retinoblastoma without retinal examination.

Familial Exudative Vitreoretinopathy

This may look like retinopathy of prematurity, but it occurs in full-term children. Eye is normal sized, and typically there is no cataract.

Myelinated Nerve Fibers

White reflex in band or arcuate formation in region of optic nerve presents here. There is no elevation of tissue or cataract association.

Norrie Disease

Norrie disease is X-linked recessive with affected males blind at birth or early infancy. It may look like PFV or retinoblastoma with retrolental mass.

Retinal Detachment

A patient with retinal detachment can have white reflex from detached retina. This may be difficult to distinguish from retinoblastoma. Eye is generally normal sized.

High Myopia

The eye is normal or longer than usual.

Vitreous Hemorrhage

Red reflex is attenuated or eliminated by blood. There is no cataract and eye is normal sized.

When to Refer

All of the differential diagnostic considerations that cause leukocoria in an infant are reasons for urgent referral to an ophthalmologist.

Treatment

The pediatric ophthalmologist is optimistic that this child's eye has primarily anterior PFV changes. It appears that the optic nerve and retina are not substantially involved. The specialist recommends surgical correction in the near future. Surgery takes place the next week, with the infant under general anesthesia. Intraoperatively the cataract and adherence of the PFV plaque to the ciliary body processes are well seen (Figure 26-4). The cataract is removed.

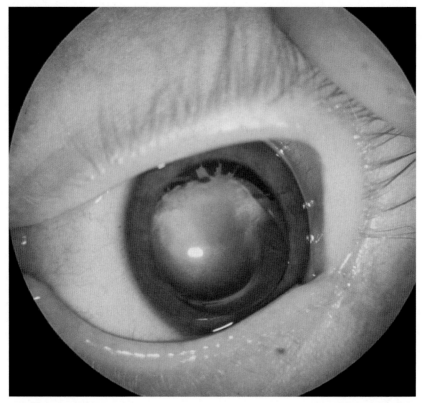

Figure 26-4. Central dense cataract changes with ciliary processes rotated anteriorly in the superior portion of the eye (note dark area between cataract and dilated iris). Courtesy of Daniel J. Karr, MD.

The infant will be given a contact lens (to do the focusing work of the natural lens, which has been removed) as soon as surgical inflammation subsides and the wound heals sufficiently. She will need patching therapy of the normal right eye to promote visual development of the affected left eye. Compliance with contact lens use and patching therapy will be the major determinants of final visual acuity. She eventually develops good vision (Figure 26-5).

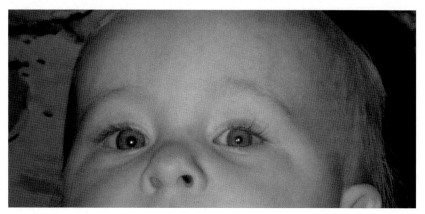

Figure 26-5. Smaller left eye. Good vision with contact lens in place. Courtesy of Daniel J. Karr, MD.

Discussion

The spectrum of ocular involvement in PFV is extensive. It ranges from minimal footprints of earlier stages of development, such as Mittendorf dot (small dot on the posterior lens capsule) and Bergmeister papilla (stalk off the optic nerve), to severely microphthalmic eyes and severe posterior segment involvement (Figure 26-6). The posterior segment health determines overall visual potential. Retinal detachment, intraocular hemorrhage, ciliary body detachment, and traction effects on the anterior segment resulting in cataract formation with anterior chamber shallowing and severe angle-closure glaucoma result from posterior PFV disease. Eyes with retinal, macular, and optic nerve involvement (attachment and traction) are less likely to have useful vision. Surgery in such eyes is limited to preservation of the globe and prevention of glaucoma from secondary changes from chronic PFV.

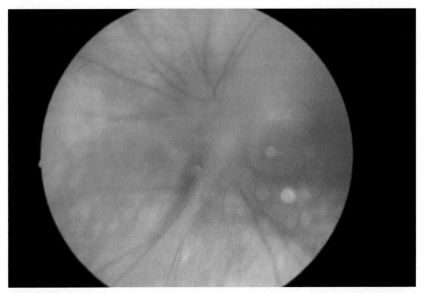

Figure 26-6. Stalk incorporated into optic nerve and macula on retinal photograph, different patient. Courtesy of Daniel J. Karr, MD.

Key Points

- Leukocoria (white pupil) is a condition in which normal red reflex is absent or reduced.
- Many of the differential diagnostic considerations that cause leukocoria in an infant are reasons for urgent referral to an ophthalmologist. These include retinoblastoma, persistent fetal vasculature (PFV), retinopathy of prematurity, cataract, toxocariasis, uveitis, and an assortment of other intraoculartumors.
- Untreated PFV usually has progressive cataract formation with the potential for later development of angle-closure glaucoma.

Suggested Reading

Goldberg MF. Persistent fetal vasculature (PFV): an integrated interpretation of signs and symptoms associated with persistent hyperplastic primary vitreous (PHPV). LIV Edward Jackson Memorial Lecture. *Am J Ophthalmol.* 1997;124(5):587–626

Karr DJ, Scott WE. Visual acuity results following treatment of persistent hyperplastic primary vitreous. *Arch Ophthalmol.* 1986;104(5):662–667

Section 5

Abnormalities of the Anterior Segment

Chapter 27

Different-Colored Eyes

Deborah K. VanderVeen, MD

Presentation

The pediatrician sees a male infant for the first time at his 6-month well-child visit. His parents report that his eyes have different colors; there is a section of dark brown in the right eye, with otherwise green eyes (Figure 27-1). The parents wonder if they should be concerned about this and if it is related to any other eye problems. They have not noticed any problems with the baby's vision. There is no other ocular history such as injury or infection to the eye, and family ocular history is unremarkable. This child has been healthy and developmentally normal, and pregnancy and birth history are unremarkable.

The pediatrician performs a routine vision screening and eye examination and does not find anything else unusual about the appearance of the infant's eyes. He shows age-appropriate visual responses.

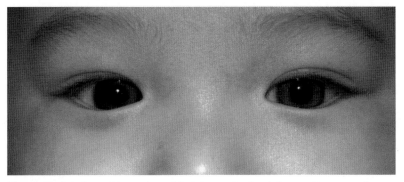

Figure 27-1. Infant with section of dark brown in the right eye. Courtesy of Rupa Krishnamurthy Wong, MD.

Diagnosis

This infant has heterochromia iridis, which is a difference of color between sectors of the iris in one eye. Thus, this condition is often termed *sectoral* heterochromia iridis. Heterochromia iridis usually refers to 2 different-colored eyes in a single individual (Figure 27-2). The general term *hetero-chromia* is commonly used when describing differences in iris coloration, and is used along with the description *sectoral* when differences are present in only one section of an eye. There is a small chance that this infant's iris may change to one color before the age of 2 years, although eye color most often becomes apparent in the first 6 months of life.

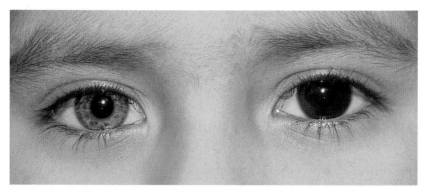

Figure 27-2. Heterochromia iridis in a different patient. Courtesy of Deborah K. VanderVeen, MD.

Heterochromia is usually an isolated finding. Familial heterochromia is transmitted in autosomal-dominant fashion, as in Waardenburg syndrome (see below). Ocular and systemic diseases, eye trauma, and certain medications may also contribute to the development of heterochromia.

Differential Diagnosis

Diagnoses besides heterochromia iridis that should be considered include the following:

Waardenburg Syndrome

This syndrome is characterized by pigmentary disturbances of the iris, hair, and skin and is associated with congenital sensorineural hearing loss. It is an autosomal-dominant disorder caused by mutations in the *PAX3* gene.

Horner Syndrome

Patients with congenital or perinatal Horner syndrome may have less iris pigmentation on the affected side because melanocytes in the iris depend on sympathetic innervation to maintain pigmentation (see Chapter 30). These patients also will often have an ipsilateral mild blepharoptosis (droopy eyelid), miosis (small pupil), and anhidrosis.

Congenital Glaucoma

Corneal haziness in one or both eyes due to glaucoma can cause iris details to appear less distinct or change color. Congenital glaucoma typically causes epiphora (excessive watering), blepharospasm (uncontrolled closure of the eyelids), and photophobia (light sensitivity). Intraocular pressure is elevated. Additionally, certain glaucoma medications may cause increased melanin production within melanocytes, leading to darkening of iris color in the treated eye.

Ocular Trauma

Eye injury, previous ophthalmic surgery, or other sources of inflammation or bleeding in the eye may permanently change iris color.

Neurofibromatosis

Patients with neurofibromatosis may develop changes in iris color. This familial condition causes multiple, benign, pedunculated soft tumors over the body associated with pigmented areas.

When to Refer

This infant does not need to see an ophthalmologist. Referral to an ophthalmologist is probably not necessary for most infants for whom, once the eye color stabilizes, no other abnormalities are seen and typical sectoral pigmentation difference or difference between the 2 eyes is noted.

Infants should be referred to an ophthalmologist if they have other eye problems (eg, droopy eyelid, small pupil, inflammation, bleeding or other signs of injury, corneal haziness) or other abnormalities (eg, congenital hearing loss, pigmentary changes of skin or hair). These signs and symptoms could indicate the presence of an ocular or systemic disease. Also, any child who has a late change in iris color (particularly after 2 years of age) should be referred for a complete ophthalmologic evaluation.

Treatment

Heterochromia in the absence of ocular or systemic disease requires no treatment.

Discussion

Usually eye color becomes apparent in the first 6 months of life, but it can continue to change during the first 2 years. Eye color depends on the amount of melanin present in the iris. Eye color is inherited as a polygenic trait, and at least 2 genes have been linked to eye color: *EYCL3*, on chromosome 15, and *EYCL1*, on chromosome 19. How these genes interact is unknown. Other genes may act on the pattern and placement of pigment in the iris.

Key Points

- Heterochromia iridis is a benign condition noted in the first year of life and is generally isolated.
- Waardenburg syndrome should be considered for children with congenital sensorineural hearing loss.
- Ocular diseases may cause acquired heterochromia, and patients with signs and symptoms of any eye disease should be evaluated and treated by an ophthalmologist.

Suggested Reading

Johns Hopkins University. OMIM: Online Mendelian Inheritance in Man. http://omim.org. Accessed April 3, 2012

Wallis DH, Granet DB, Levi L. When the darker eye has the smaller pupil. *J AAPOS*. 2003;7(3):215–216

Chapter 28

Unusual Pupil

Daniel J. Karr, MD

Presentation

An 18-month-old girl is referred to the pediatrician's practice by a county health nurse, who has followed up with the patient for general health concerns and immunizations. The only notable physical finding has been an unusual pupil in the right eye. The family is not concerned because the father's side of the family has "funny eyes," but no one has problems with seeing.

The pediatrician examines the child, and she is a happy, active, well-developed 18-month-old. She has extremely good visual attention and tracks in all directions. She has no objection when the pediatrician covers either eye and sees objects well with each eye. An iris defect is easily seen, with the right pupil appearing somewhat like a keyhole (Figure 28-1). There is good red reflex in both eyes. Both pupils respond to light.

The child is referred for pediatric ophthalmologic evaluation to document vision and explore other possible ocular findings.

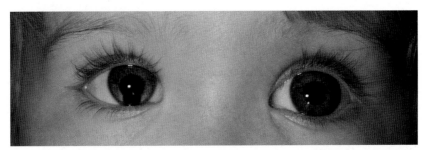

Figure 28-1. Iris defect in right pupil with classic keyhole configuration. Courtesy of Daniel J. Karr, MD.

Diagnosis

This girl has a pupillary lesion compatible with iris coloboma. The position suggests a typical coloboma because it is inferonasal. This developmental defect of ocular tissue may involve just the iris as an isolated lesion. Iris coloboma, however, may be just the tip of the iceberg, with any or all of the structures between the optic nerve and iris being involved (figures 28-2 and 28-3). If the choroid is affected, the overlying retina and underlying sclera can also be thinned or missing.

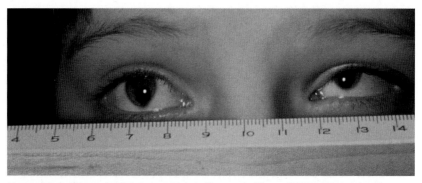

Figure 28-2. Bilateral coloboma with small eyes and loss of vision from retinal involvement. Courtesy of Daniel J. Karr, MD.

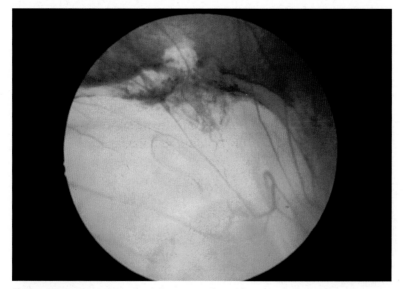

Figure 28-3. Chorioretinal coloboma involving the macula for patient shown in Figure 28-2 seen in inferior yellow-white section of image with more normal choroid/retina in superior section of image. Courtesy of Daniel J. Karr, MD.

The results of this patient's pediatric ophthalmologic evaluation show that she has bilateral changes indicating retinochoroidal colobomas (figures 28-4 and 28-5).

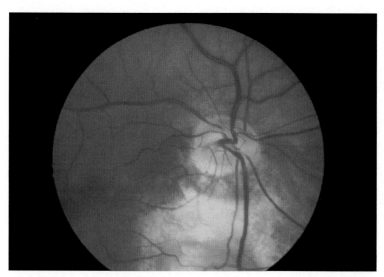

Figure 28-4. Right eye with coloboma sparing the macula and most of the optic nerve. Courtesy of Daniel J. Karr, MD.

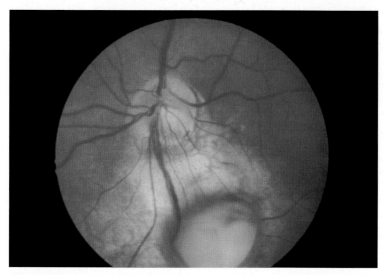

Figure 28-5. Left eye with coloboma sparing the macula and most of the optic nerve. Fortunately, the macula and optic nerve were relatively uninvolved, which explained the patient's good vision responses. Courtesy of Daniel J. Karr, MD.

The ophthalmologist also examines the girl's father, who has no obvious visual concerns but on slit-lamp examination has an iris defect (Figure 28-6). His dilated retinal examination shows bilateral colobomas, trace on the right side and more prominent on the left (Figure 28-7). Follow-up genetic evaluation documents autosomal-dominant transmission with variable expression.

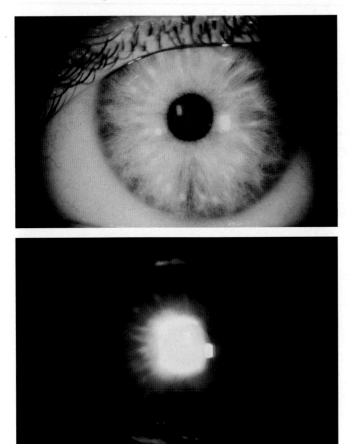

Figure 28-6. Iris defect in patient's father at the 6-o'clock position. Bottom view with transillumination demonstrates light reflection through the inferiorly thinned iris. Courtesy of Daniel J. Karr, MD.

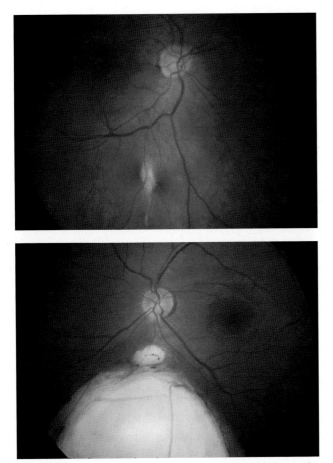

Figure 28-7. Right (top) and left (bottom) fundi of father with trace coloboma in right eye and larger coloboma in left eye. Courtesy of Daniel J. Karr, MD.

Differential Diagnosis

Diagnoses besides coloboma that should be considered include the following:

Trauma or Prior Surgery

Intraocular surgery or globe trauma can result in an abnormal or displaced pupil.

Iris Scarring/Synechiae

Iritis and congenital papillary membrane may cause distortion of the pupil, simulating coloboma. Slit-lamp examination can differentiate between these entities.

When to Refer

Vision effects from ocular coloboma are specifically related to the structures involved and can range from minimal concerns to blindness. The iris coloboma in this patient permitted normal vision development with possible increased light sensitivity from the larger pupil. When a coloboma is associated with the optic nerve and macula (central retina-fovea), it can result in profound loss of vision. Coloboma may also be associated with microphthalmia and cystic eye formation. Therefore, children with suspected coloboma should have a thorough ophthalmologic evaluation. Because colobomas may be inherited, children with this defect should receive genetic evaluation and counseling.

Treatment

Colobomas may be seen with other systemic diseases and syndromes of developmental defects. Thus, there must be good communication between the pediatrician and pediatric ophthalmologist in treating patients with associated diseases. Treatment considerations in children with coloboma depend on specific findings. Refractive error correction, amblyopia therapy with patching, cataract surgery, and retinal laser or detachment surgery may be necessary.

Discussion

Typical colobomas arise from incomplete closure of the optic fissure during early gestation. They are frequently bilateral but asymmetric in features. Colobomas may be inherited as an autosomal-dominant trait with variable expressivity and incomplete penetrance. Alternatively, a coloboma may be sporadic, autosomal recessive, or even sex-linked in transmission.

Vision prognosis depends on location and severity of the coloboma formation. Any child with coloboma, from iris to optic nerve, needs a baseline examination to rule out amblyopia, cataract, and retinal detachment. Structural findings will provide at least a rough prediction of future acuity as well as the need for intervention. Visual acuity testing is the best way to monitor for change.

Colobomas are often present in coloboma, heart anomaly, choanal atresia, retardation, and genital and ear anomalies (CHARGE) association; vertebral defects, imperforate anus, tracheoesophageal fistula, and radial and renal dysplasia (VATER) association, and Goldenhar syndrome (oculoauriculovertebral spectrum). Numerous chromosomal duplication and deletion syndromes, as well as Goltz syndrome (focal dermal hypoplasia), Walker-Warburg syndrome, and Aicardi syndrome may present with colobomas.

Key Points

- Iris coloboma may be an isolated lesion or part of a complex ocular developmental defect.
- Minor colobomas may yield normal vision but when associated with severe structural involvement, can result in profound loss of vision.
- Ocular examination of family members is extremely useful in understanding genetic implications.
- Colobomas may also be seen with other systemic diseases.
- They are often present in coloboma, heart anomaly, choanalatresia, retardation, and genital and ear anomalies (CHARGE) and vertebral defects, imperforate anus, tracheoesophageal fistula, and radial and renal dysplasia (VATER) associations and Goldenhar syndrome (oculoauriculovertebral spectrum). Thus, there must be good communication between the pediatrician and pediatric ophthalmologist.
- Numerous chromosomal duplication and deletion syndromes as well as Goltz syndrome, Walker-Warburg syndrome, and Aicardi syndrome may present with colobomas.

Suggested Reading

Mets MB, Erzurum SA. Uveal tract in infants. In: Isenberg SJ, ed. *The Eye in Infancy.* 2nd ed. St. Louis, MO: Mosby; 1994:308–317

Onwochei BC, Simon JW, Bateman JB, Couture KC, Mir E. Ocular colobomata. *Surv Ophthalmol.* 2000;45(3):175–194

Chapter 29

Brown Spot on the Eye

Deborah K. VanderVeen, MD

Presentation

A 9-year-old African American girl comes to the pediatrician's office for a routine physical examination and mentions that she has a "freckle" on her left eye. She first noticed it a couple of years ago. She has not seen an ophthalmologist. She does not have any ocular pain, itching, tearing, discharge, or visual symptoms. She is a healthy and active girl. Her family history is unremarkable for ocular or dermatologic disease.

The pediatrician checks her vision, which is normal. On examining her eye, the pediatrician sees a brownish triangular area of pigment lateral to the cornea (Figure 29-1). The eye otherwise appears normal. She does not have any unusual or generalized freckling of her skin.

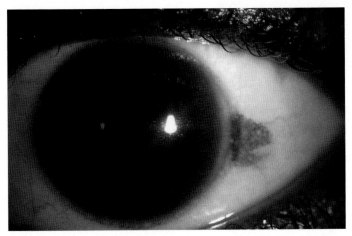

Figure 29-1. Conjunctival pigmented nevus at limbus. Courtesy of Deborah K. VanderVeen, MD.

Diagnosis

The patient has a typical pigmented conjunctival nevus. Although there is no need to refer this patient, she eventually goes to an ophthalmologist when unrelated mild myopia develops.

These benign tumors tend to come to the attention of parents or care-givers in late childhood or the teen years. Most conjunctival nevi appear near nasal or temporal quadrants of the corneal limbus, near but not involving the cornea. Nevi are rarely found in fornices of the eyelids, although nevi of the caruncle (Figure 29-2) or plica semilunaris (medial conjunctival fold) are not uncommon. Although most conjunctival nevi are brown or tan, some are amelanotic or very lightly pigmented, especially in children with light skin complexion (Figure 29-3). Amelanotic nevi are sometimes confused with focal inflammatory lesions. If a slit lamp is available, other features of nevi include intralesional microcysts, and feeder and visible intrinsic vessels.

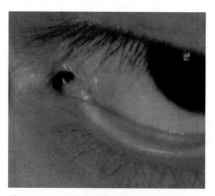

Figure 29-2. Caruncle pigmented nevus. Courtesy of Deborah K. VanderVeen, MD.

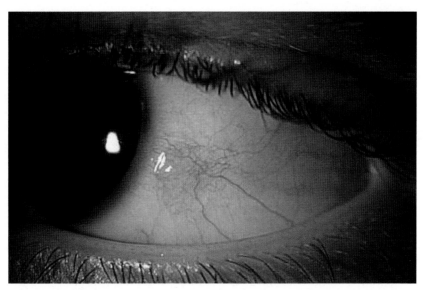

Figure 29-3. Amelanotic (nonpigmented) nevus at limbus. Courtesy of Deborah VanderVeen, MD.

Differential Diagnosis

Diagnoses other than pigmented conjunctival nevus that should be considered include the following:

Conjunctival Racial Melanosis

These benign patches of brown conjunctival pigmentation, typically bilateral and congenital, are commonly found in darkly pigmented patients.

Primary Acquired Melanosis

These patchy or irregular areas of flat tan or brown pigmentation arise on the conjunctiva and are generally found in adults.

Malignant Melanoma of Conjunctiva

Conjunctival melanoma can be melanotic or amelanotic. It should be suspected if a conjunctival lesion is raised or grows, becomes vascular, or changes color. It usually arises from preexisting areas of primary acquired melanosis, less commonly from conjunctival nevi or de novo. It is rare in children but can be lethal, with a 26% rate of metastasis and 13% death rate 10 years after diagnosis, in the adult population.

Ocular Melanocytosis

Ocular melanocytosis is congenital slate gray to brownish pigmentation of underlying sclera without involvement of overlying conjunctiva. Abnormal pigmentation may also be present in skin (oculodermal melanocytosis). It requires monitoring for glaucoma or melanoma.

When to Refer

Referral to an ophthalmologist is warranted for patients with conjunctival nevus that appears to be changing significantly or relatively quickly in size or color, or for nevus in an atypical location (eg, fornix, tarsal conjunctiva, cornea) or with atypical appearance (eg, elevation; inflammation; vascularity; changing, irregular margins). Additionally, if there are symptoms of irritation from the lesion, referral should be considered. Any patient with generalized nevus syndrome in addition to conjunctival nevus should also be referred for a complete ophthalmologic evaluation.

Treatment

For typical conjunctival nevus, observation is usually recommended. If the patient complains of surface irritation, artificial tears may be recommended for lubrication on an as-needed basis. If there is a question about the diagnosis, unusual features, or growth, an ophthalmologist may document the lesion via photography and reevaluate in 6 months. For patients with no unusual features or symptoms, follow-up may be advised on an as-needed basis. If the patient's concerns or bothersome symptoms persist or if the lesion develops atypical features, excision of the lesion by the ophthalmologist may be recommended. Nevi may become enlarged and can be affected by hormonal changes such as puberty, pregnancy, and oral contraceptive use.

Excision of conjunctival nevus from a child is usually performed in the operating room so that adequate sedation or anesthesia can be administered. These lesions should be sent for pathologic study. Typical histopathology features include thickening of the conjunctiva and increased cellularity, with variable amounts of pigment and inflammatory cells (Figure 29-4).

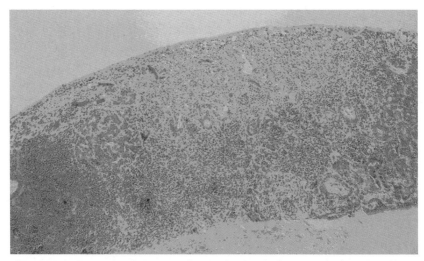

Figure 29-4. Conjunctival pigmented nevus histopathology section, hematoxylin, and eosin stain. Low power of surface shows nests of small blue cells and epithelial cyst formation, a common feature in conjunctival nevi. Minimal amounts of melanin are seen in this section. Courtesy of Richard Robb, MD.

Once a nevus is removed, the remaining conjunctiva generally heals quickly, and recurrence is unusual.

Discussion

Conjunctival nevus is the most common type of conjunctival tumor in children. Once identified, most conjunctival nevi do not change greatly, although 5% to 7% have been documented over years to change in color (usually darkening) or increase in size.

Other benign conjunctival tumors may be choristomas, vascular, lymphoid, or inflammatory types. Even in a large tertiary referral center for ocular oncology, 97% of conjunctival lesions prove to be benign, and only 3% are malignant. Evolution of a conjunctival nevus into malignant melanoma is less than 1%.

Key Points

- More than 97% of conjunctival tumors in children are benign; the most common type is conjunctival nevus.
- Less than 1% of conjunctival nevi evolve into malignant melanoma.
- Conjunctival nevi can vary in color from dark brown to amelanotic, but they have a typical appearance near the nasal or temporal limbus.

Suggested Reading

Shields CL, Fasiuddin AF, Mashayekhi A, Shields JA. Conjunctival nevi: clinical features and natural course in 410 consecutive patients. *Arch Ophthalmol.* 2004;122(2):167–175

Shields CL, Shields JA. Conjunctival tumors in children. *Curr Opin Ophthalmol.* 2007;18(5):351–360

Chapter 30

Pupil Asymmetry

Ken K. Nischal, FRCOphth
Will Moore, BSC, FRCOphth

Presentation

Case 1

A 7-year-old boy is brought to the pediatrician's office because his mother noticed that his pupils are different sizes. On direct questioning it transpires that this was noticed after a bout of chickenpox. On examination the pediatrician finds that the larger pupil fails to constrict in bright light. The pediatrician then asks the boy to look at a near target and notes that the larger pupil takes a long time to constrict.

The pediatrician believes this is Adie pupil due to ciliary ganglionitis, most likely because of the chickenpox. The pediatrician tests pharmacologically with 0.125% pilocarpine (by diluting 1% pilocarpine with sterile water or balanced salt solution).

The test result is positive for Adie pupil. The pediatrician reassures the mother but asks an important question: "Does your child have any difficulties reading?" Generally the affected eye can no longer accommodate (focus at near) normally. The child has asthenopia (headaches or eyestrain) and just "won't" read, according to the parent.

The boy is sent to a pediatric ophthalmologist for evaluation of the focusing system (dynamic retinoscopy).

Case 2

A 7-month-old boy is brought to the pediatrician's office. His mother has noted unequal pupils and different-colored eyes (iris heterochromia). She reports a clear history of birth trauma. (A traumatic birth with history of a stretched arm during delivery may indicate trauma to the region of C2-T8.) Iris heterochromia is especially relevant if the infant is brown eyed and the affected eye is now lighter because the sympathetic system is needed to maintain melanin.

The pediatrician tests the infant in bright and dark ambient light (figures 30-1 and 30-2). Anisocoria (different size pupils) increases in dim light, suggesting Horner syndrome. The pediatrician looks again and realizes the baby has very mild blepharoptosis (droopy eyelid),

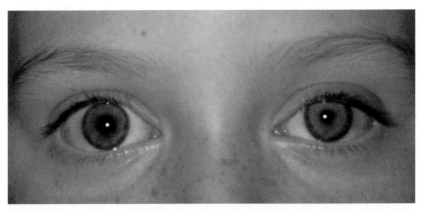

Figure 30-1. Anisocoria with right pupil larger than left in light conditions. Also mild left upper eyelid ptosis. Representative photo courtesy of David B. Granet, MD.

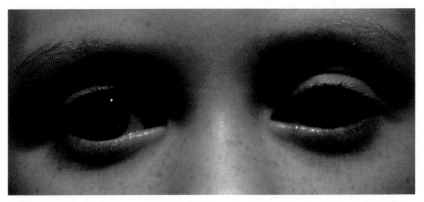

Figure 30-2. Anisocoria with right pupil larger than left exacerbated in dark conditions. Also mild left upper eyelid ptosis. Representative photo courtesy of David B. Granet, MD.

which the mother had not mentioned. Remembering the triad of miosis (small pupil), eyelid ptosis, and anhidrosis in Horner syndrome, the pediatrician asks the mother if the baby's face looks funny when he cries. She notes that one side does not flush the same as the other.

The infant is referred to a pediatric ophthalmologist for further testing to confirm Horner syndrome.

Diagnosis

Anisocoria is a difference in pupil size greater than 1 mm. The most common cause is completely normal and benign: simple or physiologic anisocoria, which affects 17% to 20% of the affected population. However, less common secondary causes can be serious. The main secondary causes are described in "Differential Diagnosis" on the next page.

Because of the chance of a potentially serious cause of anisocoria, examination and medical history are important. The child should be examined in bright light and then in a darkened room. As shown in figures 30-3 and 30-4, the difference between the pupils will

- Remain the same if the cause is physiologic, simple anisocoria, or pharmacologic
- Be more apparent in the dark, with the smaller pupil at fault, and a sympathetic nervous system lesion affecting the dilator pupillae muscle, which fails to dilate the pupil in dim light (Horner syndrome)
- Be more apparent in the light, with the larger pupil at fault, and a parasympathetic nervous system lesion affecting the pupil constrictor muscle, which fails to constrict the pupil in bright light (Adie pupil)

In case 2, if the pediatric ophthalmologist diagnoses Horner syndrome, the specialist will send the child back to the pediatrician to exclude cervical and abdominal masses on examination. Other cranial nerve palsies should also be excluded. In patients without surgical history, the pediatrician should order magnetic resonance imaging (MRI), with and without contrast medium, of the brain, neck, and chest as well as urinary catecholamine metabolite testing.

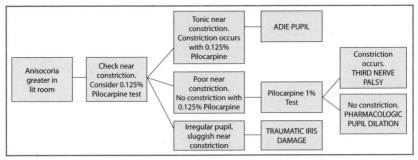

Figure 30-3. Flow diagram for larger pupil (suspected Adie pupil). Adie pupil has a denervation supersensitivity to 0.125% pilocarpine compared with normal pupil observed 10 to 15 minutes after instillation into both eyes. Courtesy of Ken K. Nischal, FRCOphth.

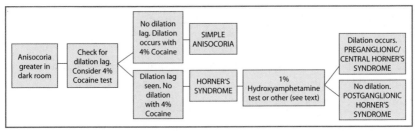

Figure 30-4. Flow diagram for smaller pupil (suspected Horner syndrome). Courtesy of Ken K. Nischal, FRCOphth.

If there is a history of birth trauma, as in case 2, the pediatrician can hold off on imaging and monitor the patient. Although a urinary catecholamine metabolite test (looking for evidence of neuroblastoma) may seem like a good precaution, it is not as sensitive as imaging. Any increasing heterochromia or development of associated cranial nerve palsy or cervical mass should prompt MRI of the head, neck, and chest, with and without contrast medium.

Differential Diagnosis

Secondary causes of anisocoria that should be considered include the following:

Horner Syndrome

Miosis, partial ipsilateral eyelid ptosis with or without lower eyelid elevation (apparent enophthalmos), and ipsilateral hemifacial anhidrosis and reduced flushing (first- or second-order neuron) are present. There may be iris heterochromia (affected iris is lighter) if the condition is congenital or long-standing. Eyelid ptosis occurs because Müller muscle, a smooth muscle, is innervated by the sympathetic nervous system. The main muscle of the eyelid, the levator, is innervated by the third cranial nerve and is not affected. In dim light the pupil fails to dilate.

Adie Pupil (Ciliary Ganglionitis)

There is often accommodative (focusing) paresis, with reduced and slow pupil reaction to accommodation with a tonic, slow dilation after near-vision effort. Sectorial vermiform iris movements (iris response asymmetry in different sectors) may be seen on microscopic slit-lamp evaluation. In bright light the pupil fails to constrict.

Traumatic Iris Damage

Damage to the iris will cause anisocoria to be greater in bright light, with sluggish constriction.

Posterior Synechiae/Persistent Pupillary Membrane

Posterior synechiae (scarring between lens and iris) usually seen in anterior uveitis and persistent papillary membrane is congenital.

Cranial Third Nerve Palsy

Anisocoria is greater in bright light, and constriction occurs. There is pupillary constriction on the 1% pilocarpine test.

Topical Medication

The cause is unilateral use of mydriatic or miotic eyedrops typically in patients with glaucoma. Anisocoria is greater in bright light. The pupil does not constrict on the 1% pilocarpine test.

When to Refer

When pupil asymmetry is 1 mm or greater in bright light or darkness, the cause is more consistent with abnormality of the parasympathetic or sympathetic nervous system. Such patients should be referred to an ophthalmologist or neurologist.

In a pediatric ophthalmologist's office, topical testing with 4% cocaine might be performed if Horner syndrome is suspected. However, 1.0%

or 0.5% apraclonidine (1 drop) with punctual occlusion (to avoid systemic absorption) may also be done. After the apraclonidine test, the infant must stay in the office for at least 1 hour to check respiratory rate and pulse. Apraclonidine test result is positive in Horner syndrome. Other tests may be done, as described in Box 30-1.

Box 30-1. Topical Tests

Cocaine 4%

After instilling 1 to 2 drops into both pupils, the tester observes the patient 15 minutes later. Cocaine blocks reuptake of noradrenaline at nerve endings of the postganglionic sympathetic nerves in the iris, potentiating its action. If the sympathetic pathway is not intact (anywhere along its path), no noradrenaline is released and cocaine will have no effect. Therefore, a negative response (no change in pupil size) will demonstrate the presence of Horner syndrome.

Hydroxyamphetamine 1%

If this test is performed, it must be done more than 24 hours after the cocaine test. The patient is observed 30 minutes after instillation of 1 to 2 drops into both pupils. Hydroxyamphetamine potentiates the release of noradrenaline from intact nerve endings, so if dilation occurs, the third-order neuron is intact and the abnormality is in first- or second-order neurons. Hydroxyamphetamine may not be available commercially; therefore, other drops have been used in its place (adrenaline and phenylephrine, or apraclonidine).

Adrenaline 1:1,000 and 1.25% Phenylephrine

After instilling 1 to 2 drops into both pupils, the evaluator waits 20 minutes before observing the patient. Only with a postganglionic lesion will the pupil dilate because of denervation hypersensitivity to adrenergic neurotransmitters. Eyelid ptosis may also be temporarily relieved.

Apraclonidine

A relatively selective α_2 agonist, apraclonidine is used in the medical management of glaucoma. It has been used in 1% and 0.5% solutions as a diagnostic test for Horner syndrome, utilizing its α_1 effect on a pupil with denervation hypersensitivity. One or 2 drops of 0.5% apraclonidine is instilled in each eye, and the patient is observed 20 minutes later. A positive test result shows dilation of the smaller pupil if the lesion is in the third-order neuron. This eyedrop has been reported to cause systemic side effects in infants, including apnea, so it is used with caution.

Treatment

The treatment of anisocoria depends on its cause.

Adie Pupil (Case 1)

If necessary, the child with Adie pupil will be given reading eyeglass correction if symptomatic.

Horner Syndrome (Case 2)

The patient in case 2 had congenital Horner syndrome caused by stretch injury at birth. No ocular or systemic treatment is needed. There is no specific treatment for Horner syndrome, with treatment being directed at the underlying cause. No ophthalmic treatment is needed when an eyelid droops only slightly (see Chapter 18).

Discussion

Adie Pupil

Adie pupil is believed to often result from a viral or bacterial infection that causes inflammation and damage to certain neurons. Affected neurons are in the ciliary ganglion, a part of the brain that controls ocular movements, and the spinal ganglion, which plays a role in the response of the autonomic nervous system. The most common association with Adie pupil is varicella-zoster virus (chickenpox), but other viral infections can cause ciliary ganglionitis. It can also be iatrogenic or seen after trauma. Visual prognosis is usually good with treatment.

Horner Syndrome

Visual prognosis is good if amblyopia management is undertaken if necessary and if the underlying cause is treated if need be.

Acquired Horner syndrome may be the result of
- *Central (first-order neuron) lesions:* posterior hypothalamus down to the spinal cord C8-T2.
- *Preganglionic (second-order) lesions:* C8-T2 to superior cervical ganglion in the neck.

- *Postganglionic (third-order) lesions:* from superior cervical ganglion via internal carotid to cavernous sinus, then via sixth cranial nerve (abducens nerve) to nasociliary and ciliary nerves to the eye

To date, Horner syndrome has not been reported as a remote effect of abdominal neuroblastoma. This malignant tumor has caused Horner syndrome by directly invading and affecting first-, second-, or third-order neurons.

Key Points

- The most common cause of pupil asymmetry is physiologic and benign.
- Other causes of pupil asymmetry can be lethal.
- In-office examination and eyedrop testing should be performed to identify which patients have an underlying cause and to treat any associated focusing problems.
- When pupil asymmetry is 1 mm or greater in bright light or darkness, it is more consistent with parasympathetic or sympathetic nervous system abnormality, and the patient should be referred to an ophthalmologist or neurologist.

Suggested Reading

Mahoney NR, Liu GT, Menacker SJ, Wilson MC, Hogarty MD, Maris JM. Pediatric Horner syndrome: etiologies and roles of imaging and urine studies to detect neuroblastoma and other responsible mass lesions. *Am J Ophthalmol.* 2006;142(4):651–659

Watts P, Satterfield D, Lim MK. Adverse effects of apraclonidine used in the diagnosis of Horner syndrome in infants. *J AAPOS.* 2007;11(3):282–283

Chapter 31

Painful Red Eye

Steven J. Lichtenstein, MD

Presentation

A 7-month-old boy is brought to the pediatrician's office by his mother because she says he has "pinkeye." She tells the pediatrician that his left eye has been red, with pus draining from it, for the past 6 days. She also states that he has been rubbing the eye and has become very fussy over the past 2 days. He has not taken his bottle in more than 24 hours and has been keeping the eye closed most of the time he is awake. He is sleeping a lot but wakes up frequently, apparently crying in pain. The infant has been a patient since birth and until this visit has only had well-baby examinations. His immunizations are up to date, and his growth is within age-appropriate growth curves.

On examination, the patient is lying in his mother's arms, lethargic and whimpering, and appears to be in distress. The pediatrician opens the lids of his right eye, which seems completely normal. The pediatrician tries to open the lids to examine his left eye, but this causes the infant to become extremely agitated and upset (Figure 31-1). The pediatrician gets a very brief look at the infant's left globe and sees that his conjunctiva is greatly injected and there is a moderate amount of purulent discharge. The infant is forcibly closing his eyelids, but the pediatrician thinks that his cornea looks "strange." Further attempts to look at his left eye prove futile, and all the pediatrician has seen is that he does have a pink eye, as the mother has reported.

A red flag is that the infant is in distress. This makes the pediatrician think that a serious problem has affected his eye. Without a proper eye examination, empirical treatment of bacterial conjunctivitis is inappropriate. The physician, therefore, immediately refers the patient to a local pediatric ophthalmologist.

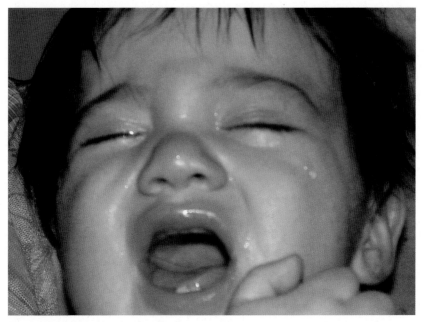

Figure 31-1. Patient immediately after eye examination attempt. Courtesy of Steven J. Lichtenstein, MD.

With the pediatric ophthalmologist, examination is again extremely difficult. Subsequently, the patient is taken to the operating room, and with the infant under mask anesthesia, a lid speculum is used to open his eyelids. During a thorough eye examination the pediatric ophthalmologist discovers that the left eye has an epithelial defect with an underlying stromal infiltrate (Figure 31-2).

Diagnosis

This infant obviously has an inflamed left eye, but it is not "pinkeye" (conjunctivitis). As shown in Figure 31-2, the infant has a corneal ulcer.

Once the diagnosis of corneal ulcer is made, identification of the etiologic organism is imperative for proper treatment. Although some corneal ulcers may be sterile, an infection is usually the cause, including bacterial, viral, fungal, and protozoan infections. Because treatments vary widely depending on the cause of an ulcer, proper cultures must first be obtained. A corneal scraping of the ulcer with Gram stain can be an invaluable asset in the differential diagnosis

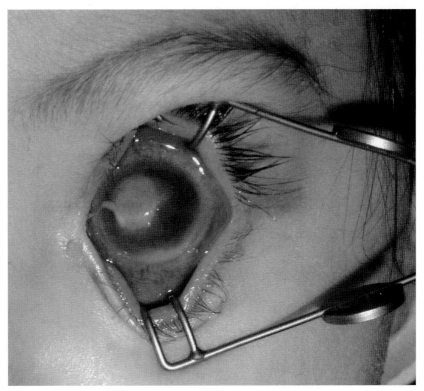

Figure 31-2. Epithelial defect with underlying stromal infiltrate. Courtesy of Steven J. Lichtenstein, MD.

and should be performed as quickly as possible. In this case, the offending organism is *Pseudomonas aeruginosa*.

Differential Diagnosis

Diagnoses besides corneal ulcer that should be considered include the following:

- Adnexal disease of the lids and lashes, including staphylococcal blepharitis
- Bacterial, viral, and allergic conjunctivitis
- Herpes simplex and zoster conjunctivitis and keratitis
- Uveitis secondary to juvenile idiopathic arthritis or trauma
- Keratoconjunctivitis sicca in children with craniofacial anomalies
- Conjunctival, corneal, or orbital foreign bodies
- Benign or malignant conjunctival neoplasms

When to Refer

A corneal ulcer has the potential to permanently impair vision or perforate the eye. It is always considered an ophthalmologic emergency and needs immediate referral. Additionally, an immediate referral to a pediatric ophthalmologist is essential in the case of apparent "conjunctivitis" that is not responding to proper therapy or in the presence of pain, photophobia (light sensitivity), or an unusual-looking cornea.

Treatment

The infant receives intensive antibiotic therapy with a topical fluoroquinolone, along with a cycloplegic drop, atropine 1% ophthalmic drops, to eliminate the ciliary spasm causing significant pain. The fluoroquinolone drop is instilled every 30 minutes, around the clock, for 36 hours. Figure 31-3 shows the infant after 36 hours of treatment. One year after the infection, the cornea shows loss of transparency (Figure 31-4). Two years after the infection, the cornea has a residual scar (Figure 31-5), which causes a major decrease in visual acuity to 20/200, even after intensive occlusion therapy to treat associated amblyopia. Even 5 years after the *Pseudomonas* infection, the corneal scar persists, and visual acuity has only improved to 20/100 with continued intensive occlusion therapy (figures 31-6 and 31-7).

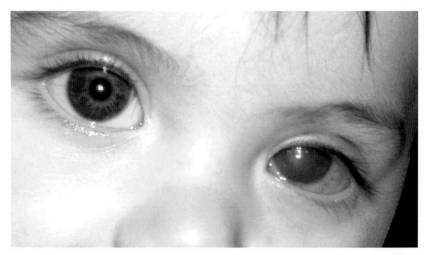

Figure 31-3. Infant after 36 hours of appropriate antibiotic treatment for corneal ulcer. Courtesy of Steven J. Lichtenstein, MD.

A topical regimen of broad-spectrum antibiotics, administered frequently, should be started as soon as the cultures and corneal scraping are performed. The goals of treatment are to eliminate the underlying cause of the ulcer, to relieve pain as quickly as possible, and to prevent or reduce scar formation. The antibiotic must be bactericidal, and frequent instillation is necessary to achieve high levels of antibiotic in the

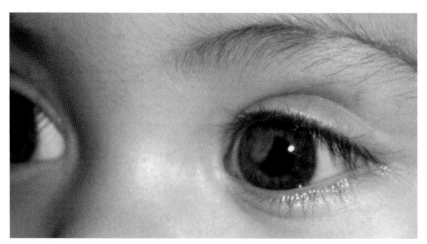

Figure 31-4. One year after corneal ulcer. Cornea shows loss of transparency. Courtesy of Steven J. Lichtenstein, MD.

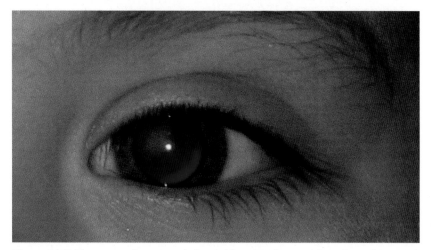

Figure 31-5. Two years after corneal ulcer with residual scar and resultant decreased vision (20/200). Courtesy of Steven J. Lichtenstein, MD.

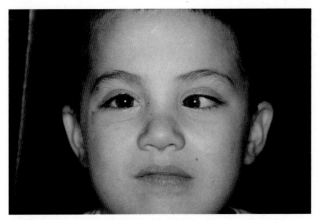

Figure 31-6. Five years after corneal ulcer with resultant decreased vision (20/100) and an esotropia due to vision asymmetry. Courtesy of Steven J. Lichtenstein, MD.

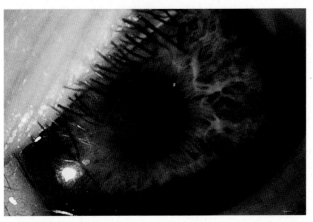

Figure 31-7. Close-up of left eye showing persistent, visually significant corneal scarring. Courtesy of Steven J. Lichtenstein, MD.

corneal stroma to rapidly kill the organism. The severe pain caused by ciliary spasm can be controlled with a cycloplegic drop, such as 1% atropine ophthalmic solution. Occasionally children need hospital admission to ensure appropriate treatment adherence for large central ulcers where poor healing can severely decrease vision.

Discussion

A corneal ulcer, also called ulcerative keratitis, is a breakdown of the epithelial layer of the cornea, with involvement of the corneal stroma. Because of this stromal involvement, the extremely orderly arrangement of the collagen fibers is disrupted, typically leading to permanent scar formation during healing and thus loss of corneal transparency. Poor visual acuity can result.

With delayed or incorrect treatment, permanent sequelae can include blindness and loss of the eye if corneal perforation occurs. Care must be taken when using any antibiotic, including topical ophthalmic preparations, in all children. Children can experience significant allergic reactions if sensitive to the antibiotic, with the drops draining from the eye to the nose through the nasolacrimal system. Also, care must be taken with the use of atropine ophthalmic drops, especially in young children. Rapid absorption of the drops through the nasal mucosa can produce toxic levels of atropine with potentially serious and even fatal reactions seen with exuberant use of topical drops.

Key Points

- A red eye in a child is most often conjunctivitis, caused by bacteria, a virus, or an allergic reaction. However, when symptoms of an apparent conjunctivitis intensify and do not start to resolve within 2 to 3 days, a more serious disease process should be considered.
- An inflammation of the conjunctiva from bacterial, viral, or allergic causes, conjunctivitis from any cause is irritating, annoying, and "a pain," but not painful.
- Immediate referral to a pediatric ophthalmologist is essential in the case of apparent conjunctivitis that is not responding to proper therapy or in the presence of pain, light sensitivity, or an unusual-looking cornea.
- A corneal ulcer misdiagnosed and mistreated as routine conjunctivitis can lead to permanent sequelae, ranging from a scar with poor visual acuity to blindness and possible loss of the eye.

Suggested Reading

Krachmer JH, Mannis MJ, Holland EJ. *Cornea: Fundamentals of Cornea and External Disease.* 1997:403–407

Leibowitz HM, Leibowitz W. *Corneal Disorders: Clinical Diagnosis and Management.* Philadelphia, PA: WB Saunders Co; 1984:353–372

Morrow GL, Abbott RL. Conjunctivitis. *Am Fam Physician.* 1998;57(4):735–746

Chapter 32

Cloudy Corneas in a Newborn

David T. Wheeler, MD, MCR
Irene Hsu-Dresden, MD

Presentation

A 3-week-old girl visits the pediatrician because her parents have noted frequent tearing (epiphora) and sensitivity to light (photophobia). The baby is unwilling to open either eye. It is the first time the pediatrician has examined this full-term newborn. According to her parents, she is otherwise healthy and there is no family history of congenital eye problems.

After turning down the room lights and cajoling the patient, the pediatrician is able to view her eyes (figures 32-1 and 32-2). The physician observes a central corneal opacity in both eyes but no conjunctival injection or discharge. The parents deny any difficulties with pregnancy or vaginal delivery. The mother has no history of sexually transmitted infection and was vaccinated against rubella as a child. Therefore, there is a low likelihood of trauma or an infectious cause. The pediatrician requests a consultation with a pediatric ophthalmologist to evaluate the eyes, determine the diagnosis, and initiate treatment.

Diagnosis

Based on the ocular findings, Peters anomaly is high on the differential diagnosis. Peters anomaly is a congenital central corneal opacity that is usually bilateral and often associated with glaucoma. The patient's symptoms of photophobia and epiphora are also suspicious for glaucoma, congenital or secondary to Peters anomaly.

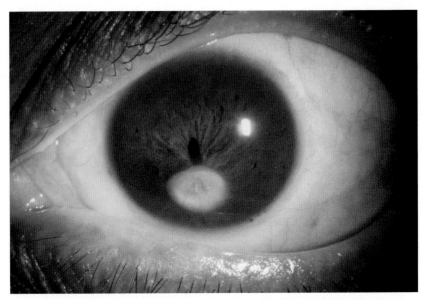

Figure 32-1. Eye showing a dense corneal opacity, or leukoma. The opacity in Peters anomaly varies in diameter and density but is present in all patients. It is usually more central than seen in this image (representative photo). Courtesy of David T. Wheeler, MD.

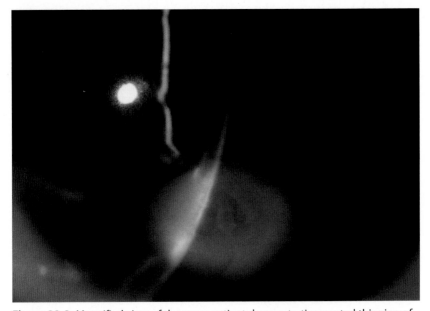

Figure 32-2. Magnified view of the same patient demonstrating central thinning of the opacified cornea. Courtesy of David T. Wheeler, MD.

In a newborn with corneal opacities, the mnemonic STUMPED is often used for the differential diagnosis.

- Sclerocornea
- Trauma (Descemet membrane tear from forceps delivery)
- Ulcer (infectious)
- Metabolic disease (mucopolysaccaroidoses)
- Peters anomaly
- Edema (glaucoma, congenital hereditary endothelial dystrophy [CHED])
- Dermoid (limbal) or dystrophy (CHED, congenital hereditary stromal dystrophy [CHSD])

The pediatric ophthalmologist diagnoses Peters anomaly and urgent corneal transplantation is performed in both eyes. The diagnosis is confirmed on histopathologic analysis of the corneas, which demonstrates defects in the posterior corneal stroma, Descemet membrane, and endothelium. After diagnosis, the newborn was returned to the pediatrician for a thorough examination to rule out systemic abnormalities, such as craniofacial anomalies, congenital heart disease, pulmonary hypoplasia, syndactyly, ear anomalies, genitourinary disorders, central nervous system abnormalities, dwarfism, chromosomal abnormalities, and fetal alcohol syndrome. A genetic consultation is recommended.

Differential Diagnosis

Diagnoses besides Peters anomaly that should be considered include the following:

Sclerocornea

Sclerocornea is an extension of opaque scleral tissue onto the peripheral cornea. A noninflammatory condition that is present congenitally, it is nonprogressive, and visual acuity is reduced only if the central cornea is involved. Patients with sclerocornea do not typically manifest with tearing and photosensitivity.

Metabolic Disease

Metabolic disease is low on the differential diagnosis for this patient because the systemic complications of metabolic disease are often diagnosed before corneal manifestations are observed. Furthermore, these deposits are usually not seen during the neonatal period.

Congenital Hereditary Endothelial Dystrophy

This dystrophy is characterized by diffuse bilaterally symmetrical corneal edema that results from severe endothelial cell dysfunction beginning late in gestation. Diffuse corneal edema affects all layers of the cornea. Intraocular pressure is normal, but photophobia and epiphora may be observed because of epithelial edema.

Congenital Hereditary Stromal Dystrophy

Congenital hereditary stromal dystrophy differs from CHED by the lack of corneal edema. Furthermore, the anterior and posterior corneal layers are relatively spared in CHSD.

Glaucoma

Newborns with congenital glaucoma not only demonstrate opaque corneas but may also present with inflammation and buphthalmos, which refers to abnormally large corneas (literally, "ox-like eye"). Parents often state that their children are very sensitive to light (photophobia), tear frequently (epiphora), and blink constantly (blepharospasm).

Corneal Dermoid

Dermoids are usually well-circumscribed, firm, solitary lesions that are adherent to sclera and cornea. They are typically present at birth, have little or no potential for growth, and are composed of displaced nests of epithelial and dermal tissue. Photophobia and epiphora are uncommon. Dermoids rarely occlude the visual axis but often cause astigmatism that can result in amblyopia if not optically corrected.

When to Refer

If Peters anomaly is suspected, referral to an ophthalmologist experienced in treating children is necessary. Many of these patients have secondary glaucoma and may have other associated ocular abnormalities that contribute to a poor visual outcome. Timely detection and management of these conditions is critical to achieving optimal visual function.

Treatment

Management of Peters anomaly is difficult. Despite early diagnosis and prompt medical treatment or surgery, many of these patients have a poor visual outcome. Glaucoma should be treated promptly with medication or surgical intervention. Early penetrating keratoplasty (corneal transplantation), within the first 3 months, can potentially offer hope for visual development, although graft rejection is common in children.

In this case, the newborn was referred for corneal transplantation in both eyes. The lenses were not involved and remained clear. Glaucoma subsequently developed in one eye and required further treatment. The child was prescribed glasses and amblyopia therapy. Despite good compliance, she developed nystagmus and significantly impaired visual function in both eyes.

Discussion

Peters anomaly, a rare congenital malformation, is defined as a congenital central corneal opacity with corresponding defects in the posterior corneal stroma, Descemet membrane, and endothelium (Figure 32-3). It represents a spectrum of morphologic abnormalities and probably results

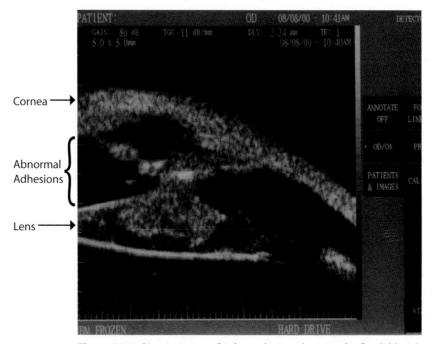

Figure 32-3. Biomicroscopy (high-resolution ultrasound) of a child with diffuse corneal opacification and adhesions from the cornea to the lens. Courtesy of David T. Wheeler, MD.

from several pathogenic mechanisms, including genetic or environmental factors. Eighty percent of reported cases are bilateral, and glaucoma develops in 50% to 70% of all cases. Many patients have a poor visual outcome because of rejection of the cornea, abnormal lens anatomy, glaucoma, and intractable amblyopia. Some patients have associated systemic abnormalities.

The family should be offered genetic counseling. Several loci have been implicated in abnormal development of anterior ocular structures (eg, *PAX6, PITX2, PITX3*), and familial transmission has been reported.

Key Points

- Peters anomaly is a congenital central corneal opacity that is usually bilateral and often associated with glaucoma.
- Photophobia (light sensitivity) and epiphora (excessive tearing) are common in Peters anomaly.
- Referral to an ophthalmologist experienced in treating children is necessary.
- The pediatrician must perform a thorough examination to rule out systemic abnormalities.

Suggested Reading

Najjar DM, Christiansen SP, Bothun ED, Summers CG. Strabismus and amblyopia in bilateral Peters anomaly. *J AAPOS.* 2006;10(3):193–197

Nischal KK. Developmental anomalies of the anterior segment and globe. In: Wright KW, Spiegel PH. *Pediatric Ophthalmology and Strabismus.* 2nd ed. New York, NY: Springer-Verlag; 2003:369–390

Taylor D, Hoyt CS. Peters anomaly. In: *Pediatric Ophthalmology and Strabismus.* 3rd ed. Edinburgh, United Kingdom: Elsevier Saunders; 2005:256–258

Chapter 33

Abnormally Large Pupils

Jenille M. Narvaez
Shira L. Robbins, MD

Presentation

A 3-day-old boy presents to the pediatrician's office because of parental concern of possible eye abnormalities. On observation, the pediatrician notes bilateral unusual red reflexes (Figure 33-1). The boy's eyes look dilated without ever receiving drops. The newborn is the product of a 39-week gestation; weighs 6 pounds, 3 ounces; and is otherwise healthy according to his family. The pediatrician refers the patient to a pediatric ophthalmologist for further evaluation.

The ophthalmologist performs a detailed ocular examination and notes only a thin rim of iris tissue present bilaterally. In some places, the lens periphery and ciliary processes are apparent (Figure 33-2). There is lack of pigmentation in the macula (the part of the retina responsible for central vision) and no macular reflex. Mild clouding of the cornea suggests possible glaucoma. However, intraocular pressures are normal. The ophthalmologist also takes photographs to document this corneal

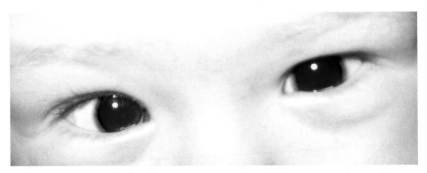

Figure 33-1. Enlarged red reflexes in representative patient. Abnormally small iris size with edge of the lens visible. This is the natural (not pharmacologically dilated) state of the pupils. Courtesy of David B. Granet, MD.

clouding at baseline. The infant's mother reports no major eye disease on either side of the family.

The ophthalmologist refers the family for a fluorescence in situ hybridization (FISH) analysis and abdominal ultrasound scan, and asks them to return in 5 days.

On the patient's return to the pediatric ophthalmologist's office, intraocular pressures remain normal, corneal clouding has cleared, and

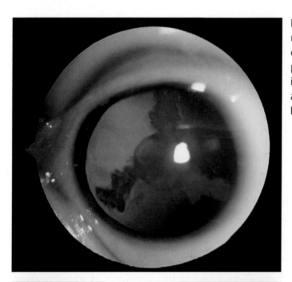

Figure 33-2. Edge of natural lens and zonules clearly seen in aniridic patient with hypoplastic iris. Associated cataracts are seen. Courtesy of Richard W. Hertle, MD.

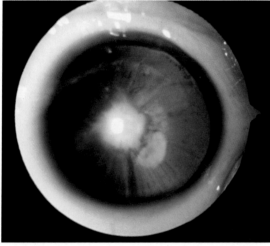

macular pigmentation is still absent. Abdominal ultrasonogram is normal. The FISH analysis, however, reveals a microdeletion of the *PAX6* ocular development gene on chromosome 11p13.

Diagnosis

This is a case of aniridia, an underdevelopment or hypoplasia of the iris. Although the name suggests a total lack of iris, a rudimentary iris or iris stump is always present. Aniridia is a congenital condition that can be sporadic or inherited, typically by autosomal dominance. *PAX6* gene mutations are found in 60% to 70% of cases. Because there is no family history, this case is most likely sporadic.

Aniridia is commonly associated with decreased vision and various ocular conditions that may complicate its presentation and diagnosis. Studies show variable incidence of decreased vision in patients with aniridia, ranging from 5% of patients with familial aniridia and visual acuity worse than 20/200 to 86% with visual acuity worse than 20/100. As this patient gets older, he will experience photophobia (sensitivity to light) and glare symptoms owing to the lack of iris, which normally limits the amount of light entering the eye.

Other ocular associations of aniridia occur later in life and include cataract, glaucoma, lens dislocation, nystagmus, optic nerve hypoplasia, macular hypoplasia, and strabismus (eye misalignment). Cataract formation occurs in 50% to 85% of patients before age 20 years. Glaucoma incidence is highly variable and typically presents in adolescence. Lens dislocation (ectopia lentis) occurs in up to 56% of patients with aniridia and is usually associated with glaucoma. Nystagmus can also occur and presents later in infancy. It appears as involuntary, rapid, and rhythmic eye movements. Optic nerve hypoplasia has been found in 75% of aniridic patients. Optic nerve hypoplasia and macular hypoplasia are what cause the decreased vision in these patients. Strabismus, specifically esotropia, is often found in patients with aniridia.

Aniridia can be associated with various systemic syndromes that must be considered during diagnosis and treatment. One major concern in patients with aniridia is Wilms tumor of the kidney. It usually occurs in patients younger than 3 years and has been seen in as many as 30% to

50% of patients with sporadic aniridia. Wilms tumor is not typically associated with familial aniridia. Large deletions of the 11p13 chromosome, which include the adjacent *PAX6* and *WT1* genes, are responsible for this association and are part of Wilms tumor, aniridia, genitourinary abnormalities, and mental retardation (WAGR) syndrome. *PAX6* mutations are associated with aniridia, and *WT1* mutations are associated with Wilms tumor. Although aniridia itself is not considered lethal, Wilms tumor is one of the most common malignant tumors in childhood and can be fatal. Even with treatment, survival rates are 50%. Abdominal ultrasonography should be repeated every 3 months to screen for Wilms tumor until it can be ruled out via genetic testing. In this patient, normal abdominal ultrasonogram and FISH analysis revealing 2 intact copies of the *WT1* gene suggest no evidence of Wilms tumor.

Differential Diagnosis

Diagnoses besides aniridia that should be considered include the following:

- Trauma
- Bilateral mydriasis (pupil enlargement) (usually iatrogenic from dilating eyedrops)

When to Refer

If an 11p13 chromosomal deletion of the *WT1* gene is confirmed, the patient should be referred to a nephrologist to manage genitourinary abnormalities of WAGR syndrome. Genetic counseling also is recommended in these cases.

Treatment

Given this patient's intact *WT1* genes, the ophthalmologist asks the family to return in 3 months for evaluation of the patient's visual function and macular pigmentation. Normal macular pigmentation increases over the first few months of life; therefore, macular hypoplasia cannot be diagnosed until that time.

Treatment of aniridia involves correction, prevention, and treatment of its associated ocular conditions. Refractive errors can be corrected with eyeglasses or contact lenses, and eye misalignment may be treated with patching, eye exercises, or eye muscle surgery. Photophobia can be treated with sunglasses, contact lenses, or intraocular lenses, which act as a false iris to limit the amount of light that enters the eye. Vision is usually poor. Treatment should also include ongoing evaluation of possible onset of glaucoma and cataract, which, if present, should prompt surgical intervention. Associated nystagmus can also be addressed surgically.

Discussion

Aniridia is rare, with an international incidence rate ranging from 1 in 64,000 to 1 in 96,000 live births; a study in Denmark estimated the incidence rate of aniridia at 1 in 40,000.

Key Points

- Aniridia is a congenital condition that causes bilateral iris hypoplasia and typically presents as partially absent irises.
- It is associated with a *PAX6* gene mutation on chromosome 11p13.
- Associated conditions, such as Wilms tumor, must be considered and screened for with abdominal ultrasonography.
- Genetic analysis can also be helpful in early detection of associated conditions.
- Ophthalmologic management includes correction of refractive errors and photophobia; evaluation for onset of cataract, corneal disease, and glaucoma; and treatment of strabismus and nystagmus.

Suggested Reading

Elsas FJ, Maumenee IH, Kenyon KR, Yoder F. Familial aniridia with preserved ocular function. *Am J Ophthalmol.* 1977;83(5):718–724

Grønskov K, Olsen JH, Sand A, et al. Population-based risk estimates of Wilms tumor in sporadic aniridia. A comprehensive mutation screening procedure of PAX6 identifies 80% of mutations in aniridia. *Hum Genet.* 2001;109(1):11–18

Kurli M, Finger PT. The kidney, cancer, and the eye: current concepts. *Surv Ophthalmol.* 2005;50(6):507–518

Nelson LB, Spaeth GL, Nowinski TS, Margo CE, Jackson L. Aniridia. A review. *Surv Ophthalmol.* 1984;28(6):621–642

Taylor D, Hoyt CS, eds. *Pediatric Ophthalmology and Strabismus.* 3rd ed. Edinburgh, United Kingdom: Elsevier Saunders; 2005

Walton DS. Aniridia (PAX6(+/-)). *J Pediatr Ophthalmol Strabismus.* 2005;42(2):128

Chapter 34

Unusual Fundus Color

Henry A. Ferreyra, MD

Presentation

A 5-year-old Hispanic boy and his 4-year-old adopted white sister come with their mother to the pediatrician's office for wellness examinations. The mother's only concern is that they "sit too close to the TV." The pediatric nurse checks their visual acuity and measures 20/60 in both children.

The pediatrician suspects nearsightedness (myopia) and examines their eyes with the direct ophthalmoscope. The pediatrician begins with the boy. The optic nerve, macula, and vessels look healthy, but the fundus seems darker than expected (Figure 34-1). Then the pediatrician examines the girl. To the pediatrician's surprise, her fundus is noticeably different. Although the optic nerve, macula, and vessels look healthy,

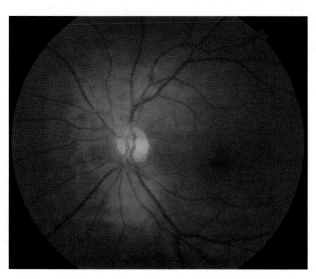

Figure 34-1. Heavily pigmented retina. Courtesy of Henry A. Ferreyra, MD.

the fundus is lightly colored, and the choroidal vessels are prominently visible (Figure 34-2).

Unsure of the clinical significance of these pigmentary variations but realizing that they probably have myopia needing correction, the pediatrician refers both children to an ophthalmologist specializing in children.

Diagnosis

Although these fundi look markedly different, the ophthalmologist deems they are both normal.

These cases illustrate the importance of being able to recognize and distinguish normal variants from true disease. This may seem straightforward, but as seen by these examples, "normal" describes a range, rather than a specific set of values or features. For example, like hair color and skin complexion, the amount of ocular fundus pigmentation exists along a continuum. Generally, the amount of fundus pigmentation

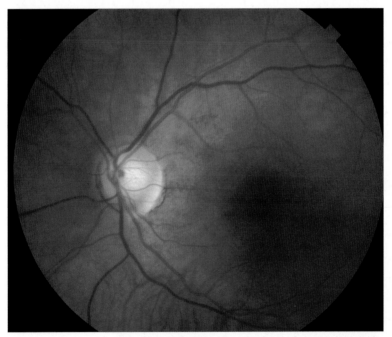

Figure 34-2. Blonde fundus with choroidal blood vessels seen through lightly pigmented retina, especially seen inferiorly. Courtesy of Henry A. Ferreyra, MD.

parallels skin and hair pigmentation. The darker fundus in Figure 34-1 is expected in an individual with a dark complexion, whereas the lighter fundus in Figure 34-2, often called a blonde fundus, is seen in someone with a fair complexion. Although the fundi look much different from each other, they are both normal variants found on opposite ends of the pigmentation fundus spectrum.

The definition of *normal retina* is contextual and depends on such factors as age and ethnicity. For instance, the lightly pigmented fundus of Figure 34-2 would be normal for someone of fair complexion but would be abnormal for someone of dark complexion and could indicate disease, such as ocular albinism (see "Differential Diagnosis").

The technique for performing a thorough fundus examination using the direct ophthalmoscope is detailed in Box 34-1.

Differential Diagnosis

Diagnoses that should be considered for a hypopigmented fundus include the following:

Albinism (Oculocutaneous, Ocular)

An albinotic fundus lacks pigment in the retinal pigment epithelium and choroid, which permits clear visualization of the choroidal blood vessels.

Retinal and Choroidal Dystrophies

The end stage of many hereditary retinal and choroidal degenerations may result in diffuse loss of fundus pigmentation. Examples of retinal dystrophies include retinitis pigmentosa, cone-rod dystrophy, Stargardt dystrophy, and Sorsby dystrophy, while examples of choroidal dystrophies include choroideremia and gyrate atrophy.

Toxic Retinopathies

Diffuse loss of fundus pigmentation can be seen with toxic retinopathies in the advanced stage. Examples include chloroquine, hydroxychloroquine, thioridazine, and chlorpromazine.

Inflammatory Diseases

If their involvement was extensive, inflammatory diseases, such as Vogt-Koyanagi-Harada syndrome and sympathetic ophthalmia, as well as infectious causes, such as herpetic retinitis (known as acute retinal necrosis) and cytomegalovirus retinitis, can result in diffuse fundus hypopigmentation once inflammation resolves.

Box 34-1. Fundus Examination

The direct ophthalmoscope is the instrument that pediatricians primarily use to examine the ocular fundus. It has the advantages of being portable and providing a highly magnified (approximately 15X depending on the patient's refractive error) upright image. However, the view is monocular and lacks stereopsis (3-D), and the direct ophthalmoscope cannot be used to examine the far peripheral retina, even with pupillary dilation.

Ideally, direct ophthalmoscopy should be performed in a darkened room and the patient's pupils should be dilated. However, dilation should be avoided in patients under observation by a neurologist and also in patients with shallow anterior chamber angles so as not to induce angle-closure glaucoma.

The pediatrician should begin the examination by holding the direct ophthalmoscope in front of the eye that corresponds to the patient's eye being examined. (For instance, if examining the patient's *right* eye, the pediatrician holds the ophthalmoscope with the *right* hand in front of his or her *right* eye). The physician sets the lens dial to zero diopters to examine the red reflex from a distance of approximately 2 feet. Media opacities or cataracts will be seen as dark shadows, and vitreous floaters will move when the patient moves the eye. If the pupils are not dilated, the pediatrician instructs the patient to focus on a distant target to keep the pupil as large as possible. Then the pediatrician approaches the patient's eye until reaching the optimal working distance of 2 to 3 cm from the patient's eye. Keeping the other eye open or imagining looking at a distant target helps relax the accommodation of the tester's eye and produces a clearer view. While drawing closer to the patient's eye, the pediatrician turns the lens dial to focus the fundus image until it is sharp.

The major features of the ocular fundus should always be examined in a stepwise fashion. It helps to begin with the optic nerve. As the evaluator aims the ophthalmoscope approximately 15° nasal to central fixation, the optic nerve should come into view. All the major vessels "begin" at the nerve and branch off from there. If the pediatrician follows these vessels back to their origin (thinner to thicker), they lead to the optic nerve. The physician evaluates the optic disc cup, optic disc rim, and surrounding area. The optic nerve should be assessed for color, size, and edema of the optic nerve border. The pediatrician follows the retinal vessels and evaluates their caliber, patency, and arteriovenous crossing sites.

Then the physician evaluates the appearance of the macula and looks for the foveal light reflex. Finally, the evaluator examines the fundus beyond the vascular arcades and looks for hemorrhages, exudates, or other lesions.

When to Refer

There is little downside to referring a patient with a suspected fundus abnormality to an ophthalmologist. For example, if the white retinal lesion a pediatrician is concerned about turns out to be a benign finding like myelinated nerve fiber layer, no harm was done. However, if it turns out to be retinoblastoma, the delay in diagnosis and treatment can have lethal consequences.

Some retinal diseases have subtle abnormalities in the fundus or even a normal fundus appearance. If a patient presents with visual symptoms but the fundus appears normal on examination, the pediatrician should maintain a high index of suspicion and refer the patient to an ophthalmologist.

If there is a concomitant decrease in visual acuity, the patient should be referred to an eye care provider.

Treatment

No treatment is needed for a normal retinal variant, as seen in these cases.

Discussion

Besides the spectrum of normal retinal variation, there are nonpathogenic anomalies. These are often incidental findings and are usually a developmental anomaly without major clinical consequence. An example would be mild cases of myelinated nerve fibers, which appear as a flat, white, feathery retinal lesion, usually but not exclusively near the optic nerve. Myelinated nerve fibers are retinal ganglion cell axons that are abnormally myelinated anterior to the normal boundary of development, the lamina cribrosa. The list of nonpathogenic findings is lengthy and beyond the scope of this chapter. There are a number of good ophthalmic atlases that show nonpathogenic variants as well as ocular disease (see "Suggested Reading").

Key Points

- The appearance of the ocular fundus exhibits a spectrum of normal variation as well as nonpathogenic anomalies that must be distinguished from true disease.
- When examining the ocular fundus, the pediatrician should look for variations from normal rather than attempt to specifically diagnose a disease.
- Some retinal diseases have subtle abnormalities in the fundus or even a normal fundus appearance.
- If a patient presents with visual symptoms but the findings of the fundus examination are normal, the pediatrician should maintain a high index of suspicion and refer the patient to an ophthalmologist.
- Failure to diagnose a change in retinal color, such as the white lesions in retinoblastoma, can have lethal consequences.

Suggested Reading

Spalton DJ, Hitchings RA, Hunter P. *Atlas of Clinical Ophthalmology.* 3rd ed. St. Louis, MO: Mosby; 2004

Yannuzzi LA. *The Retinal Atlas: Expert Consult.* Philadelphia, PA: Saunders; 2010

Chapter 35

Acute Visual Loss

Avery H. Weiss, MD

Presentation

A 7-year-old boy is seen on an emergent basis in the pediatrician's office for evaluation of a 1-day history of blurred vision in his left eye. He has no history of eye problems and denies recent trauma, fever, rash, headache, or neurologic signs. Three weeks ago he received a diagnosis of paranasal sinusitis and was treated with an oral cephalosporin. He has otherwise been healthy. The pediatric nurse confirms that visual acuity is reduced in the left eye.

The eye does not look inflamed, and neurologic findings are normal. The pediatrician checks the pupils and finds that the left pupil does not react the same as the right. On examination with a direct ophthalmoscope, the optic nerve looks normal on the right eye but very different than normal on the left (Figure 35-1). This abnormality prompts a referral to a pediatric ophthalmologist.

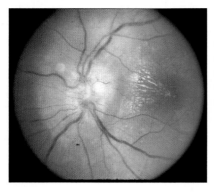

Figure 35-1. Fundus examination reveals optic disc swelling, neuroretinal edema, splinter hemorrhages, and evolving macular exudate. Patient described in chapter had similar optic nerve findings. Courtesy of Avery H. Weiss, MD.

Eye examination by the pediatric ophthalmologist reveals a visual acuity of 20/20 in the right eye and hand motion at near in the left eye. Eye alignment and ocular excursions are normal. Pupils measure 6 mm and react to light, but there is a relative afferent pupillary defect on the left eye. Slit-lamp examination reveals no evidence of corneal opacification, iridocyclitis, or cataract. Dilated fundus examination shows a hyperemic and mildly swollen optic disc on the left with no macular abnormalities, retinal infiltrates, arterial occlusion, or perivascular sheathing. Visual field testing reveals loss of central vision in the left eye and a normal visual field in the right eye. Color discrimination and interocular comparison of brightness perception are reduced in the left eye.

Diagnosis

The combination of acute unilateral visual loss, ipsilateral afferent pupillary defect (Marcus Gunn pupil), and hyperemic optic disc swelling is highly suggestive of optic neuritis. Collectively, decreased visual acuity, central visual field loss, and reductions in color discrimination and brightness are conclusive evidence of visual loss.

Results of the ophthalmologic examination exclude other causes of acute visual loss related to media opacities (eg, corneal disease, cataract, intraocular hemorrhage) as well as retinal vascular occlusion and retinal detachment. Other possibilities in the differential diagnosis of optic neuritis are excluded as well (see "Differential Diagnosis"). Because acute optic neuritis can be the initial manifestation of a demyelinating disease, the neurologic history and physical examination are critical components in the evaluation of optic neuritis in childhood.

After confirmation that the diagnosis is optic neuritis, the child returned to the pediatrician, who ordered magnetic resonance imaging (MRI). The MRI demonstrates multifocal white-matter lesions and signal enhancement of the left optic nerve (Figure 35-2). These findings are consistent with acute disseminated encephalomyelitis (ADEM). In patients with optic neuritis, MRI is preferable to computed tomography imaging because the latter fails to delineate white-matter abnormalities. Lumbar puncture is performed to rule out meningitis and encephalitis. For exclusion of multiple sclerosis, quantitative and qualitative analysis of IgG in the cerebrospinal fluid is ordered and found to be normal.

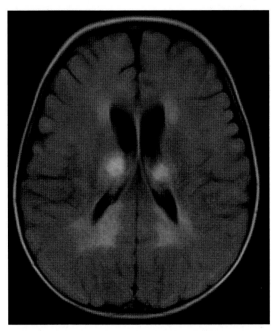

Figure 35-2. Brain magnetic resonance imaging shows increased flair signal in periventricular white matter. Courtesy of Avery H. Weiss, MD.

Concurrence of optic neuritis and transverse myelitis would prompt serologic testing for the aquaporin-4–specific water channel autoantibody, neuromyelitis optica (NMO)-IgG antibody. A complete blood cell count with differential white blood cell count is normal in the child. Serologic testing for respiratory viruses, Epstein-Barr virus, *Borrelia,* herpesviruses, and mycoplasma may be indicated if there is an antecedent history of an infectious illness. Systemic lupus erythematosus is an important consideration in adolescent females with skin rash, arthralgias, cytopenias, and associated neurologic signs. Visual evoked potentials (VEPs) show moderate to severe reduced and delayed responses. Visual fields can show central or generalized sensitivity losses. Although VEPs and visual fields improve, the presence of persistent abnormalities are evidence of irreversible optic nerve damage. Optical coherence tomography (OCT) confirms swelling of the optic disc and nerve fiber layer in the acute phase. The OCT can quantify the axonal loss and thereby index the severity of optic nerve damage that results.

Unilateral visual loss localizes the underlying abnormality to the eye or afferent visual pathway (optic nerve and visual radiations). Although this child has unilateral disease, optic neuritis is frequently bilateral. When visual loss is bilateral, visual cortical disease due to abnormalities of the occipital region (migraine, tumors, stroke, hemorrhage) must be considered.

Differential Diagnosis

Optic neuritis is an exclusionary diagnosis that is reliably made only when other causes of optic neuropathy such as trauma, compression, ischemia, nutritional deficiency, metabolic disease (especially mitochondrial), and genetic and toxic causes have been excluded. Diagnoses besides acute disseminated encephalomyelitis that should be considered in children with optic neuritis include the following:

Neuroretinitis

Neuroretinitis is characterized by optic neuritis combined with retinal infiltrates due to toxoplasma or cat-scratch disease. It is excluded by a normal-appearing retina.

Cat-scratch Disease

Recent exposure to a cat, lymphadenopathy, and segmental optic nerve swelling suggest cat-scratch disease.

Lyme Disease

A history of tick bite, rash (erythema migrans), and facial palsy implicate Lyme disease.

Multiple Sclerosis

Acute optic neuritis can be the initial manifestation of multiple sclerosis (MS). Early symptoms of MS seldom occur before the age of 15 years. The pediatrician should question whether the patient has symptoms of MS, including fatigue, weakness, pain, tingling or numbness in the arms and legs, incoordination, and bladder and bowel dysfunction.

Neuromyelitis Optica

Neuromyelitis optica is an inflammatory disorder defined by the combination of optic neuritis and transverse myelitis. The NMO antibody in serum helps establish the diagnosis.

Systemic Lupus Erythematosus

Systemic lupus erythematosus is a relevant consideration in adolescent girls who present with optic neuritis.

When to Refer

Visual loss with or without an abnormal-appearing optic nerve should prompt the pediatrician to refer the patient to an ophthalmologist or neurologist.

Treatment

The child is hospitalized and treated with intravenous methylprednisolone (30 mg/kg) for 3 days. He is discharged on an oral regimen of prednisone with a tapering dose. Visual acuity in the left eye recovers to 20/20. This child has experienced no recurrences.

Many clinicians choose to treat children with acute optic neuritis using systemic corticosteroids, especially in bilateral cases with severe visual loss. This is in accordance with the findings of the Optic Neuritis Treatment Trial, although the study excluded children.

If this child had developed recurrent optic neuritis or other neurologic signs more than 6 months after initial presentation, he would have been reevaluated for MS, multiphasic ADEM, and mitochondrial myopathy. Acute visual loss caused by optic nerve disease can uncommonly be a manifestation of mitochondrial encephalomyopathy.

Discussion

Optic neuritis affects far fewer children than teenagers and adults. It usually occurs in isolation and is most frequently related to an antecedent infectious illness, as in this case (Table 35-1). Visual loss has an abrupt onset and can be severe but often improves within a few days. Acute optic neuritis can be painless or painful with eye movement. Presumably the offending pathogen initiates an immune-mediated inflammation or directly invades the optic nerve. Headache, malaise, irritability, and fever can be signs of concurrent meningitis, encephalitis, or paranasal sinusitis, necessitating the proper diagnostic testing and treatment.

Table 35-1. Causes of Optic Neuritis in Childhood

Infections, parainfectious, or postinfectious
  Epstein-Barr, herpes simplex, and varicella zoster viruses
  Mycoplasma influenza and other respiratory viruses
  Bartonella, Borrelia burgdorferi, measles, mumps, rubella, *Chlamydia,*
    Mycobacterium tuberculosis, and *Cryptococcus*

Contiguous inflammation
  Extraocular: meningitis, encephalitis, orbital cellulitis/pseudotumor, and
    paranasal sinusitis
  Intraocular: uveitis

Demyelinating disease
  Acute disseminated encephalomyelitis
  Multiple sclerosis
  Neuromyelitis optica

Systemic lupus erythematosus
  Immunization (rare)

Acute disseminated encephalomyelitis, the cause in this case, is typically a monophasic inflammatory disorder of the central nervous system following a viral or bacterial prodrome. It is characterized by multifocal neurologic deficits on the MRI. This rare neurologic disorder affects children more often than adults.

Immunizations are rarely associated with optic neuritis.

Key Points

- Optic neuritis presents with acute visual loss, afferent pupillary defect, and a variable presence of optic nerve swelling.
- Optic neuritis in children is usually due to an antecedent or concurrent infectious disease but can be a manifestation of a demyelinating disease.
- Laboratory evaluation of optic neuritis should include magnetic resonance imaging to exclude a demyelinating disease.

Suggested Reading

Beck RW, Cleary PA, Anderson MM Jr, et al. A randomized, controlled trial of corticosteroids in the treatment of acute optic neuritis. The Optic Neuritis Study Group. *N Engl J Med.* 1992;326(9):581–588

Krupp LB, Banwell B, Tenembaum S; International Pediatric MS Study Group. Consensus definitions proposed for pediatric multiple sclerosis and related disorders. *Neurology.* 2007;68(16 Suppl 2):S7–S12

Tenembaum S, Chitnis T, Ness J, Hahn JS; International Pediatric MS Study Group. Acute disseminated encephalomyelitis. *Neurology.* 2007;68(16 Suppl 2):S23–S36

Wilejto M, Shroff M, Buncic JR, Kennedy J, Goia C, Banwell B. The clinical features, MRI findings, and outcome of optic neuritis in children. *Neurology.* 2006;67(2):258–262

Chapter 36

Infant With Increasing Head Size

Ryan W. Shultz, MD
Terry Schwartz, MD

Presentation

A 6-month-old girl is brought to the pediatrician's office for a routine examination. The parents state that "her head looks odd." They observe that she has been gazing downward for extended periods over the past few weeks. The parents note that she is eating less than usual, but they deny malaise, emesis, lethargy, or irritability. The perinatal and general medical history is unremarkable. Height, weight, and head circumference have been at about the 50th percentile for age at all previous visits.

The pediatrician notes on examination that although the patient remains at the 50th percentile for height and weight, her head circumference is at the 98th percentile for age. She is afebrile and in no distress. Palpation reveals a tense, bulging anterior fontanelle. Results of the neurologic examination are appropriate for age. Extraocular movements seem to be limited in upgaze, and she persistently gazes downward during the examination. A brief look at the optic nerve through non-dilated pupils reveals elevated optic disc margins with no other gross abnormality. The pediatrician requests consultation with a pediatric neurologist and orders a neuroimaging study. Although magnetic resonance imaging (MRI) or computed tomography (CT) scan would be appropriate for the suspected condition, in this case MRI was unavailable without a significant delay, so a CT scan was scheduled (Figure 36-1).

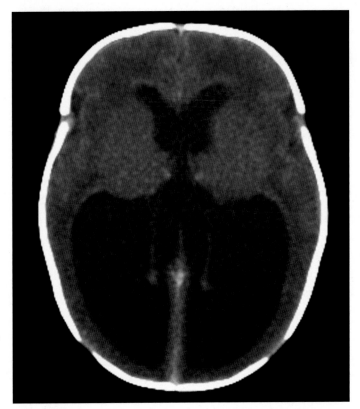

Figure 36-1. Axial computed tomography scan demonstrating ventriculomegaly. Note separation of coronal and sagittal sutures. Courtesy of Terry Schwartz, MD.

Diagnosis

Imaging shows ventriculomegaly, indicating that hydrocephalus is the diagnosis. Hydrocephalus is a condition in which there is enlargement of the ventricles from increased cerebrospinal fluid (CSF). It can be associated with increased intracranial pressure (ICP). It results most commonly from hypersecretion or impaired reabsorption of CSF but can also be caused by abnormal circulation of CSF (Box 36-1).

Disproportionately increasing head circumference may be the presenting sign in children younger than 2 years in whom cranial sutures have not yet fused. Irritability, nausea, vomiting, full fontanelle, and failure

Box 36-1. Most Common Causes of Pediatric Hydrocephalus

Aqueduct stenosis	Intrauterine infection
Posterior fossa neoplasm	Choroid plexus papilloma
Chiari malformation	Neonatal meningoencephalitis
Intracranial hemorrhage	Vein of Galen malformation
Dandy-Walker malformation	Congenital
Craniosynostosis	Idiopathic

to thrive are common findings when ICP is increased. In infants and young children, a relative paresis of upgaze can result in the setting-sun sign, or persistent downgaze. This finding can be present in up to 40% of children with hydrocephalus. Limited abduction of the eye (inability to move the eye toward the ear) and acquired esotropia (crossed eyes) from sixth cranial nerve palsy can be associated with increased ICP or traction on the sixth nerve, or following treatment with a shunt. Downward-beating nystagmus (rapid, involuntary movement of the eyeball) and esotropia can be associated with increased ICP from Chiari malformation.

Elevated ICP can result in increased CSF pressure in the dural sheath surrounding the optic nerves. Edema of the optic nerve head, called papilledema or disc edema, is the clinical finding. Examination with the direct ophthalmoscope can reveal blurred optic disc margins, engorged retinal vessels, and hemorrhages (Figure 36-2). Increased ICP from any cause can result in papilledema, but not all patients with increased ICP experience papilledema. Optic nerve edema caused by increased ICP cannot be distinguished on clinical examination from optic nerve edema due to other causes.

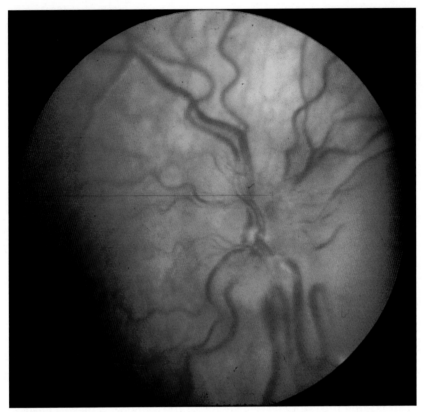

Figure 36-2. Photograph of optic disc edema. The disc is elevated, retinal veins are dilated and tortuous, and there is blurring of the disc margin. Courtesy of Terry Schwartz, MD.

Differential Diagnosis

Diagnoses besides hydrocephalus that should be considered include the following:

Familial Megalencephaly

These patients are asymptomatic with normal neurologic development.

Neurocutaneous Disorders

Evaluate for signs and symptoms consistent with neurofibromatosis type 1, tuberous sclerosis, linear sebaceous nevus syndrome, and hypomelanosis of Ito.

Autism Spectrum Disorder

Autism spectrum disorders are associated with difficulties with social interactions, communication, and behavioral issues.

Achondroplasia

This is the most frequent form of dwarfism.

Cerebral Gigantism

Fragile X Syndrome

Fragile X syndrome occurs in males with mental retardation. Characteristics such as long face, prominent ears, large jaws, and macro-orchidism appear after puberty.

PTEN Hamartoma Syndromes

Leukodystrophies

Lysosomal Storage Disorders

Bone Marrow Expansion

Patients with thalassemia major may have bone marrow expansion.

Primary Bone Disorders

These can be skeletal or cranial dysplasias.

When to Refer

Consultation with specialists in pediatric ophthalmology, neurology, and neurosurgery are all warranted in a patient with diagnosed or suspected hydrocephalus.

Treatment

Ventriculoperitoneal shunt and lumboperitoneal shunt are the surgical treatment options for lowering ICP. Medical management using diuretics (eg, furosemide, acetazolamide) may be an option if the infant is too unstable to undergo surgery.

Persistent fever may be a sign of shunt infection, and recurrence of symptoms as mentioned previously can occur with shunt infection or mechanical failure of the shunt. Suspicion of shunt failure requires urgent referral to the pediatric subspecialist.

Discussion

Papilledema can persist after successful lowering of ICP. Resolution of papilledema after lowering of ICP is variable and not a reliable indicator of treatment response, especially in the presence of optic nerve atrophy.

Visual acuity is usually normal with early papilledema but can be severely reduced as it becomes chronic. Persistent and severe increased ICP can result in atrophy of the optic nerve, with permanent and irreversible loss of visual acuity and visual field. After the optic nerve becomes atrophic, papilledema will not occur, even in the presence of substantial pressure elevation. Vision can also be reduced from damage to the posterior visual pathway (eg, optic radiations, visual cortex).

Key Points

- Hydrocephalus may result in irreversible visual and neurologic deficits.
- Impaired outflow or reabsorption of cerebrospinal fluid is the most common cause of increased intracranial pressure (ICP).
- Papilledema is swelling of the optic nerve caused by increased ICP and is not present in all patients with increased ICP.
- Papilledema can persist after resolution of increased ICP and is not a reliable sign of early treatment success.
- Ocular findings in infants and young children with hydrocephalus include cranial nerve palsy, setting-sun sign, nystagmus, decreased visual acuity, visual field loss, and papilledema.

Suggested Reading

Brodsky MC, Baker RS, Hamed LM. *Pediatric Neuro-ophthalmolgy.*
New York, NY: Springer; 1996:76–80, 87, 426–440

National Institute of Neurological Disorders and Stroke. Hydrocephalus
fact sheet. http://www.ninds.nih.gov/disorders/hydrocephalus/detail_
hydrocephalus.htm. Updated December 16, 2011. Accessed March 14,
2012

Nazir S, O'Brien M, Qureshi NH, Slape L, Green TJ, Phillips PH.
Sensitivity of papilledema as a sign of shunt failure in children.
J AAPOS. 2009;13(1):63–66

Steffen H, Eifert B, Aschoff A, Kolling GH, Völcker HE. The diagnostic
value of optic disc evaluation in acute elevated intracranial pressure.
Ophthalmolgy. 1996;103(8):1229–1232

Tzekov CT, Cherninkova S, Gudeva T. Neuroophthalmological symptoms
in children treated for internal hydrocephalus. *Pediar Neurosurg.*
1991–1992;17(6):317–320

Chapter 37

Headache With Double Vision

Michael X. Repka, MD, MBA

Presentation

A 16-year-old girl comes to the pediatrician's office with recent onset
of binocular horizontal double vision. She has complained of episodic
blurred vision for the last month and even stopped driving because of
this. She complains of nonspecific global headaches, which also began
1 month ago. There has been no nausea or vomiting. There is no history of eye problems or decreased vision. There is no family or personal
history of strabismus. Her mother has a history of classic migraine
since she was a teenager. The patient's current medications include
minocycline for management of acne over the last 4 months.

On examination she weighs 45 kg and is 5 feet, 5 inches tall. Vision is
20/25 in each eye without correction. The right eye is noticeably deviated
inward (Figure 37-1). Fundus examination is difficult, but the optic disc
border is not sharp and there may be a hemorrhage on its surface.

Urgent ophthalmologic consultation is requested, which confirms the
presence of bilateral swollen optic discs (Figure 37-2). The ophthalmologist also notes hemorrhages on the optic disc as well as limitation of
abduction (outward movement) of the left eye. Because vision is normal
and both eyes are affected, this most likely represents papilledema (optic
disc swelling) rather than bilateral optic papillitis, in which vision would
be greatly reduced. The presence of optic disc swelling and abducens
nerve paresis strongly suggests increased intracranial pressure.

Neuroimaging is urgently requested to rule out a space-occupying
lesion. Although computed tomography can be done emergently,
magnetic resonance imaging (MRI) is preferred. The MRI is normal,
without evidence of a mass. The neuroradiologist also obtains a
magnetic resonance venogram of the cerebral venous sinuses.

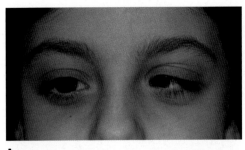

A

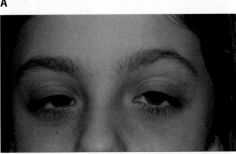

B

Figure 37-1. Esotropia. There is inward deviation of the right eye along with inability to fully abduct that eye to the right. **A,** Right gaze with failure of the right eye to abduct. **B,** Right esotropia in primary position. **C,** Full abduction of the left eye. Courtesy of Michael X. Repka, MD, MBA.

C

Diagnosis

Sudden onset of an esotropia in a teenager is alarming. Differential diagnosis includes decompensation of a preexisting strabismus, increased intracranial pressure, or abducens nerve (sixth cranial nerve) paresis (see "Differential Diagnosis" on page 256).

The most likely diagnosis in this case is intracranial hypertension, commonly termed pseudotumor cerebri (PTC). This condition is defined as follows:

- Elevated intracranial pressure (normal <250 mm for patients aged 8 to 18 years and <200 mm for older than 8 years)

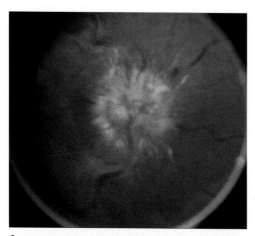

Figure 37-2. Both optic nerves demonstrate swelling, hemorrhage, and ischemia. Vision in each eye was normal in spite of this appearance. **A,** Right. **B,** Left. Courtesy of Michael X. Repka, MD, MBA.

A

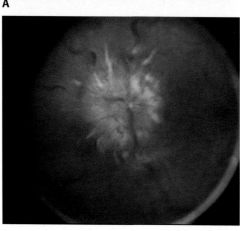

B

- Normal brain on imaging
- Normal-sized or small ventricles of the brain
- Normal cerebrospinal fluid (CSF) composition

Findings of the neurologic examination are usually normal. Some patients may have ocular motor problems (usually a sixth cranial nerve paresis), as in this case, or other minor neurologic symptoms. A diagnosis cannot be made until the criteria listed previously are satisfied. Thus, a lumbar puncture is performed in the emergency department following the MRI to examine CSF and measure intracranial pressure. The CSF analysis shows normal findings, but opening pressure is 350 mm H_2O.

Often PTC is idiopathic, but it may be associated with a systemic condition. Many medications have been associated with PTC, including corticosteroid use or withdrawal, tetracycline-type drugs (including minocycline and doxycycline), cyclosporine, medroxyprogesterone, nalidixic acid, lithium, excessive vitamin A, retinoic acid, and recombinant growth hormone. Lyme infection and various nephropathies have also been associated with PTC.

Differential Diagnosis

Diagnoses besides PTC that should be considered include the following:

Decompensation of Preexisting Strabismus

Eye misalignment can worsen over time. If the condition was not identified originally, it can be confused with an acute onset condition. One of the hallmarks of decompensated strabismus is the symmetry of the misalignment in all fields of gaze.

Abducens Nerve (Sixth Cranial Nerve) Paresis

Paresis of the abducens nerve should be considered in all patients with blurred or double vision. Acute bilateral sixth nerve paresis is often posttraumatic but may be a presenting sign of intracranial tumor or increased intracranial pressure.

Hypertension

This condition can lead to optic nerve edema as well as cranial nerve palsy–induced strabismus.

Anterior Ischemic Optic Neuropathy

These are swollen discs with nerve fiber layer infarcts associated with loss of vision.

Pseudopapilledema

Vision is usually normal. Optic disc drusen or calcifications may be seen in optic nerves.

Optic Neuritis

Vision will be reduced with optic neuritis. The condition is often bilateral in young children and unilateral in teenagers.

When to Refer

In the absence of personal history of strabismus, sudden-onset esotropia in a teenager warrants urgent neuroimaging to exclude a space-occupying lesion of the brain. If the optic disc is considered to be possibly abnormal, as in this case, consultation with an ophthalmologist should be urgently requested.

Treatment

Management is coordinated with an ophthalmologist to monitor visual function, which is a marker for optic nerve health. For drug-associated PTC, the first and most important step is removal of the potentially causative agent; in this case it is presumed to be minocycline. Generally this is sufficient to reverse the problem, and it does in this case. Because there is no optic neuropathy, the patient is followed up without treatment.

If there had been evidence of mild or moderate optic nerve dysfunction, the child would also be treated with acetazolamide (15 mg/kg/day). If visual loss were severe, serial lumbar punctures are often prescribed in the short term; however, their effectiveness has not been proven. If pressure remains high and optic disc swelling persists, lumboperitoneal shunt or optic nerve sheath fenestration is warranted to rapidly reduce intracranial pressure. These surgical decompressions allow more normal perfusion of the optic nerve, protecting it from further damage.

For those children and teens in whom PTC is associated with obesity, a similar treatment algorithm is followed while encouraging weight loss, which also seems to be curative.

Discussion

Pseudotumor cerebri is relatively rare in childhood, but incidence increases after puberty. Prior to puberty, gender ratio is 1:1, whereas after puberty, girls outnumber boys by 2 to 1. Obesity is noted in about 50% of patients with PTC after puberty.

The most common symptom is headache, often posterior, which occurs in up to 86% of cases. In young children and infants irritability and apathy have been noted, rather than headache. Other common symptoms are nausea, transient visual loss, vomiting, and fatigue. Fatigue is frequent in younger children. Less frequent symptoms include ataxia, dizziness, neck pain, paresthesias, facial and limb numbness, and tinnitus. Occasionally children are asymptomatic.

The most common ocular symptom is decreased vision, followed by horizontal double vision. Both symptoms may be intermittent or constant. However, transient visual obscuration and visual loss are rarely presenting symptoms in children, most likely because of inability of a child to describe the problem. Many children do not present for examination until there is substantial and irreversible visual loss.

Key Points

- Headaches of pseudotumor cerebri (PTC) or drug-associated intracranial hypertension are not localized.
- High index of suspicion for PTC should be maintained for patients receiving one of the medications known to be associated with this condition.
- Early detection of PTC prevents permanent visual loss.

Suggested Reading

Balcer LJ, Liu GT, Forman S, et al. Idiopathic intracranial hypertension: relation of age and obesity in children. *Neurology.* 1999;52(4):870–872

Cinciripini GS, Donahue S, Borchert MS. Idiopathic intracranial hypertension in prepubertal pediatric patients: characteristics, treatment, and outcome. *Am J Ophthalmol.* 1999;127(2):178–182

Phillips PH, Repka MX, Lambert SR. Pseudotumor cerebri in children. *J AAPOS.* 1998;2(1):33–38

Thuente DD, Buckley EG. Pediatric optic nerve sheath decompression. *Ophthalmology.* 2005;112(4):724–727

Chapter 38

Night Blindness

Henry A. Ferreyra, MD

Presentation

A 12-year-old boy presents to the pediatrician's office with a complaint of difficulty seeing at night. His parents acknowledge that he appears clumsy at night and bumps into things. Although he wears glasses for myopia (nearsightedness), his best-corrected visual acuity was 20/20 during his most recent eye examination by his optometrist. He is healthy and does not have any known medical problems.

The pediatric nurse checks his visual acuity with a Snellen chart and measures 20/20 in each eye. Using a penlight, the pediatrician examines the boy's pupils and records normal responses.

Then the pediatrician examines the patient's anterior segment with a direct ophthalmoscope and notices small central lens opacities in each eye, especially evident with retro-illumination (red reflex). Still using the direct ophthalmoscope, the pediatrician examines the posterior segment and at first glance, the fundi appear essentially normal. The patient is cooperative, allowing the pediatrician to perform a more thorough fundus examination. On closer examination, the pediatrician detects some subtle abnormalities. The retinal arteries appear thin, and the fundi have an abnormal, almost granular appearance outside the maculae. A few "bone-spicule" pigment deposits are seen in the midperiphery of the retina (Figure 38-1).

The pediatrician asks the parents if anyone in the family has similar eye problems. The mother recalls that her maternal grandfather reportedly had night blindness when he was younger and eventually became blind.

The pediatrician realizes the patient needs additional workup and refers the boy to an ophthalmology group specializing in retinal diseases.

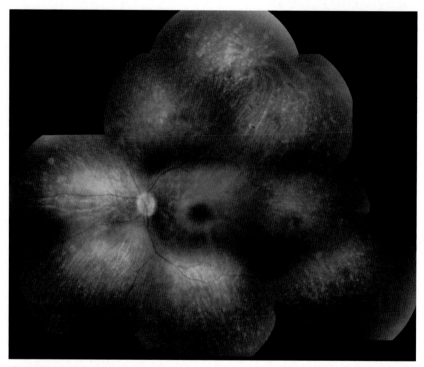

Figure 38-1. Retinal photograph showing thin retinal arteries, granular appearance outside of the maculae, with several "bone-spicule" pigment deposits in the midperiphery. Courtesy of Henry A. Ferreyra, MD.

There the boy undergoes formal perimetry (peripheral vision test) and full-field electroretinography (photoreceptor function test).

Diagnosis

Perimetry shows peripheral visual field constriction in both eyes (figures 38-2 and 38-3). The full-field electroretinogram (ERG) is extinguished (no recordable electrical activity of the retina to light stimuli). These findings indicate retinitis pigmentosa (RP).

Retinitis pigmentosa refers to a group of diseases that cause degeneration of the retina. There are currently 40 identified genes that can cause RP,

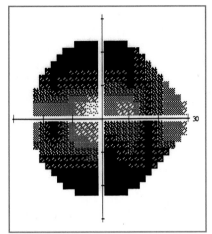

Figure 38-2. Visual field demonstrating peripheral field depression as shown by the darker areas, left eye. Courtesy of Henry A. Ferreyra, MD.

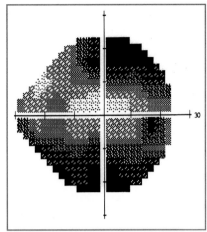

Figure 38-3. Visual field demonstrating peripheral field depression as shown by the darker areas, right eye. Courtesy of Henry A. Ferreyra, MD.

and it can be inherited in an autosomal-dominant, autosomal-recessive, or X-linked manner. It is a progressive dystrophy of primarily the rod photoreceptor cells. The first symptom of RP is night blindness. Also characterized by progressive loss of peripheral vision, RP ultimately leads to tunnel vision. The classic clinical description of RP includes "bone-spicule" intraretinal pigment deposits, attenuation of retinal arteries, and optic nerve pallor. Posterior subcapsular cataracts are also common with RP.

Differential diagnosis for night blindness in children includes acquired and hereditary causes. In the developing world, vitamin A deficiency from malnourishment is the most common cause of night blindness. Vitamin A is necessary for the production of visual pigment 11-cisretinal, and deficiency presents with night blindness, ultimately leading to blindness. In the developed world, vitamin A deficiency is uncommon but can occur in the setting of fat malabsorption, celiac sprue, cystic fibrosis, pancreatic insufficiency, cholestasis, and inflammatory bowel disease, and following gastric bypass or small-bowel surgery. Nocturnal myopia can occur from uncorrected refractive error and should be distinguished from night blindness. Nocturnal myopia refers to blurred vision under low-light conditions, even though daytime vision is normal.

Differential diagnosis of hereditary causes of night blindness includes a variety of diseases, such as RP, congenital stationary night blindness (CSNB), choroideremia, gyrate atrophy, and Goldmann-Favre syndrome. The 2 most important entities are RP and CSNB, which can be distinguished from each other by clinical appearance (see "Differential Diagnosis"). Early cases of RP may be difficult to clinically distinguish from CSNB because the fundus may appear essentially normal. However, ERG can usually help distinguish RP from CSNB.

Differential Diagnosis

Diagnoses besides RP that should be considered include the following:

Congenital Stationary Night Blindness

Unlike RP, CSNB is not progressive; it is caused by a number of different genes and can be inherited in an autosomal-dominant, autosomal-recessive, or X-linked manner. Congenital stationary night blindness can have different clinical appearances, although a normal fundus appearance is most common. Rarer forms of CSNB with an abnormal fundus appearance may have white dots (fundus albipunctatus), flecks (fleck retina of Kandori), or an abnormal golden sheen (Oguchi disease).

Choroideremia

Choroideremia is an X-linked progressive choroidal degeneration caused by a mutation in the *CHM* gene that encodes for Rab escort protein-1. Choroideremia also presents with night blindness and peripheral vision loss but is distinguished from RP by its clinical appearance. Unlike patients with RP that have "bone-spicule" pigment deposits and diffuse retinal pigment epithelium (RPE) atrophy, patients with choroideremia have severe degeneration of the retina, RPE, and choroid.

Gyrate Atrophy

Gyrate atrophy is a rare autosomal-recessive choroidal degeneration caused by mutations in the *OAT* gene resulting in deficiency in ornithine aminotransferase activity. Patients with gyrate atrophy also present with night blindness and peripheral vision loss, but they have a characteristic fundus appearance consisting of peripheral chorioretinal atrophy with well-delineated scallop-like borders. Diagnosis can be confirmed by measuring elevated plasma levels of ornithine (typically 10–20 times higher than normal). Restricting dietary arginine, a precursor of ornithine, has been shown to slow progression. In addition to dietary restriction, in patients with a pyridoxine-responsive form of gyrate atrophy, supplementation with pyridoxine has also been shown to be effective at lowering ornithine levels.

When to Refer

Night blindness may be a sign of a serious disease. Therefore, a patient presenting with night blindness should be referred to an ophthalmologist specializing in the retina who can perform specialized tests, such as an ERG.

Treatment

This patient needs monitoring by a retinal specialist. Although there is no cure for RP, it does not mean that nothing can be done. Patients with RP can benefit from something as simple as correction of refractive error or use of low-vision aids. In addition, treatable ocular complications may develop, such as cataracts or cystoid macular edema (Figure 38-4). There is some evidence that nutritional supplementation with vitamin A, lutein, or docosahexaenoic acid may slow progression.

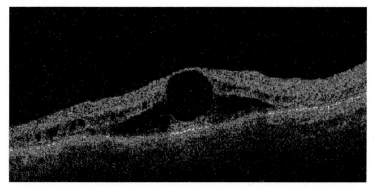

Figure 38-4. Optical coherence tomography of cystoid macular edema in retinitis pigmentosa. The central dark areas are edema disrupting normal macular structure and function. Courtesy of Henry A. Ferreyra, MD.

More encouraging are the recent results of a gene therapy trial for a severe form of RP called *RPE65*. Clinical results demonstrated only modest improvements in vision. As a proof-of-principle experiment, however, the study showed that gene therapy is possible and may be a promising treatment for RP and other hereditary retinal diseases.

Discussion

Parents of children diagnosed with RP usually have many questions and concerns, and the physician's role as an educator becomes particularly important. Most parents want to know about their children's visual prognosis and will ask when their child will "go blind." Unfortunately this is not an easy question to answer because RP is a genetically a heterogeneous disease composed of at least 40 different genes. Clinical course of RP may even show significant variation among members of the same pedigree. With so many factors affecting the natural history and rate of progression, even estimates by experienced clinicians can undoubtedly be wrong. It is better to reassure parents that RP is a chronic condition and patients do not suddenly go blind, a commonly feared misconception. It is also important to refer to a genetic counselor when there is a family history of RP, especially if parents are planning to have more children. Finally, remain positive and remind parents that although there is no cure, it does not mean that nothing can be done. There are some treatable aspects of the disease, such as refractive error, cataracts, and cystoid macular edema, and for more advanced cases, low-vision evaluation may help.

Key Points

- Retinitis pigmentosa (RP) is a clinical entity consisting of at least 40 different genetic diseases.
- The hallmark of RP is night blindness, although it is not pathognomonic.
- Retinitis pigmentosa must be distinguished from congenital stationary night blindness because prognoses are very different.
- Usually, clinical examination and electroretinogram testing are sufficient to distinguish the 2 entities. Documentation of progressive peripheral visual field loss provides definitive diagnosis.

Suggested Reading

Hartong DT, Berson EL, Dryja TP. Retinitis pigmentosa. *Lancet.* 2006;368(9549):1795–1809

Weleber RG, Gregory-Evans K. Retinitis pigmentosa and allied disorders. In Ryan SJ, ed. *Retina.* Philadelphia, PA: Elsevier; 2006:395–498

Chapter 39

Eye Problems in a Premature Infant

Lance M. Siegel, MD
Shira L. Robbins, MD

Presentation

An 8-month-old boy is brought to the pediatrician's office because the mother reports that the infant does not seem to see well and has "shaking" of his eyes. She reports that the baby was born at 26 weeks of age and spent "a long time" in the neonatal intensive care unit (NICU). She thinks the baby has been doing "well" since discharge but was unable to keep any of the outpatient follow-up appointments because she has no transportation.

On examination, the pediatrician finds leukokoria (white pupil) in one eye and poor to no visual behavior in both eyes. Concerned, the pediatrician advises and documents—in the strongest terms possible, emphasizing risk of blindness—that the mother return with the infant to the pediatric ophthalmologist for follow-up of prematurity and decreased visual behavior.

Diagnosis

The pediatrician is called later that day and informed by the ophthalmologist that the patient's lack of red reflex is due to a retinal detachment secondary to retinopathy of prematurity (ROP). The poor health of the eye has led to the eye not growing (microphthalmos) and to decompensation of the cornea, with white band keratopathy (calcium deposition) increasing the white appearance of the pupil. The eye is also esotropic (turned in toward the nose) because of loss of vision. The pediatrician follows this child for many years and takes the photograph in Figure 39-1 at age 6 years.

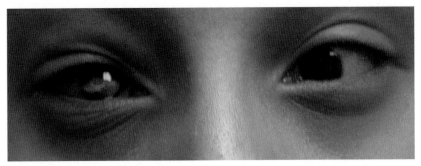

Figure 39-1. White calcific deposition on the right cornea, band keratopathy, as a result of involution of the eye after retinal detachment. There is also associated esotropia. Courtesy of Lance M. Siegel, MD.

Despite the prematurity, at the current corrected gestational age (CGA), the infant should have been able to fix and follow with each eye. An infant with normal vision should follow horizontal movement by approximately 2 months CGA and vertical movement by about 4 months CGA. The 8-month-old infant, now approximately 5 months CGA, should have a social smile as well.

Leukokoria is always concerning. Differential diagnosis includes corneal opacity, cataract, retinal detachment, glaucoma, tumor (eg, retinoblastoma), and other conditions that are beyond the scope of this chapter. In premature infants, retinal detachment with associated cataract (ROP with retrolental fibroplasia) is of primary concern.

Current guidelines suggest that all premature newborns with a gestational age younger than 30 weeks or weighing less than 1,500 g, or those with other high risks of retinopathy, must be examined and followed up by an ophthalmologist specializing in ROP. The more severe the prematurity, along with difficult newborn course (high oxygen requirements, sepsis, intraventricular hemorrhage, and other stressors), the greater the likelihood of more aggressive ROP. The initial eye examination in premature newborns is usually performed in the hospital at 4 or 5 weeks of age with sequential repeated examinations until retinal blood vessels have developed past the risk of ROP. The examining ophthalmologist determines when the next retinal examination needs to be performed based on physical findings. Because of the natural history of ROP, specific intervals of examination need to be strictly adhered to;

otherwise, retinal detachment and blindness can occur quickly and be irreversible.

Ocular sequelae of prematurity are common. In more than 25% of babies born younger than 32 weeks of age, strabismus will develop, and up to 50% of children born prematurely may require glasses in the first 2 years of life. Myopia is frequent and can be severe. Severity of myopia often correlates with severity of ROP and whether laser treatment was performed. Most retinal disease occurs from 4 weeks after birth to 4 weeks CGA. By 0 to 8 weeks CGA, retinal vessels usually finish growing, and a mature retinal vasculature can be documented.

Eye problems can, and often do, occur in the first 2 years of life. These problems include strabismus, amblyopia, cataracts, retinal traction or retinal detachments, and need for eyeglasses with subsequent prescription changes as eyes grow. Late retinal detachments can occur throughout and beyond the teenage years in patients with ROP. Those with more severe neonatal disease have a higher risk of late problems. Follow-up ROP examinations are more frequent in the first 2 years of life, after which they should be performed at least annually, especially in those who had severe ROP as a neonate.

Differential Diagnosis

Diagnoses besides ROP that should be considered in an infant with abnormal retinal vascularization and detachment include the following:

Familial Exudative Vitreoretinopathy

A genetic disorder occurring in full-term infants that disrupts retinal vascularization.

Persistent Hyperplastic Primary Vitreous

Caused by persistent embryologic structure formation, this can cause a traction retinal detachment difficult to differentiate but typically unilateral.

When to Refer

Any newborn, infant, or child with leukocoria should be referred to an ophthalmologist for dilation of the pupils, fundus examination, and perhaps further testing. Premature newborns (born younger than 30 weeks or weighing less than 1,500 g) must be examined and followed up by an ophthalmologist specializing in ROP. Babies over this weight and gestational age with unstable clinical course and at the discretion of the neonatologist should be screened as well.

Treatment

When central vascular plus disease occurs in the presence of peripheral ROP, laser therapy may be required to halt disease progression. The goal of laser treatment is to decrease risk of further disease progression and retinal detachment. In cases of severe ROP not meeting requirements for laser treatment, the disease can still occasionally worsen or more often will regress naturally with normalization of retinal vasculature.

Experimental treatments of intraocular injections of anti-angiogenesis agents are currently being studied and seem best suited to the most posterior cases of zone 1 disease. These agents seem promising, but their long-term safety on other developing organs has not been established. When these agents are used the time frame for acute progression of retinal disease is prolonged.

Discussion

Classification of ROP uses zone, stage, and clock hours. Zone refers to how far from the optic nerve the vessels have grown. Stage refers to how severe the disease is, and clock hours refer to how large an area the disease covers. Classification of the disease is presented in Table 39-1 and depicted in figures 39-2 through 39-5. Central retinal vessel dilation and tortuosity is an ominous sign, termed plus disease (Figure 39-4).

Table 39-1. Classification of Retinopathy of Prematurity

Stage	Retinal Findings
1	Retinal vessels are greatly perturbed and stop growing, and a demarcation line divides vascular from avascular retina.
2	More severe progression; retinal vessels end with an elevated line (ridge).
3	Ridge with abnormal neovascularization or fibrovascularization
4	Partial retinal detachment
5	Complete retinal detachment, usually due to tractional or scar forces

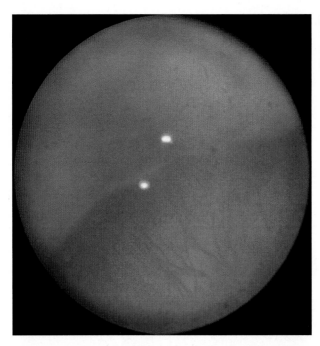

Figure 39-2. Stage 1 retinopathy of prematurity. Courtesy of Shira L. Robbins, MD.

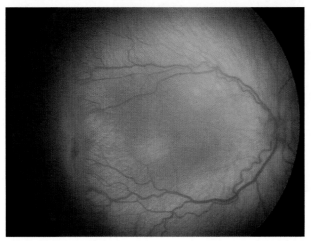

Figure 39-3. Stage 3 retinopathy of prematurity. Courtesy of Shira L. Robbins, MD.

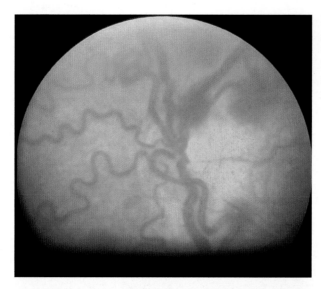

Figure 39-4. Plus disease (central retinal vessel dilation and tortuosity). Courtesy of Shira L. Robbins, MD.

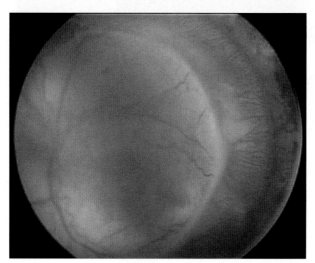

Figure 39-5. Stage 4 and 5 retinopathy of prematurity: retinal detachment with traction. Courtesy of Shira L. Robbins, MD.

Even with appropriate laser treatment, severe ROP may have poor outcomes. In addition, because this disease develops over time, 34 to 37 weeks is the most common time frame during which laser treatment would need to be done. This is often the time these patients are sent home, and in the United States these high-risk populations often have poor follow-up. Even a 1-week delay of laser treatment after criteria are met can result in complete and total loss of vision and the eye. It is incumbent on the NICU to ensure families understand the serious nature of this disease to facilitate follow-up compliance.

Vision can be reduced in premature babies because of ocular and central nervous system (CNS) disease. Conditions affecting the CNS that lead to decreased vision include cortical visual impairment, nystagmus, and periventricular leukomalacia with associated optic nerve cupping. Nystagmus can be present at birth due to radiographically evident cerebral abnormalities or occult CNS abnormalities (congenital), or it can develop later, as in this case, resulting from severe sensory deprivation (retinal detachment with subsequent eyeball involution).

Understanding the pathology of ROP is important to treat and prevent problems. The eye is curved like a satellite dish. Vessels of the retina start growing at 16 to 22 weeks along the back of the eye, originating their growth at the optic nerve. Vessels reach the edge of the retina (ora serrata, just behind the lens) at approximately 39 to 42 weeks CGA. Thus, the younger the baby, the less the vessels have grown along the back of the eye. Oxygen, stressors, infection, intraventricular hemorrhage, necrotizing enterocolitis, severe respiratory problems, and problems with physical stability all contribute to increased risk of more severe disease by interrupting the normal vascularization process. On a chemical level, growth hormones, vascular endothelial growth factor, insulin-like growth factors, oxygen, and hypercapnia all play a role in pathogenesis of ROP. Additional research is needed and ongoing to more fully understand the factors leading to this disease and its natural history.

Key Points

- Retinopathy of prematurity (ROP) is an abnormality of retinal vascular growth, which can lead to retinal detachment.
- Retinopathy of prematurity has been found to respond relatively well to early treatment.
- While laser treatment is the treatment of choice for those babies meeting criteria for ROP treatment (threshold), there is some evidence that intra-vitreal immune therapy (eg, anti-vascular endothelial growth factor) may have some role in treatment in the future.
- Additional cutting retinal surgery is sometimes needed in cases refractory to laser.
- Most cases of ROP will regress naturally and not require treatment.
- Timely retinal examinations are imperative because retinal detachment and subsequent blindness can occur quickly.
- Ocular sequelae of prematurity include ROP, need for glasses as a child, amblyopia, strabismus, glaucoma, cataracts, optic neuropathy, and nystagmus.

Suggested Reading

American Academy of Pediatrics Section on Ophthalmology, American Academy of Ophthalmology, American Association for Pediatric Ophthalmology and Strabismus. Screening examination of premature infants for retinopathy of prematurity [published correction appears in *Pediatrics*. 2006;118(3):1324]. *Pediatrics*. 2006;117(2):572–576

Suggested Resource

Association for Retinopathy of Prematurity and Related Diseases. http://www.ropard.org. Accessed April 26, 2012

Chapter 40

Nystagmus and Poor Vision Since Birth

Elias I. Traboulsi, MD

Presentation

On the vision screening of a 6-year-old Middle Eastern girl, a pediatric nurse finds that her vision is extremely poor and her eyes shake. Her consanguineous parents, who recently immigrated to the United States, tell the pediatrician that her vision has been poor since birth. Previous eye examinations failed to yield a specific diagnosis because her retinal findings were normal. Because of her nystagmus, a brain magnetic resonance image was obtained and was normal. The child is intelligent and has no known medical or neurologic problems.

On eye examination, the pediatrician finds that the patient has pendular nystagmus (constant rhythmic movements) and poor vision. She is able to identify only hand movements in both eyes. Pupils are sluggishly reactive. There is good red reflex.

The pediatrician refers the girl to a pediatric ophthalmologist for further testing.

Diagnosis

The pediatric ophthalmologist examines the girl and sees no sign of optic nerve hypoplasia on ophthalmoscopy, as shown in another patient in Figure 40-1. History rules out many other differential diagnoses (see "Differential Diagnosis" on page 277). The patient's retinal fundus has pigmentary changes, suggesting Leber congenital amaurosis. Although the retinal fundus may be normal in some patients with Leber congenital amaurosis, most have some degree of pigmentary changes (Figure 40-2).

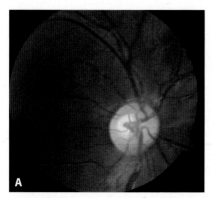
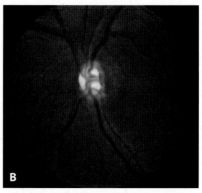

Figure 40-1. Optic nerve hypoplasia. **A,** Normal optic nerve head. **B,** Very small optic nerve head and almost total absence of nerve fiber tissue (white reflective sheen). Courtesy of Elias I. Traboulsi, MD.

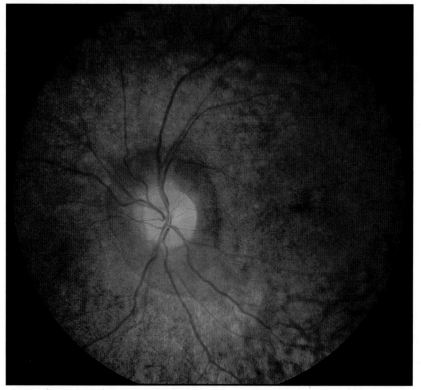

Figure 40-2. Fundus of patient with Leber congenital amaurosis. Note optic atrophy (pale color), attenuated blood vessels, and pigmentary changes (dark speckled appearance). Courtesy of Elias I. Traboulsi, MD.

Diagnosis of retinal dystrophy requires an electroretinogram (ERG). This test measures the response of retinal rods and cones (photoreceptors) to light stimulation under light (photopic) and dark-adapted (scotopic) conditions. On this patient's ERG, the photopic and scotopic responses are not recordable, indicating poor functioning of rods and cones. In Leber congenital amaurosis, photopic and scotopic electrical responses are non-recordable. Therefore, clinical diagnosis is Leber congenital amaurosis, which is recessively inherited.

Differential Diagnosis

Diagnoses in an infant or young child with poor vision and nystagmus that should be considered besides Leber congenital amaurosis include the following:

Cortical Visual Loss

Lack of prematurity or history of perinatal problems generally rules out cortical blindness.

Bilateral Optic Nerve Hypoplasia

Optic nerve hypoplasia is easily diagnosed using ophthalmoscopy (see Figure 40-1). It can be associated with central nervous system and endocrinologic abnormalities, such as absence of the septum pellucidum (septo-optic dysplasia or de Morsier syndrome), schizencephaly, and growth hormone deficiency or hypothyroidism. Optic nerve hypoplasia is frequently found in patients with fetal alcohol syndrome. Therefore, the pediatrician should look for other physical signs of this condition and ask about a history of maternal ingestion of alcohol during pregnancy.

Achromatopsia

Monochromatic vision, or achromatopsia, is recessively inherited. The ERG shows that only photopic responses are abolished, pointing to cone dysfunction.

Albinism With Foveal Hypoplasia

Patients with albinism are usually very fair in complexion or lack skin and hair pigment altogether. Slit-lamp examination shows iris transillumination defects. Retinal examination shows decreased retinal pigment, particularly in the macula.

Congenital Cataracts Causing Visual Deprivation

Congenital cataracts can be diagnosed with direct ophthalmoscope, as they produce leukocoria (white pupil) or a black reflex against the red reflex of the fundus. There may be a history of congenital cataracts in one parent in dominant cases.

Infantile Nystagmus Syndrome (Congenital Motor Nystagmus)

All other findings are normal in children with this form of nystagmus. This type of nystagmus is almost a diagnosis of exclusion and is generally a familial X-linked condition.

When to Refer

Children with nystagmus should be referred to a pediatric ophthalmologist. When optic nerve hypoplasia is present, a pediatric neurologic consultation is in order because central nervous system abnormalities occur in up to 50% of these patients. Consultation with a pediatric endocrinologist may also be necessary in patients with optic nerve hypoplasia because hypopituitarism may be present.

Treatment

This girl undergoes genetic testing. Management of patients with Leber congenital amaurosis includes genetic testing to determine the exact genetic defect, genetic counseling, and after the exact genetic defect is identified, possible referral for gene or other types of vitamin A derivative supplements. More than 15 genes have been identified to date that cause about two-thirds of cases. Only those cases that result from mutations in the *RPE65* gene are currently being considered for gene replacement therapy under research protocols. It is hoped that therapy becomes available for other forms of this disease.

Any child with nystagmus may obtain visual improvement with eyeglasses and possible eye muscle surgery. All children with substantial reduction of vision need a low vision evaluation and special accommodations in school. They also should be referred to local services for people who are blind.

Discussion

One in every 1,000 children has nystagmus. In 80% to 90% of cases, nystagmus results from vision loss due to eye diseases. It can be the first sign of vision loss. Pendular nystagmus (as opposed to jerk nystagmus, which has a slow and fast refixation component) is the type of nystagmus that most often occurs because of vision loss during childhood. Pendular nystagmus can be congenital or acquired. Congenital nystagmus, such as occurs with albinism, often spontaneously improves slightly as the infant or child gets older.

Key Points

- Some early cases of retinal dystrophies can have normal-appearing retinas.
- Retinal dystrophies and optic nerve hypoplasia can have other systemic disease associations that require evaluation.
- All children with substantial reduction of vision need low vision evaluation and special accommodations in school.
- Pediatricians should be familiar with local resources and services for people who are blind.

Suggested Reading

Chung DC, Traboulsi EI. Leber congenital amaurosis: clinical correlations with genotypes, gene therapy trials update, and future directions. *J AAPOS.* 2009;13(6):587–592

Garcia ML, Ty EB, Taban M, David Rothner A, Rogers D, Traboulsi EI. Systemic and ocular findings in 100 patients with optic nerve hypoplasia. *J Child Neurol.* 2006;21(11):949–956

Lee AG, Brazis PW. Localizing forms of nystagmus: symptoms, diagnosis, and treatment. *Curr Neuorol Neurosci Rep.* 2006;6(5):414–420

Traboulsi EI. The Marshall M. Parks memorial lecture: making sense of early-onset childhood retinal dystrophies—the clinical phenotype of Leber congenital amaurosis. *Br J Ophthalmol.* 2010;94(10):1281–1287

Chapter 41

Swelling of the Optic Nerve

G. Robert LaRoche, MD

Presentation

A 12-year-old girl tells the pediatrician that she has had almost daily headaches for 3 months. They occur at any time of day, mainly at school; are not accompanied by any other symptoms; and can be alleviated by acetaminophen. Her examination shows normal neurologic findings but a decreased visual acuity of 20/40 at distance in both eyes. She had not complained about her vision. Both parents are mildly myopic and wear glasses to drive. A fundus examination shows what appears to be very asymmetric optic nerve swelling.

Despite the lack of other symptoms or signs and the apparent benign nature of her headaches, an urgent ophthalmologic evaluation of the child is requested because of possible papilledema. The worry is that increased intracranial pressure is causing swelling of the optic nerve heads. Examination of the optic nerves by the ophthalmologist shows mild blurring of the optic nerve margins, low visibility of the small vessels at the edge of the optic nerve, and no retinal hemorrhages, without exudates or retinal surface wrinkling, marked dilation, or tortuosity of retinal vessels (Figure 41-1).

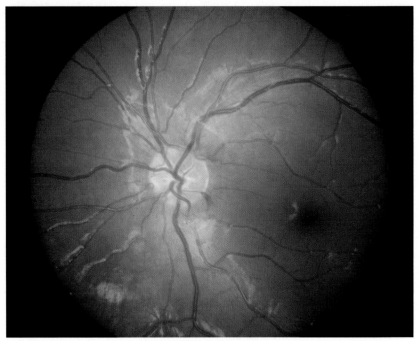

Figure 41-1. Suspected optic nerve edema, nerve drusen. Courtesy of G. Robert LaRoche, MD.

Diagnosis

The ophthalmologist reports the same day and sends other photographs to help illustrate his findings of autosomal-dominant optic nerve drusen (Figure 41-2A, B). Diagnosis is also confirmed by ultrasonography of the optic nerve head (Figure 41-2C). The same findings are found in the mother. The child is also mildly myopic, as are both parents.

There are many causes of optic nerve swelling. However, the term *papilledema* is reserved for swelling of the optic nerve head caused by raised intracranial pressure. Other causes of optic nerve swelling are typically inflammatory, infiltrative, or ischemic.

Drusen of the optic nerve are congenital, and most childhood cases present as questionable papilledema. They are refractile bodies inside the optic nerve head. Affected optic nerves tend to be smaller with small optic cups. Drusen become more visible as patients age, typically

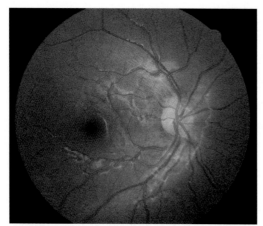

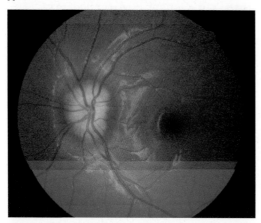

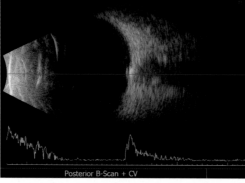

Figure 41-2. A, Right eye, normal appearance. **B,** Left eye, buried optic nerve drusen. **C,** Ultrasound B-scan of left disk; bright white signal at optic nerve head is consistent with drusen calcific deposits. Courtesy of G. Robert LaRoche, MD.

during early adolescence. Symptoms are rare and usually occur when the condition has become advanced. Optic nerve drusen are frequently autosomal dominant in inheritance and bilateral in 75% of cases. Drusen cause an irregular, often "lumpy-bumpy" contour to edges of the optic nerve when buried, later becoming visible as yellowish, globular, discrete bodies at the surface of the optic nerve. They are more common on the nasal aspect of the optic nerve. Presentation on fundus photographs is variable, as demonstrated by another case (Figure 41-3).

High-magnification photography and ultrasound imaging are helpful in making the diagnosis. The margin of the optic nerve does not show actual obscuration of surface vessels, whereas this finding is highly characteristic of early papilledema. Exudates, cotton-wool spots, and hyperemia are all absent in drusen but are typical of papilledema.

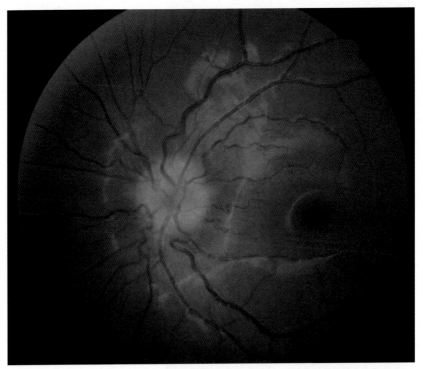

Figure 41-3. Another case of early optic nerve drusen in a 9-year-old girl. Courtesy of G. Robert LaRoche, MD.

Ultrasound image shows well-isolated, high-reflective foci at the surface of optic nerves. Autofluorescence of the drusen shows with photographic techniques using specific filters. Newer imaging techniques like optical coherence tomography can also be very useful. Visual field testing eventually shows peripheral visual field defects in 75% of cases. Computed tomography scan can sometimes show calcification foci at the optic nerve head later in the child's life.

Differential Diagnosis

Diagnoses besides optic nerve drusen that should be considered include papilledema, neuroretinitis, cancerous invasion of the nerve, and very rarely in children, ischemic optic neuropathy. A hallmark of these, except for papilledema, is decrease in vision.

Papilledema

This swelling of the optic nerve head is caused by raised intracranial pressure. In early papilledema, the margin of the optic nerve shows obscuration of surface vessels. Exudates, cotton-wool spots, hyperemia, and venous congestion are all typical.

When to Refer

A patient should be urgently referred to an ophthalmologist if the optic nerve appears swollen. While optic nerve drusen are not an urgent problem to deal with, other causes of optic nerve swelling are.

Treatment

There is no standard treatment for optic nerve drusen. However, annual examinations are warranted to identify early and treat possible sequelae. Photographs of the optic nerve drusen can assist in following these patients.

Discussion

Symptoms of optic nerve drusen usually do not occur unless enough axons have been involved (peripheral visual field defects), or vascular erosion has caused hemorrhages or neovascularization of surrounding adjacent retina. This, in turn, can cause scars with visual consequences.

For these reasons, patients are followed up regularly for life by an ophthalmologist to try to manage any treatable complications as soon as possible.

Key Points

- Optic nerve drusen are a cause of optic nerve fullness that can be mistaken for swelling.
- The condition is often familial, so parents should be questioned about their ocular history and examined by an ophthalmologist.
- This condition requires a detailed ophthalmologic examination as well as supporting tests to confirm the diagnosis, including ultrasound image of the optic nerve head to search for the classic highly reflective concretions.
- Patients require lifelong follow-up because of possible visual complications, some of which are amenable to treatment to prevent significant visual loss.

Suggested Reading

Brodsky M. Congenital optic disc anomalies. In: Taylor D, Hoyt CS, eds. *Pediatric Ophthalmology and Strabismus.* 3rd ed. Edinburgh, United Kingdom: Elsevier Saunders; 2005:625–645

American Association for Pediatric Ophthalmology and Strabismus. Optic nerve drusen. http://www.aapos.org/terms/show/82. Accessed April 26, 2012

Chapter 42

Excavated Optic Nerve

Cameron F. Parsa, MD

Presentation

A 7-year-old girl comes to the pediatrician's office for a routine examination. Her family history includes renal failure in her father, paternal uncle, and paternal grandmother. She has no trouble reading the eye chart; because she appears cooperative, the pediatrician examines her ocular fundus with an ophthalmoscope.

The pediatrician notes a somewhat excavated appearance of both optic discs, but after further reflection suddenly realizes that the normal central blood vessels are entirely missing. Instead, there is a multiplicity of cilioretinal vessels making hairpin turns about the periphery of these otherwise "vacant" optic discs (Figure 42-1). (A normal ocular fundus with central retinal vessels is depicted for comparison in Figure 42-2).

Because the patient's father accompanies her, the pediatrician asks to look into his eyes to see if this might be a hereditary anomaly. The pediatrician notes that in the father the central retinal vessels, although attenuated, appear present. The discs do seem a bit excavated, but more specifically, there again are numerous cilioretinal vessels, far more than the one, or none, often present. Each of these vessels, which stay outside the dural sheath of the optic nerve, emerges from the periphery of the disc and makes a characteristic loop or hairpin turn over the neural rim of the disc to course over and supply the retina (Figure 42-3).

Diagnosis

The pediatrician is not familiar with this anomaly and refers to an atlas of ophthalmology kept in the office. The pediatrician examines fundus photographs in a chapter titled "Congenital Optic Disc Anomalies."

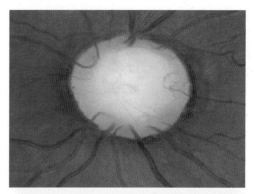

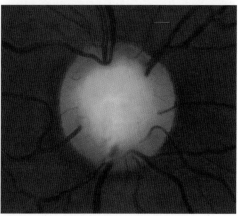

Figure 42-1. Absent of central retinal vessels within each optic disc, with exclusive peripheral cilioretinal blood supply to the retina. Courtesy of Cameron F. Parsa, MD.

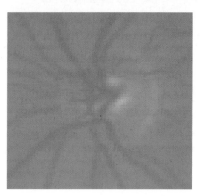

Figure 42-2. Normal optic nerve with smaller excavation and retinal vessels emerging from disc center. Courtesy of Cameron F. Parsa, MD.

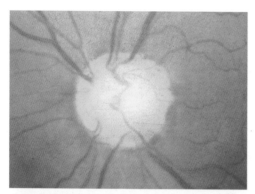

Figure 42-3. Father's optic nerves with large cups with attenuated central disc vessels but multiple peripheral cilioretinal vessels. Courtesy of Cameron F. Parsa, MD.

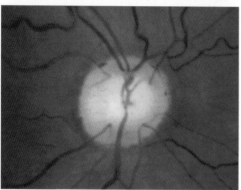

Many are listed under the rubric coloboma (see "Differential Diagnosis" on page 293). The pediatrician reads and understands that all true colobomas, whether in the anterior or posterior segment of the eye, are the result of an incomplete closure of the embryonic optic vesicle. This vesicle first forms superotemporally, invaginating and rotating about the axis of the optic nerve. Any defect in closure thus always causes a tissue defect that is situated inferonasally, to be subsequently filled in by fibrous tissue proliferation (Figure 42-4). (This tissue defect can involve not only the optic disc but also a substantial portion of inferonasal choroid and retina, as seen in figures 42-4 and 42-5.) Chorioretinal microanastomotic channels enlarge therein, to develop into visible cilioretinal vessels that supply the retina to the periphery of this area devoid of neural tissue. Concomitant lack of normal optic nerve–retinal intermediary tissue barriers leaves many such patients prone to eventual retinal detachments.

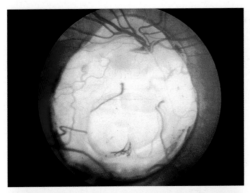

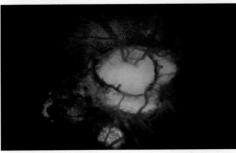

Figure 42-4. Posterior coloboma variants. Note relative normality of the discs superotemporally, with predominant defects always inferonasal. Courtesy of William F. Hoyt, MD.

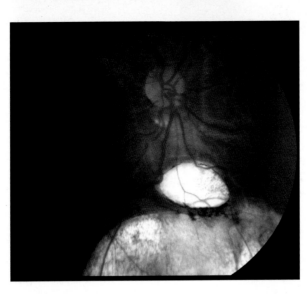

Figure 42-5. Posterior coloboma variant affecting choroid and retina inferonasally but sparing the optic disc. Courtesy of David B. Granet, MD.

When making the proper diagnosis of a coloboma, no matter how large the inferonasal tissue defect might be, it is important to remember that the superotemporal aspect of the fundus, from where the optic vesicle first develops, is always relatively normal. The pediatrician takes note, however, that in the girl and her father, the anomalies are symmetrical and are not inferonasally focused, effectively ruling out diagnosis of a typical or true posterior coloboma.

Photographs in the atlas depict "excavated optic disc anomalies" such as posterior staphyloma (Figure 42-6), also sometimes erroneously called posterior coloboma. With posterior staphyloma, there is symmetry about the disc center and may be central excavation. However, nearly all vessels can be seen to originate from a normal central retinal vasculature in an optic disc that is simply more depressed within the surrounding evaginating scleral shell. Discoloration of surrounding retina is secondary to stretching and thinning, which in turn is due to outpouching of the thinned and weakened posterior scleral shell, giving rise to the aptly named posterior staphyloma. Such defects are almost always unilateral and not hereditary.

Concentrating on the specific finding of multiple cilioretinal vessels in both eyes of the patient, the pediatrician notices that vessels described in the morning glory anomaly (so named because it resembles the flower) also appear distinct without any central origin, emerging

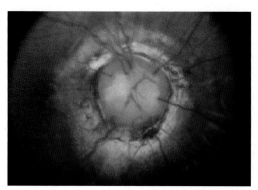

Figure 42-6. Excavated optic disc anomaly with normal central origin of vessels—peripapillary optic disc staphyloma. Courtesy of Cameron F. Parsa, MD.

from the nerve periphery (Figure 42-7). Occasionally called an atypical coloboma, the morning glory anomaly is also unilateral, often left-sided, nonhereditary, and often in females and usually associated with poor vision because of associated retinal maldevelopment. Interestingly, when there is associated discoloration of the retina focused inferiorly, this may point to the presence of a transsphenoidal defect with basal encephalocele compressing the pituitary gland and producing hormonal deficiencies. The patient has none of these issues.

Perplexed yet undaunted, the pediatrician accesses a computer. Searches for "vacant discs" and "multiple cilioretinal vessels" link to what was sometimes described as renal-coloboma syndrome but now more appropriately is termed papillorenal syndrome. The pediatrician reads that there is no coloboma present in this syndrome, as the disc morphology of the girl also clearly indicates. However, both optic papillae have a characteristic finding of multiple cilioretinal vessels, as in this case. The pediatrician then realizes that the patient has this autosomal-dominant disorder, which at times has a detectable mutation in the *PAX2* homeobox developmental gene. The previously unrecognized hallmark of this disorder, bilateral absence of the central retinal vasculature (with multiple compensatory cilioretinal vessels), led these discs to be labeled as colobomas or atypical colobomas until recently. This lack of normal central vasculature instead signifies a systemic defect of angiogenesis (as opposed to vasculogenesis), which also affects development of the kidneys and urinary tract.

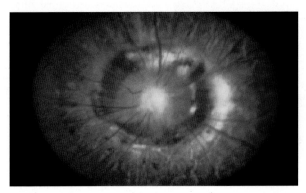

Figure 42-7. Central funnel-shaped excavation with overlying glial tuft and peripheral vessels to retina—morning glory optic disc anomaly. Courtesy of Irene H. Maumenee, MD.

Although it is now evident that the girl's diagnosis is papillorenal syndrome, the pediatrician rightly sends the patient to a pediatric ophthalmologist for confirmation and photographic documentation. Just as with colobomas that may affect the optic nerve, if a defect exists in barrier intermediary tissue between retina and optic nerve, this can allow for cerebrospinal fluid (CSF) seepage to eventually produce retinal detachment.

Differential Diagnosis

Diagnoses besides papillorenal syndrome that should be considered include the following:

- Typical coloboma
- Posterior staphyloma
- Atypical coloboma (morning glory anomaly)

When to Refer

Referral to an ophthalmologist should be made for any patient suspected of having a congenitally excavated optic nerve when neural rim is missing in a meridian, such as may occur with colobomas (inferonasally), in the papillorenal syndrome (often centrally excavated, but which may reach the disc laminar edge), or even with small but deep optic pits where the excavation may reach intermediary tissue by laminar edge. An ophthalmologist is needed to assist in diagnosis and assess and monitor for infrequent but potentially severe complications, such as serous retinal detachments or superimposed glaucoma, and refer to a nephrologist if papillorenal syndrome is present.

Treatment

After diagnosis of papillorenal syndrome is confirmed by an ophthalmologist, the patient undergoes a comprehensive renal workup. In this girl, the neural rim at the edge of the optic disc was present in all meridians, with no risk for developing serous retinal detachments, and she was also found to have normal kidneys. Her father, on the other hand, was found to have previously unsuspected microproteinuria. He was placed on an angiotensin-converting enzyme (ACE) inhibitor as a renal protective measure. Other relatives were also examined, and the father's sister was found to have similar ocular findings along with small kidneys and borderline hypertension. She too was placed on an ACE inhibitor to defer renal failure.

Patients with ocular findings of papillorenal syndrome should be examined for potential renal anomalies, and referral to a nephrologist should be considered. Family members should also be examined for this autosomal-dominant entity. Ultrasonography may reveal renal hypoplasia. Doppler ultrasonography can be used to determine hydrodynamic resistive indices of parenchymal blood flow in young children, which may be predictive of chances of renal failure eventually developing. Proteinuria can be effectively detected in its early stages by microalbuminuria testing prior to any changes in serum urea nitrogen and creatinine. With early diagnosis, aggressive blood pressure control to the low end of normal values has the potential to add many decades to useful kidney life.

Discussion

Excavated optic discs in the pediatric population, rather than being a sign of early glaucoma as in adults, indicate embryonic malformation from a variety of causes. Specific identifiable features allow one to classify them as colobomas, papillorenal syndrome, posterior staphylomas, morning glory anomaly, or smaller optic pits. Whatever the embryologic cause, should the excavation extend to the laminar disc edge abutting retina, it may also encompass intermediary tissue that otherwise serves as a barrier between the perineural CSF compartment and subretinal space. Such individuals are then prone to developing serous retinal detachments if intracranial pressures exceed intraocular pressures. Later in life, there is also risk of congenitally malformed laminar optic disc tissue to become further depressed in response to elevated intraocular pressures. Such deformation can kink nerve axons and lead to superimposed glaucoma.

Identified individuals should be followed by an ophthalmologist. It is important to recognize the pathognomonic feature of bilateral multiplicity of cilioretinal vessels with variably attenuated central retinal vessels (pinpointing systemically defective angiogenesis), particularly when there is known family history of idiopathic renal or genitourinary disorders such as vesicoureteral reflux, indicative of papillorenal syndrome. When diagnosis is made, many otherwise unsuspected family members with this autosomal-dominant entity can be treated much earlier with effective renal protective measures, potentially adding decades to useful kidney life.

Key Points

- Nomenclature of congenital posterior anomalies is often confused and grouped together as various "colobomatous" defects.
- Anomalous disc laminar tissue can sometimes lead to secondary problems such as serous retinal detachments and eventually, glaucoma.
- Not rare, papillorenal syndrome remains greatly underdiagnosed because of a lack of awareness of its characteristic optic disc findings.
- Most cases of papillorenal syndrome cannot be detected by current genetic analysis. Hence, it is important to recognize the pathognomonic optic papillary anomaly of bilateral multiplicity of cilioretinal vessels, particularly when there is known family history of idiopathic renal or genitourinary disorders.
- Patients should be evaluated for potential renal anomalies.

Suggested Reading

Johnson TM, Johnson MW. Pathogenetic implications of subretinal gas migration through pits and atypical colobomas of the optic nerve. *Arch Ophthalmol.* 2004;122(12):1793–1800

Parsa CF. Congenital optic disc anomalies. In: Albert DM, Miller JW, eds. *Albert and Jacobiec's Principles and Practice of Ophthalmology.* 3rd ed. Philadelphia, PA: Saunders Elsevier; 2007:4271–4275

Parsa CF, Goldberg MF, Hunter DG. Papillorenal ("renal coloboma") syndrome. *Am J Ophthalmol.* 2002;134(2):300–301

Parsa CF, Parsa A. Diagnosing papillorenal syndrome: see the optic papilla. *Pediatr Nephrol.* 2008;23(10):1893–1894

Chapter 43

White Mass on the Optic Nerve

Zane F. Pollard, MD

Presentation

A 6-year-old boy comes to the pediatrician's office with a 5-month history of his left eye turning intermittently toward his nose. In the past week the crossing has become constant, and the boy complains of decreased vision in this eye. A brief medical history related from the parents reveals the child to be in excellent health, with no non-ocular complaints. The mother admits to having 2 puppies, born 1 year ago, in the house as pets.

Examination of the child shows a greatly crossed left eye. On ophthalmoscopy a white mass appears to be protruding off the left optic nerve, but because the boy is moving, it is difficult to obtain a good view. Lens of the eye is clear, and nothing is blocking the view of the retina.

Diagnosis

More common differential diagnoses of a white reflex include cataract, retinoblastoma (malignant tumor), persistent fetal vasculature (formerly called persistent hyperplastic primary vitreous), Coats disease, toxoplasmosis, and *Toxocara* (roundworm) infection.

The pediatrician should refer this case to a pediatric ophthalmologist promptly to rule out life-threatening retinoblastoma. However, this child has no retinal lesions. The lens of the eye is clear, and it is easy to see the retina; therefore, no cataract is present. This child's mass does not extend to the lens and the boy is older than the usual age at presentation of persistent fetal vasculature. His retina has no exudates, as is typical of Coats disease. This presentation is not characteristic of toxoplasmosis, which does not present with a mass but usually with an inflammation in the retina and choroid.

This child has ocular toxocariasis. The mass coming off the optic nerve is the most common ocular presentation of infection with this parasite (Figure 43-1). A peripheral retinal granuloma with retinal detachment (Figure 43-2) is the second most common presentation, and endophthalmitis (Figure 43-3) is a less common presentation.

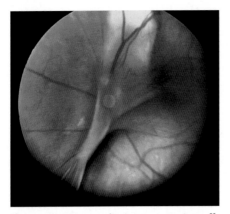

Figure 43-1. Large gliotic mass coming off of the optic nerve and obscuring details. Courtesy of Zane F. Pollard, MD.

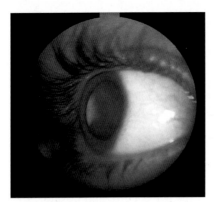

Figure 43-2. A white gliotic mass is seen in the temporal peripheral retina of this child's left eye. Courtesy of Zane F. Pollard, MD.

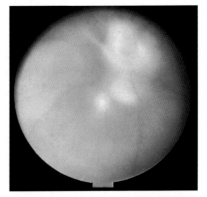

Figure 43-3. Toxocara endophthalmitis. We can barely make out a gliotic mass coming off the optic nerve. Anatomy of the optic nerve is quite obscured as the vitreous is very hazy because of endophthalmitis. The patient was treated with thiabendazole and steroids systemically. Courtesy of Zane F. Pollard, MD.

The enzyme-linked immunosorbent assay (ELISA) for *Toxocara* has a very high specificity. Ophthalmologists formerly thought that a high titer for *Toxocara* was necessary for diagnosis, but current clinical understanding is that any positive titer with clinical correlation is clinically significant. With time, titers will fall. Therefore, in a patient who was infected 1 or 2 years prior to diagnosis, titers may be positive but low. Although very uncommon, it is possible to have a titer positive for *Toxocara* in a patient with retinoblastoma. Prior to the development of the ELISA test for *Toxocara*, diagnosis was made clinically and confirmed by examining the eye after enucleation, which used to be performed so as not to miss retinoblastoma. Because the larva that causes ocular toxocariasis does not complete its life cycle in the human, there are no eggs in the stool by which diagnosis can be made. That is the reason the ELISA test is so valuable.

The visceral form of this disease, called visceral larva migrans, occurred in only a few patients in a series of 300 patients. Immunology of this infection is such that the patient usually presents with ocular toxocariasis or visceral larva migrans. Table 43-1 lists differences in presentation.

Table 43-1. Comparison of Ocular Toxocariasis With Visceral Larva Migrans

	Ocular Toxocariasis	Visceral Larva Migrans
Average age of patient	7.5 y	2 y
White blood cell count	Normal	Elevated
Eosinophilia	Normal (rarely elevated)	Elevated (can be 30%)
Hepatomegaly	None	Usually present
Splenomegaly	None	Usually present
Ocular findings	Posterior pole granuloma, peripheral granuloma, endophthalmitis	Usually none

Differential Diagnosis

Diagnoses besides ocular toxocariasis that should be considered include the following:

Cataract

A white or gray opacity is present on the lens, which can obstruct vision. Red reflex is absent or abnormal.

Retinoblastoma

This congenital malignant tumor is most often diagnosed before age 5 years. Retinoblastoma originates in the retina and could invade the optic nerve. Leukokoria, or white pupil, is present on examination.

Persistent Fetal Vasculature (Persistent Hyperplastic Primary Vitreous)

This condition usually occurs in a microphthalmic, or small, eye (90% of the time) and typically has a stalk emanating from the optic nerve to the posterior surface of the lens. Usually the diagnosis is made at birth or shortly thereafter in the workup of a child with a small eye.

Coats Disease

Usually seen unilaterally in young males, Coats disease can produce a localized macular lesion. However, Coats disease has exudates in the retina and dilated peripheral vessels that leak serum.

Toxoplasmosis

Toxoplasmosis can involve the optic nerve. Usually, however, infection is confined to the retina, with involvement of the underlying choroid, because it is inflammatory retinochoroiditis. It is uncharacteristic in toxoplasmosis to see a mass in the eye.

When to Refer

The pediatrician should promptly refer a patient with a white mass on the eye to a pediatric ophthalmologist to rule out life-threatening retinoblastoma. A white pupil can also be the presentation of a cataract.

Treatment

Visual prognosis in an eye infected with *Toxocara* is very poor. By making the correct diagnosis with the use of the retinal presentation and the ELISA test, the clinician can save the patient from an unnecessary enucleation. Once the mass is determined to not be cancerous, a vitrectomy (removing debris in the vitreous) as well as cutting any inflammatory, cicatricial bands, which might have caused a retinal detachment, may help. If the eye is quiescent and needs surgery, it can be performed without prior medical treatment. If active inflammation is present, anthelmintics are used prior to surgery. If the retina is not extensively involved, as in this case, the pediatric ophthalmologist can treat amblyopic visual loss by patching the good eye. Strabismus surgery can be performed to straighten the eye if misalignment has occurred. In this child, the uninvolved eye was patched 6 hours a day for 6 months until maximal improvement was obtained, and then 4 hours per day until age 9 years to maintain improvement. After age 9, patching is no longer needed.

The anthelmintic albendazole is the recommended drug for treatment of toxocariasis. The author also has treated several children with other anthelmintics, such as diethylcarbamazine and thiabendazole. Because death of larva from anthelmintic agents causes an inflammatory reaction, the author recommends concurrent systemic corticosteroids. If there is active uveitis, topical steroid drops can also be used.

The best approach is prevention. All children should be advised by their parents and pediatricians not to put dirt, sticks, or blades of grass in their mouths. This is the common pathway to infection when dog feces laden with *Toxocara* eggs are mixed in soil. Other preventive measures, such as properly disposing dog or cat feces and covering a sandbox when not in use, should be recommended.

Discussion

Visceral larva migrans typically occurs in children 1 to 4 years of age. Ocular invasion usually occurs in older children and adolescents. In ocular toxocariasis, systemic signs and symptoms most often are absent. It is typically unilateral.

Toxocara species are common in dogs and cats, especially puppies and kittens. Most cases of toxocariasis in the United States result from *Toxocara canis.*

Key Points

- *Toxocara* is most often confused with retinoblastoma, cataract, persistent fetal vasculature, and toxoplasmosis.
- The enzyme-linked immunosorbent assay test for *Toxocara* has a very high specificity, and any positive titer with clinical correlation should be considered clinically significant.
- Anthelmintics and corticosteroids are used as well as vitrectomy to treat ocular toxocariasis.
- The patient and family should be counseled on measures to prevent future infections.

Suggested Reading

Hagler WS, Pollard ZF, Jarrett WH, Donnelly EH. Results of surgery for ocular Toxocara canis. *Ophthalmology.* 1981;88(10):1081–1086

Pollard ZF. Long-term follow-up in patients with ocular toxocariasis as measured by ELISA titers. *Ann Ophthalmol.* 1987;19(5):167–169

Pollard ZF, Jarrett WH, Hagler WS, Allain DS, Schantz PM. ELISA for diagnosis of ocular toxocariasis. *Ophthalmology.* 1979;86(5):743–752

Schantz PM, Weis PE, Pollard ZF, White MC. Risk factors for toxocaral ocular larva migrans: a case-control study. *Am J Public Health.* 1980;70(12):1269–1272

Chapter 44

Trauma Leading to Pain, Photophobia, and Small Pupil

Arlene V. Drack, MD

Presentation

A 6-year-old boy presents to the pediatrician's office 2 days after Christmas. His older brother received a pellet gun, and he was inadvertently struck in the right eye the day before as he walked by the area where his brother was shooting. He had immediate pain and tearing and complained of nausea but eventually went to bed and fell asleep for the night. On awakening, the pain was intense and he would not open the eye. Therefore, the parents brought him to the pediatrician's office.

On examination, the child will barely open either eye. When a glimpse is obtained of the eyes, the right eye is diffusely injected (red), with tearing. The pupil is smaller than the left eye and minimally reactive. The child is very photophobic (light sensitive), and dimming the room lights aids in examination. Red reflex is present in each eye with direct ophthalmoscope but appears somewhat dull in the affected right eye. Distance visual acuity is 20/60 in the right eye and 20/25 in the left eye.

Topical proparacaine (anesthetic) is instilled in the right eye. The child says this reduces the pain somewhat, but light is still very painful. Fluorescein stain is instilled, and when a blue light is shone on the eye, a circular corneal abrasion can be seen across the center of the cornea.

Diagnosis

The pediatrician prescribes erythromycin eye ointment for the corneal abrasion, but because of the intense level of pain refers the child promptly to an ophthalmologist for evaluation that same day.

The ophthalmologist rechecks the boy's vision in a dim room and finds a distance acuity of 20/60, right eye, and 20/25, left eye.

Slit-lamp microscopic examination reveals subconjunctival hemorrhage at the nasal conjunctiva, near the limbus (the area where cornea meets sclera). A corneal abrasion can be seen, along with many cells (all white blood cells) and mild flare (protein) in the anterior chamber of the right eye. There is no hyphema (blood in the eye) or cataract, and the anterior chamber is well formed. However, the conjunctiva is diffusely injected, with more intense injection around the limbus (Figure 44-1). There is a mild ptosis of the right eyelid. The pupil is miotic (small), without sphincter tears. The left eye is totally normal.

Intraocular pressure is 9 mm Hg in the right eye and 14 mm Hg in the left, which is normal on the left but low in the right (affected) eye. Extraocular movements are full, and there is no strabismus (eye mis-alignment) at distance or near. Results of dilated fundus examination show normal optic nerve, macula, retina, and vitreous in both eyes.

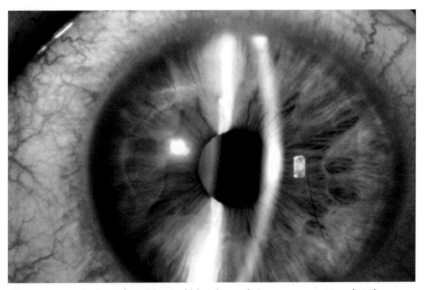

Figure 44-1. Injection of conjunctival blood vessels is more pronounced at the limbus. Courtesy of Shira L. Robbins, MD.

Corneal abrasion is common due to blunt trauma if the object moves too quickly for the person to blink the eye in defense. Corneal abrasion, however, may be only the tip of the iceberg with blunt trauma, especially of the small projectile variety (Box 44-1). Miotic (small) pupil in this patient is a warning sign that there likely is iritis as well as corneal abrasion. Also, the fact that topical anesthetic does not completely relieve the pain is a sign that iritis is probably present. That the intra-ocular pressure in the affected eye is lower than in the unaffected eye is another sign that iritis is occurring. Corneal abrasion will not affect intraocular pressure, whereas iritis usually lowers it.

Iritis is an inflammation of the iris, the colored part of the eye. The iris is a sphincter muscle, and like any muscle, when inflamed, it causes a deep, aching pain. When the pupil is small, the most likely diagnosis is simple iritis, with spasm of sphincter muscle. If the pupil is large, a condition called traumatic mydriasis, the cause may be iritis, but there is the possibility of a sphincter tear or optic nerve damage also causing the pupil to react abnormally. An afferent pupillary defect on the swinging flashlight test, in which the affected pupil dilates and the unaffected pupil constricts from an enlarged state when light is rapidly switched from the affected pupil to the other, suggests optic nerve damage. If the pupil is irregular, there may be damage to the iris itself from the impact. This makes it more likely that there are also other issues now or as future sequelae, such as a dislocated lens or cataract.

Blunt trauma with a projectile smaller than bones of the orbital rim can cause a myriad of potentially serious and usually painful injuries. Larger objects such as baseballs often have some of the impact absorbed by orbit bones, providing relative protection to the globe (eye). Orbital fracture may occur, with relatively little severe damage to the eye. Projectiles that are smaller than the orbital rim usually cause more severe injuries to the eyeball, some of which can be seen immediately, and some of which are realized later.

Box 44-1. Possible Sequelae of Blunt Trauma

Blunt trauma may cause retinal detachment, which can be blinding if not detected and treated in a timely fashion. Traumatic optic neuropathy is also not uncommon. Retinal and optic nerve sequelae of blunt trauma can usually be diagnosed only by an ophthalmologist using special equipment such as indirect ophthalmoscope and lenses at slit-lamp microscope.

Posterior vitreous detachment, in which vitreous gel of the eye separates from the retina, may occur anytime within approximately 6 weeks of blunt ocular trauma. In some cases it occurs gradually; in others it is acute. Flashes and floaters often accompany vitreous detachment, and retinal holes and detachments may occur. Because of potentially delayed onset of vitreous detachment, a second dilated retinal examination is usually recommended about 6 weeks after blunt trauma, and urgently at any point before then if symptoms occur.

Differential Diagnosis

In a patient with pain and photophobia and mildly decreased vision following blunt trauma, differential diagnosis includes corneal abrasion, traumatic iritis, hyphema, and traumatic lens subluxation. If vision loss is severe (eg, vision less than or equal to 20/200), differential expands to include commotio retinae, retinal detachment, vitreous hemorrhage, ruptured globe, choroidal rupture, traumatic cataract, and traumatic optic neuropathy. It is important to remember that these conditions often coexist. If the primary care physician can confirm that only corneal abrasion is present, conservative treatment is often sufficient. If other entities are suspected, referral to an ophthalmologist is recommended.

When to Refer

Diagnosis of traumatic iritis requires slit-lamp microscopic examination; thus, patients with suspected traumatic iritis should be referred to an ophthalmologist.

Treatment

With blunt trauma, especially from a high-velocity projectile such as a BB, pellet, paintball, or finger, there are often multiple coexisting injuries that must be treated concomitantly, yet separately. In this case, corneal abrasion should be treated with antibiotic drops or ointment and possibly a pressure patch for 24 hours, then reevaluated. Yet the traumatic iritis, which this child also has, may be causing more pain than the abrasion and must be treated at the same time.

Mainstays of treatment of traumatic iritis are cycloplegia (dilating and paralyzing the iris and ciliary muscle to decrease pain from muscle movement and to help healing) and topical corticosteroids. For this reason, referral to an ophthalmologist is essential. Topical steroids may retard healing of a corneal abrasion, so the 2 injuries must be balanced if they coexist. In this case, a long-acting cycloplegic agent such as 1% atropine (1 drop) could be applied to the affected eye. Then a combination eye ointment containing an antibiotic, such as tobramycin or neomycin, plus the steroid dexamethasone could be applied. The eye could then be pressure patched (patched tightly with the eye closed under the patch so it cannot inadvertently open, which would cause worse damage because of friction from the patch). A patient with a patch should be told to return to the ophthalmologist the following day.

Once the abrasion has healed, a more aggressive steroid such as 1% prednisolone acetate eyedrops can be instilled (1 drop 4 times a day) along with 1 drop of 1% atropine daily. The patient should follow up with the ophthalmologist every few days until there are no more cells in the anterior chamber. At that point, the prednisolone dosage is slowly tapered to avoid rebound effects, and the atropine dosage is discontinued or tapered.

Topical steroids such as prednisolone raise intraocular pressure in some susceptible individuals and may cause glaucoma. For this reason, patients on topical steroids must be followed closely by an ophthalmologist during treatment. The goal is to use steroids for the shortest time at the lowest dose possible. If inflammation is severe, the inflammation itself or trauma to the lens may cause glaucoma, or the mechanism may be mixed. If topical steroids are required for treatment of severe inflammation but intraocular pressure is above 21 mm Hg, a glaucoma medicine may be added to allow steroids to be continued safely.

Atropine will paralyze the pupil and ciliary muscle for at least 24 hours, and often for days, with just 1 drop, and it does not burn on instillation. This makes it a very useful cycloplegic for children, who often fight eyedrops. Cycloplegic agents help with the pain of corneal abrasions and iritis. However, atropine must be used with caution. It has anticholinergic side effects, including dry mouth, tachycardia, flushing, and in rare cases, death. Teaching must be done when atropine is prescribed to tell parents to use only 1 drop at a time and to wipe away excess from the face. Atropine should be kept away from children and pets. Parents should be reminded to wash their hands after instilling the drops; many parents have accidentally rubbed their eyes after instilling atropine in a child's eye and discovered a dilated pupil with blurry vision the following day and for several days afterward.

Cyclopentolate is a cycloplegic drop with fewer side effects and less toxicity, but the duration of action is only 8 hours, so it must be instilled 3 times a day, and it burns on application. The pros and cons of each medicine must be weighed in individual cases.

Discussion

Due to the grave diagnoses associated with ocular trauma, these cases need to be evaluated carefully. In addition, ocular trauma can produce sequelae that are not apparent in the acute setting. For this reason, cases of ocular blunt trauma require annual follow-up examinations by an ophthalmologist.

Key Points

- Blunt trauma from small projectiles often causes serious eye injury. Always get a good history and be suspicious that there is more than just an abrasion with this method of injury.
- A small pupil, light sensitivity, and pain not relieved with a topical anesthetic, such as proparacaine eyedrops, are warning signs of traumatic iritis.
- Topical cycloplegics, such as 1 drop of 1% atropine daily, and topical steroids, such as 1% prednisolone eyedrops, are mainstays of treatment for traumatic iritis. These medications often must be given and monitored over 1 to 2 weeks. Atropine can have serious systemic side effects in children, so careful parental counseling must be done. Cyclopentolate has fewer side effects but burns on instillation, making compliance an issue.
- Referral to an ophthalmologist is usually necessary because of the wide range of pathologic conditions that can result from injuries that cause traumatic iritis and because of the need to monitor treatment response at slit-lamp microscope.

Suggested Reading

Hargrave S, Weakley D, Wilson C. Complications of ocular paintball injuries in children. *J Pediatr Ophthalmol Strabismus*. 2000;37(6): 338–343

Hink EM, Oliver SC, Drack AV, et al. Pediatric golf-related ophthalmic injuries. *Arch Ophthalmol*. 2008;126(9):1252–1256

Lueder GT. Air bag-associated ocular trauma in children. *Ophthalmology*. 2000;107(8):1472–1475

Weitgasser U, Wackernagel W, Oetsch K. Visual outcomes and ocular survival after sports related ocular trauma in playing golf. *J Trauma*. 2004;56(3):648–650

Wirbelauer C. Management of the red eye for the primary care physician. *Am J Med*. 2006;119(4):302–306

Chapter 45

Vomiting After Eyelid Trauma

Lynnelle Smith Newell, MD
Bobby S. Korn, MD, PhD
Don O. Kikkawa, MD

Presentation

A 14-month-old boy was brought to the pediatrician's office because of swelling of the right upper eyelid (Figure 45-1). Swelling was noted after an episode of unsupervised play at home with his siblings 2 days earlier. His mother also reported several episodes of vomiting since the injury.

The pediatrician checks the boy's eye alignment and visual fixation. Because of the posttraumatic vomiting, the pediatrician refers the patient to a pediatric ophthalmologist, who performs a comprehensive

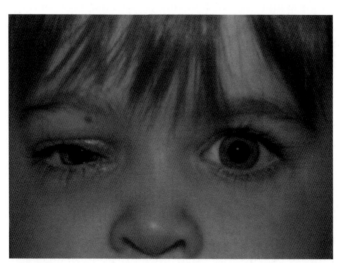

Figure 45-1. A 14-month-old boy presents with swelling in his right upper lid with associated nausea and vomiting. Courtesy of Don O. Kikkawa, MD.

ophthalmic examination, including dilated fundus examination, as well as orbital and brain imaging.

Diagnosis

Computed tomography (CT) imaging reveals an intraorbital foreign body that penetrates into the intracranial cavity. The ophthalmologist diagnoses a trapdoor orbital fracture.

Orbital fractures can present differently in children than adults. Children's bones are less ossified than adults, making them prone to greenstick fractures. These types of fractures in the orbit can create a trapdoor that entraps orbital soft tissues, including extraocular muscles or orbital fat, before snapping back to their original position. Such fractures are termed white-eyed blowout fractures (WEBOFs) because they are often small and can present with relative absence of visible external trauma. Criteria for clinical diagnosis of a WEBOF are an orbital fracture associated with nausea and vomiting, diplopia (double vision), pain with eye movement, and restrictive external ophthalmoplegia (grossly restricted eye movements). It is critical to be able to diagnose a WEBOF because it can trigger the oculocardiac reflex, resulting in life-threatening bradycardia and vasovagal symptoms. Additionally, delayed diagnosis of the WEBOF can result in ischemia, contracture, and permanent dysfunction to entrapped muscles.

Mechanism of trauma, presence of diplopia, pain with eye movement, and associated nausea and vomiting should all be specifically inquired about when orbital trauma history is given or suspected. Initial examination should include testing for visual acuity, measurement of ocular alignment, and extraocular muscle movement. Infraorbital facial sensation should also be tested because of the proximity of the infraorbital nerve to the orbital floor. Non-trapdoor fractures may present with diplopia but are less likely to have associated pain with eye movement or vomiting. Particularly among preverbal children, a history of vomiting in the setting of orbital trauma alone warrants orbital and brain imaging. A large number of patients with orbital fractures also sustain ocular injury, and initial evaluation should include a comprehensive ophthalmic examination, including dilated fundus examination.

Orbital CT scan with axial and coronal views with bone and soft-tissue windows should be performed to evaluate all suspected orbital fractures and foreign bodies (figures 45-2–45-4). Medial and inferior orbital walls are most vulnerable to fracture in children, and there is increased risk of

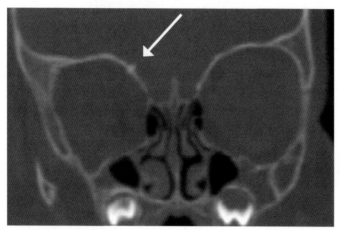

Figure 45-2. Computed tomography imaging reveals intraorbital foreign body that penetrates into the intracranial cavity, right superonasal orbit. Courtesy of Don O. Kikkawa, MD.

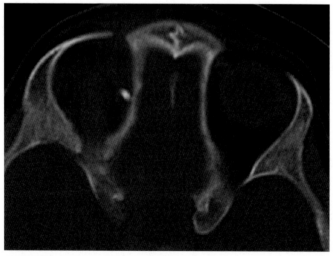

Figure 45-3. Computed tomography axial view of right intraorbital foreign body. Courtesy of Don O. Kikkawa, MD.

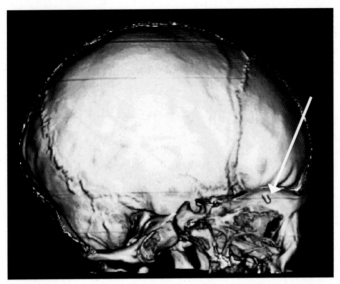

Figure 45-4. Three-dimensional computed tomography image shows vertical orientation of foreign body. Courtesy of Don O. Kikkawa, MD.

orbital roof fractures in infants. Trapdoor fractures are particularly difficult to diagnose because they can present as relatively subtle radiologic findings, such as hairline fractures or small, nondisplaced fractures on CT. Magnetic resonance imaging of the orbit should be avoided when there is suspicion of a metallic foreign body, making CTs the preferred imaging modality in these cases despite radiation exposure.

Differential Diagnosis

Diagnoses besides orbital trapdoor (white-eyed blowout) fracture that should be considered include the following:
- Preseptal cellulitis
- Orbital cellulitis
- Hordeolum/chalazion
- Rhabdomyosarcoma

When to Refer

A history of vomiting in the setting of orbital trauma, particularly among preverbal children, warrants referral to an ophthalmologist with a high likelihood of orbital and brain imaging.

Treatment

This patient is scheduled for urgent surgical repair and removal of the intraorbital foreign body. On removal, the foreign body is identified as a piece of pencil lead (Figure 45-5).

Children with a WEBOF have the best chance for full clinical recovery if surgical repair and release of entrapped orbital contents is completed within 72 hours of injury. If the oculocardiac reflex has been triggered, surgical repair is an emergency and should be performed immediately. Most often the greatest obstacle to prompt surgical repair of WEBOF is a delay in diagnosis and referral. Conventional orbital fractures are usually repaired within 2 weeks of injury for the following indications: substantial extraocular muscle restriction with diplopia, fractures greater than 50% of the orbital floor, and enophthalmos (backward displacement of the eyeball into the orbit) greater than 2 mm. Delay in repair allows for resolution of edema and hemorrhage (bleeding inside the eye).

Orbital foreign bodies can be divided into 2 categories, organic and nonorganic. Organic foreign bodies should be removed because of risk of bacterial or fungal infection. Nonorganic foreign bodies should

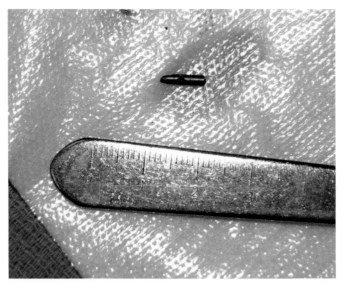

Figure 45-5. Intraorbital foreign body (pencil lead) after removal. Courtesy of Don O. Kikkawa, MD.

be removed if they are causing symptoms such as pain, diplopia, or globe displacement, but patients can be merely observed if they are asymptomatic.

Most eye injuries can be prevented with better education, reduction of risk factors, and appropriate use of eye protection. This includes improved use of eye protection while playing at-risk sports, recreational activities, and any activities at school or in the workplace that could harm the eyes. Parents should be educated on the importance of supervising their children during recreation.

Discussion

Traumatic eye injury is the leading cause of monocular blindness in children. Most injuries are sustained during recreational and sports events. The most common traumatic mechanisms are from domestic accidents, foreign bodies, projectiles, motor vehicle accidents, and an increasing frequency of injuries from bungee cords and paintball air guns. Pediatric patients most often present with contusions and foreign bodies. Eye injuries requiring hospitalization more often involve open wounds to the adnexa and orbital floor fractures.

Key Points

- All pediatric orbital trauma warrants evaluation for visual acuity, diplopia, pain with eye movements, and associated nausea or vomiting.
- All patients with suspected orbital fractures or retained foreign bodies should undergo orbital computed tomography with coronal and axial views.
- Patients with a white-eyed blowout fracture require urgent surgical release of entrapped orbital contents, immediately if the oculocardiac reflex has been triggered.
- Conventional orbital fractures are usually repaired 2 weeks after initial injury.
- All organic and symptomatic nonorganic foreign bodies in the orbit and eyelid should be removed.

Suggested Reading

Brophy M, Sinclair SA, Hostetler SG, Xiang H. Pediatric eye injury-related hospitalizations in the United States. *Pediatrics.* 2006;117(6):e1263–e1271

Lane K, Penne RB, Bilyk JR. Evaluation and management of pediatric orbital fractures in a primary care setting. *Orbit.* 2007;26(3):183–191

Prevent Blindness America. The scope of the eye injury problem. http://www.preventblindness.org/sites/default/files/national/documents/fact_sheets/FS93_ScopeEyeInjury.pdf. Published July 2010. Accessed March 14, 2012

Salvin JH. Systematic approach to pediatric ocular trauma. *Curr Opin Ophthalmol.* 2007;18(5):366–372

Chapter 46

Trauma and Double Vision

David R. Weakley, MD

Presentation

A 5-year-old boy comes to the pediatrician's office after injuring himself jumping on a trampoline. He states he was jumping with his friend, whose head hit him in the left eye. He says he can see normally with the eye but is having double vision when both eyes are open.

On examination, the pediatrician notices a problem with movement of the left eye. Figure 46-1 demonstrates the patient's eyes looking straight and up. The pediatrician refers the patient to an ophthalmologist.

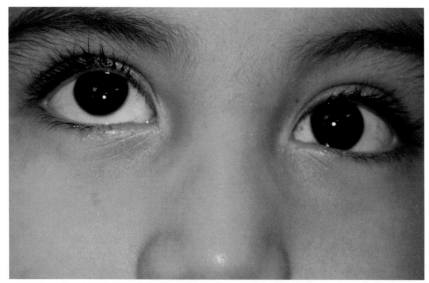

Figure 46-1. Limitation of elevation on attempted upgaze, left eye. Asymmetry of inferior scleral show (white tissue inferior to the iris) can be indicative of extraocular muscle limitation. Courtesy of Shira L. Robbins, MD.

Diagnosis

The ophthalmologist rules out injury to the globe during examination and orders a magnetic resonance imaging (MRI) or computed tomography (CT) scan of the orbit with coronal views.

This is a case of blowout fracture of the orbital floor. Direct trauma to the eye and orbit should alert one to the possibility of orbital fracture. As is true for any such injury, careful ophthalmologic examination is necessary to rule out injury to the globe. In this case, although the globe is uninjured, inability to elevate the eye should alert one to orbital floor fracture with tissue entrapment in the fracture.

Radiographic imaging should be undertaken to confirm diagnosis and assess extent of injury. Although plain films of the orbit can demonstrate the fracture (orbital rim discontinuity, air-fluid level in the maxillary sinus), a CT or MRI scan with coronal views of the orbit is the best way to demonstrate the extent of the fracture and any tissue entrapment (Figure 46-2).

Additional signs and symptoms of orbital floor, or blowout, fracture include enophthalmos (backward displacement of the eyeball into

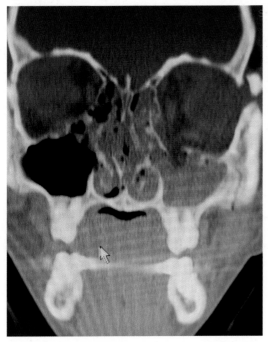

Figure 46-2. Magnetic resonance imaging demonstrating left orbital floor blowout fracture. Note displacement of soft tissue and blood in left maxillary sinus. In addition, there is a left zygomatic fracture. Courtesy of David R. Weakley, MD.

the orbit) from tissue displacement into the maxillary sinus, and numbness above the teeth and below the eye from damage to the infraorbital nerve, which runs along the orbital floor. Bradycardia can be triggered because of stimulation of the oculocardiac reflex when extraocular muscles are displaced into orbital fractures. (See Chapter 45.) Although the orbital floor is commonly fractured during eye and facial trauma due to the thinness of the orbital floor, medial wall fractures can also occur from this mechanism, and tissue can prolapse into the ethmoid sinus as well.

Differential Diagnosis

Diagnoses besides orbital floor fracture that should be considered include previous strabismus and cranial nerve palsy. These entities can be differentiated by absence of fracture or entrapment on radiographic imaging.

When to Refer

Any trauma that results in alteration of ocular motility, double vision, or decreased vision must be referred to an ophthalmologist.

Treatment

This patient underwent surgical repair of fracture with release of entrapped tissue.

After any direct globe injury is addressed, a decision must be made as to whether the fracture needs surgical repair. Small or nondisplaced fractures without tissue entrapment may heal adequately without intervention. Larger fractures, however, especially with substantial bone displacement or tissue entrapment, will generally require surgical repair. Repair involves repositioning of bone and soft tissue and, where possible, with repair of the defect with material such as absorbable gelatin film, MEDPOR, titanium, or autologous bone.

Timing of repair is somewhat controversial but generally should be done within 1 or 2 weeks to avoid difficulty due to scarring. Urgent intervention may be indicated in some cases. (See additional discussion in Chapter 45.)

Falls onto the head or unrestrained motor vehicle accidents with blunt head trauma are other causes of orbital fractures, and these fractures are often more severe than a blowout fracture. These injuries may result in orbital roof fractures as well as more extensive fractures involving multiple orbital bones. Orbital roof fractures usually do not displace bone and entrapment of tissue is very rare; thus, these fractures usually do not require surgical intervention.

Discussion

Motility deficits may remain even after good anatomic repair, and eye muscle surgery may then be required to treat any residual motility deficits. Most patients regain full mobility.

Key Points

- Any trauma that results in alteration of ocular motility must be investigated by an ophthalmologist.
- Signs and symptoms of an orbital floor fracture include inability to elevate the eye, double vision, enophthalmos, and numbness above the mouth and below the eye.
- Children with orbital floor fractures are at risk of bradycardia when the oculocardiac reflex is triggered by entrapment of orbital contents.
- Orbital floor fractures do not all need to be surgically repaired, but that decision should be made within 2 weeks of injury.

Suggested Reading

American Academy of Ophthalmology. Section 6. Pediatric ophthalmology and strabismus. In: *Basic and Clinical Science Course*. San Francisco, CA: American Academy of Ophthalmology; 2006:138–140

American Academy of Ophthalmology. Section 7. Orbit, eyelids, lacrimal system. In: *Basic and Clinical Science Course*. San Francisco, CA: American Academy of Ophthalmology; 2006

Burnstine MA. Clinical recommendations for repair of isolated orbital floor fractures: an evidence-based analysis. *Ophthalmology.* 2002;109(7):1207–1213

Chapter 47

Light Flashes, Floaters, and Visual Loss

Amy K. Hutchinson, MD

Presentation

A 9-year-old girl presents to the pediatrician's office complaining of loss of vision in her left eye. She states that she initially noted some "flashing lights" and "black floating spots" in her vision. Later she noticed a blind spot, which started in her lower visual field and then progressively enlarged. Over the past hour or so, she has noticed a dramatic worsening of the vision in her left eye. She is a healthy girl but has been wearing thick glasses for correction of myopia (nearsightedness) since she was 18 months old (Figure 47-1). There are several other family members who wear thick glasses and have had retinal detachments.

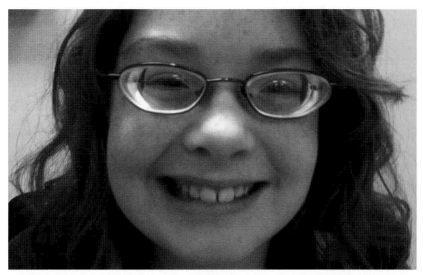

Figure 47-1. This patient has myopia, which is apparent because of the way her biconcave corrective lenses make her eyes look smaller. Severity of the myopia is indicated by thickness of the lenses. Courtesy of Amy K. Hutchinson, MD.

The pediatrician tests distance visual acuity and finds the patient to have 20/400 visual acuity in the right eye without glasses, but vision improves to 20/30 with glasses. In the left eye, however, the patient is unable to see the largest letter on the eye chart with or without glasses. The pediatrician tests the patient's pupils and suspects that a left afferent pupillary defect is present. The pediatrician is able to visualize a good red reflex and obtain views of the optic nerve and macula with direct ophthalmoscope in the right eye but is unable to obtain red reflex in the left eye.

The pediatrician decides to refer this patient to an ophthalmologist immediately; the ophthalmologist arranges to see the patient that day.

Diagnosis

The ophthalmologist calls the pediatrician the next day and tells the pediatrician that the patient had a retinal detachment and that emergency surgery was performed to reattach the retina.

This patient's history and clinical findings are highly suggestive of rhegmatogenous retinal detachment (arising from a retinal tear). Although trauma is the most common cause of retinal detachment in children, axial myopia is the most frequent predisposing factor to nontraumatic pediatric retinal detachments. Axial myopia occurs when the eye is too long such that light coming from an object is focused in front of, rather than on, the retina, resulting in a blurred image. The retina in patients with axial myopia is stretched very thin, which can result in a hole or tear (rhegma) in the peripheral retina. Vitreous fluid can dissect behind the retina and separate the retina from the underlying retinal pigment epithelium (Figure 47-2).

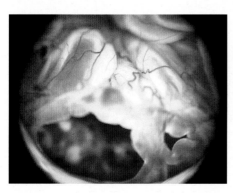

Figure 47-2. Rhegmatogenous retinal detachment in the left eye of a patient with Stickler syndrome. Note multiple peripheral tears of the retina and total detachment from underlying retinal pigment epithelium. Courtesy of Amy K. Hutchinson, MD.

There are 3 types of retinal detachment: rhegmatogenous, tractional, and exudative (Box 47-1). Rhegmatogenous retinal detachments arise from a tear in the retina and are usually associated with trauma, prior eye surgery, or high myopia (often in the setting of a hereditary vitreoretinopathy such as Stickler syndrome or a past history of severe retinopathy of prematurity).

Tractional retinal detachments are caused by centripetal mechanical forces being exerted on the retina. They usually are associated with proliferative vitreoretinopathies most commonly seen in infancy, such as retinopathy of prematurity, familial exudative vitreoretinopathy, or Norrie disease. Although less common in children than adults, proliferative retinopathy can also occur in the setting of diabetes mellitus, sickle cell disease, or prior exposure to radiation. Tractional and rhegmatogenous retinal detachments are often seen together, as tractional forces can give rise to retinal tears.

Exudative or serous retinal detachments are caused by accumulation of fluid in the subretinal space as a result of hydrostatic forces, inflammation, or neoplastic effusions. In children, exudative retinal detachments can be seen associated with tumors such as retinoblastoma and leukemia or in the setting of exudative retinopathies such as Coats disease.

Early signs of retinal tears or traction include photopsia (flashing lights and floating spots). Later, as the retina detaches, patients notice an enlarging blind spot, which they may describe as a "shadow" or "curtain" over their vision. When retinal detachment extends to involve the macula, there is a noticeable loss of central vision with corresponding reduction in visual acuity.

Unfortunately, in children, diagnosis of retinal detachment is often delayed. A high index of suspicion is necessary in children at risk of retinal detachment (Box 47-1). Because underlying pathology is often bilateral, the fellow eye must always be carefully examined.

Box 47-1. Risk Factors for Retinal Detachment in Children

Rhegmatogenous
Trauma
High myopia
History of prior ocular surgery (cataract, glaucoma, retinopathy of prematurity)
Stickler syndrome

Tractional
Acute retinopathy of prematurity
Diabetic retinopathy
Sickle cell retinopathy
Radiation retinopathy

Exudative
Retinoblastoma
Leukemia
Coats disease

Multiple types
Norrie disease
Familial exudative vitreoretinopathy
Congenital malformations of eye
Inflammation or infection of eye

Differential Diagnosis

Diagnoses besides retinal detachment that should be considered include the following:

Posterior Vitreous Detachment

Detachment of the vitreous from its connection to the optic nerve head can accompany or precede retinal detachment. Although symptoms of photopsia and floaters may occur, generally visual acuity remains intact, but patients must be evaluated by an ophthalmologist to rule out associated retinal tear or peripheral detachment.

Migraine

Ocular migraine may present with photopsia and may or may not be associated with headache and transient visual loss.

Hypotension

Photopsia or brief episodes of visual loss can be associated with postural changes, especially in dehydrated individuals. Visual recovery usually returns within seconds to minutes.

Optic Neuritis

Photopsias and transient visual loss can occur in optic neuritis, which is often accompanied by visible optic nerve head edema.

Vascular Occlusion

Occlusion of retinal vessels can result in loss of visual field. Characteristic findings on fundus examination (eg, retinal hemorrhages, cotton-wool spots, retinal whitening) are usually apparent.

Uveitis

Floaters are common in patients with uveitis and are usually accompanied by photophobia. Slit-lamp examination is required to identify the presence of white blood cells in the anterior chamber or vitreous.

When to Refer

Children with signs and symptoms of retinal detachment, including loss of vision, should be referred to an ophthalmologist.

Treatment

In the case of rhegmatogenous retinal detachment, as in this patient, urgent treatment is needed to prevent the macula from detaching. Macular detachment can result in permanent loss of central vision. While the patient is under anesthesia to surgically reattach the retina, the consultant retinal surgeon performs a careful examination of the peripheral retina of the fellow eye and finds several small holes, which are treated with laser (Figure 47-3).

Although exudative retinal detachments usually resolve with successful treatment of underlying disease, surgical procedures are required to repair rhegmatogenous or tractional retinal detachments. Procedures include placement of a scleral buckle to indent the wall of the eye and reapproximate the retina to the retinal pigment epithelium, cryotherapy or laser photocoagulation to close holes or tears in the retina, and intraocular surgery to remove vitreous traction and scar tissue from the retina. In some cases, a gas bubble or silicone oil is left in the eye at the end of the procedure to hold the retina in place.

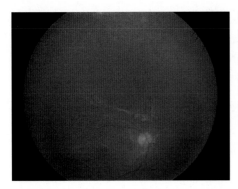

Figure 47-3. Right eye of patient shown in Figure 47-1. Note laser treatment in the retinal periphery (superior), which was administered prophylactically at the time of treatment of retinal detachment in the patient's left eye. Courtesy of Amy K. Hutchinson, MD.

Discussion

Visual prognosis is best in patients whose retinal detachment is treated before the macula detaches. Patients with conditions that predispose them to retinal detachment should be examined frequently. Patients with a family history of high myopia and retinal detachment should be examined regularly by an ophthalmologist to screen for retinal tears. Prophylactic laser photocoagulation can be used to prevent retinal detachment in patients who are found to have high-risk peripheral retinal abnormalities.

Key Points

- Flashing lights, floaters, and an enlarging blind spot are signs of retinal detachment.
- Timely treatment of retinal detachment can often restore normal vision; delayed diagnosis and treatment can result in permanent visual impairment.
- Because retinal detachments are uncommon in children, a high index of suspicion is required for patients at risk.

Suggested Reading

Bhagat N. Retinal detachments in the pediatric population: part I. *J Pediatr Ophthalmol Strabismus.* 2007;44(1):13–23

Bhagat N. Retinal detachments in the pediatric population: part II. *J Pediatr Ophthalmol Strabismus.* 2007;44(2):86–92

Fivgas GD, Capone A Jr. Pediatric rhegmatogenous retinal detachment. *Retina.* 2001;21(2):101–106

Gariano RF, Kim CH. Evaluation and management of suspected retinal detachment. *Am Fam Physician.* 2004;69(7):1691–1698

Chapter 48

Bleeding in an Eye Hit With a Ball

David R. Weakley, MD

Presentation

A 12-year-old boy presents to the pediatrician's office after having been hit in the eye with a tennis ball. The child reports some mild eye pain and a slight decrease in vision. The pediatrician tests visual acuity and finds it to be 20/40. When the pediatrician examines the eye, there is a collection of blood in the inferior aspect of the anterior chamber, the area between the back of the cornea and front of the lens (Figure 48-1).

Diagnosis

This patient has a hyphema, a collection of blood in the anterior chamber of the eye. The most common cause is blunt trauma to the eye, which results in a tear in the fine blood vessels at the root of the iris. Hyphemas also can occur from penetrating injuries or, in rare cases, spontaneously. Intraocular tumors can present with spontaneous hyphema and should be considered in the absence of trauma.

Bleeding may be partial, as seen in Figure 48-1, or in rare cases may fill the entire anterior chamber, a so-called 8-ball hyphema (Figure 48-2).

Differential Diagnosis

Diagnoses that should be considered when trauma does not appear to be the cause of hyphema include the following:

Juvenile Xanthogranuloma

This benign, usually self-limited disorder of infants and children causes cutaneous lesions but may also affect the eye. It rarely can cause nontraumatic hyphema. Elevated intraocular pressure may be present.

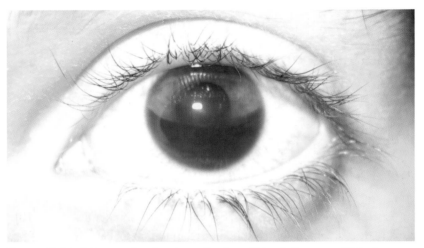

Figure 48-1. Inferior anterior chamber collection of blood. Courtesy of Shira L. Robbins, MD.

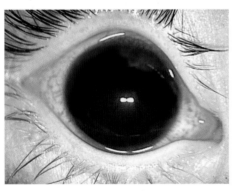

Figure 48-2. Eight-ball hyphema; heme fills the entire anterior chamber. Courtesy of David R. Weakley, MD.

Retinoblastoma

The most common malignant intraocular tumor of childhood, retinoblastoma often presents with leukokoria (white pupil), glaucoma, strabismus (eye misalignment), or vision loss. Rarely, it presents with hyphema.

When to Refer

A hyphema is considered an ocular emergency and should be seen by an ophthalmologist as soon as possible. It is important that potential associated ocular injuries be evaluated.

Treatment

Treatment often differs by size of the hyphema. For small hyphemas, such as in Figure 48-1, outpatient management may be appropriate. Standard treatment includes a topical corticosteroid drop 4 to 6 times a day, a cycloplegic drop to dilate and rest the pupil, bed rest with elevation of the head, and use of a shield over the eye for protection. The ophthalmologist generally will examine the patient every 1 to 2 days until the hyphema resolves, watching for potential complications. These include elevation of intraocular pressure as the blood works its way out of the eye and rebleeding, which is most likely to occur around the fifth day as the clot retracts. Elevation in intraocular pressure is treated with appropriate topical or oral antiglaucoma medications as needed. Both of these complications are more common among African American children with sickle cell hemaglobinopathy increasing the risk of glaucoma.

Patients with larger hyphemas (generally more than 20% or 30% of the anterior chamber filled with blood) or those with difficulty controlling intraocular pressure will usually be hospitalized and receive more aggressive therapy. Some ophthalmologists advocate the use of systemic corticosteroids or aminocaproic acid (to facilitate clot lysis), although these are generally not indicated in most hyphemas.

In some instances when intraocular pressure cannot be controlled with medication or the blood begins to stain the cornea, surgical washout of the blood or removal of a large clot may be necessary. Figure 48-3 shows the patient in Figure 48-2 immediately after surgical removal of the clot.

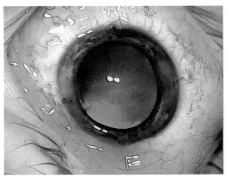

Figure 48-3. Eye after surgical clot removal; note small peripheral areas of residual heme. Courtesy of David R. Weakley, MD.

Usually the child will need periodic follow-up with an ophthalmologist, especially if the hyphema was severe, to monitor for glaucoma in the future.

Discussion

Most patients with traumatic hyphema but no associated ocular injuries recover with vision intact.

Key Points

- A hyphema (a collection of blood in the anterior chamber of the eye) is considered an ocular emergency and should be seen by an ophthalmologist as soon as possible.
- The most common cause of hyphema is blunt trauma to the eye.
- In the absence of trauma, investigation for intraocular abnormalities such as tumors is essential.
- Patients with hyphema need close ophthalmologic monitoring for potential sequelae, such as raised intraocular pressure and secondary bleeding.

Suggested Reading

American Academy of Ophthalmology. Section 6. Pediatric ophthalmology and strabismus. In: *Basic and Clinical Science Course.* San Francisco, CA: American Academy of Ophthalmology; 2006:447–449

Taylor D, Hoyt CS, eds. *Pediatric Ophthalmology and Strabismus.* 3rd ed. Edinburgh, United Kingdom: Elsevier Saunders; 2005:760

Chapter 49

Eye Burn

Jean Shein, MD

Presentation

On July 5, a 10-year-old boy is seen in the pediatrician's office because his left eye is sore and painful. The night before presentation, the patient was playing with some fireworks when one flew directly into his left eye.

The pediatrician immediately checks the patient's visual acuity, which is 20/20 in the right eye and 20/200 in the left eye. According to the boy's mother, his vision was 20/20 in both eyes before the accident.

On external examination, the patient demonstrates a first-degree burn of the left medial canthal eyelid skin. The pediatrician does not note any blisters. Tips of the eyelashes are singed. Pupils are equally round and reactive to light. The pediatrician places fluorescein dye into the patient's left eye and appreciates a large area of conjunctival uptake (Figure 49-1) as well as an adjacent corneal abrasion that involves the visual axis (Figure 49-2). The remainder of the left anterior segment appears normal. The right eye looks normal. The pediatrician also checks the boy's hands to make sure his fingers were not burned.

Diagnosis

The patient has suffered a thermal injury to his left eye. Careful history and examination are required to help determine if there is a possible rupture of the globe (eyeball), presence of a foreign body, or chemical irritant.

Signs of a possible globe rupture include massive subconjunctival hemorrhage (bleeding on the surface of the eye), eyelid laceration, chemosis (swelling of the conjunctiva), distorted pupil, limitation of extraocular motility, or blood in the anterior chamber. Occasionally,

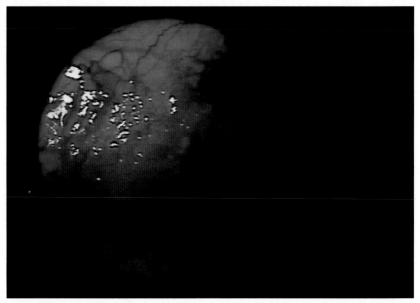

Figure 49-1. Fluorescein dye uptake of conjunctiva (left side) and adjacent cornea (right side). Courtesy of Jean Shein, MD.

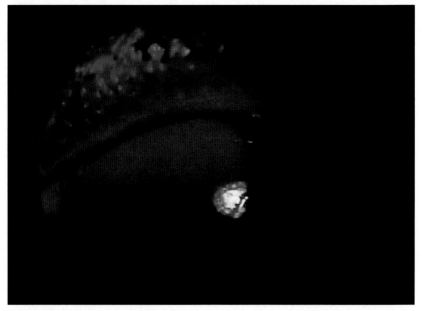

Figure 49-2. Fluorescein uptake of cornea denoting loss of epithelium. Courtesy of Jean Shein, MD.

foreign bodies on the cornea or conjunctiva can be seen with a penlight. Fluorescein dye testing is very helpful in determining the extent of an epithelial defect in the cornea or conjunctiva.

Differential Diagnosis

Diagnoses besides thermal injury that should be considered include mechanical trauma and chemical exposure. Usually history is very helpful in determining etiology of the injury.

When to Refer

A pediatric ophthalmologist should be called at once if the pediatrician suspects or sees a globe rupture, eyelid laceration, embedded foreign body, or chemical exposure. Failure of the patient to improve while on therapy is another indication for a subspecialist referral.

Treatment

For this patient, the injury is relatively superficial. He is started on a treatment regimen of broad-spectrum antibiotic ointment applied 4 times a day to the eyelid, cornea, and conjunctiva. The ointment will promote good wound healing and decrease scar formation and contracture. Cycloplegic (dilating) eyedrops may help with pain and photophobia (light sensitivity). Placing a shield over the affected eye may be necessary if the child is unable to resist touching the site of the injury. The patient should return every 1 or 2 days at first, and then weekly until vision returns to baseline and epithelial defects are healed. If there is evidence of extensive denuding of the periorbital epithelium, or distortion of the eyelids resulting in lagophthalmos (exposure of the eyeball), consultation with an oculoplastics specialist is warranted. Oral analgesics may also be indicated.

If the pediatrician suspects a ruptured globe in addition to thermal injury, the involved eye should be protected with a hard eye shield and the patient should be instructed not to eat or drink. The pediatrician should then call an ophthalmologist immediately for an emergent consultation.

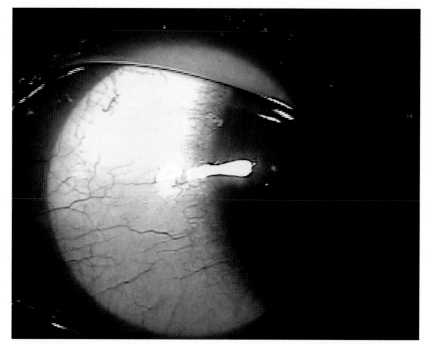

Figure 49-3. Three weeks post-injury with no corneal scarring. Courtesy of Jean Shein, MD.

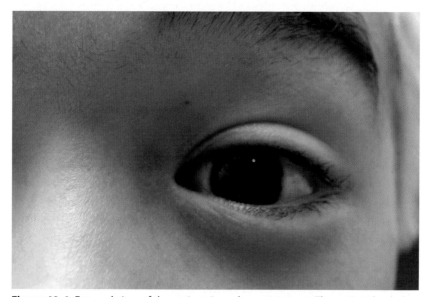

Figure 49-4. External view of the patient 3 weeks post-trauma. The patient healed well with proper treatment and had 20/20 vision. Courtesy of Jean Shein, MD.

Visible foreign bodies can be removed with topical anesthetic and a cotton-tip applicator if the pediatrician is certain they are superficial. Occasionally, foreign bodies can become deeply embedded in the cornea or lodged under eyelids, or may rupture corneal layers entirely. Removing a deeply embedded corneal foreign body typically requires examination with slit-lamp microscope. If a ruptured globe is suspected, the patient needs to be examined under sedation in an operating room setting.

In the event of possible chemical injury in addition to thermal injury, copious irrigation of the involved eye should be performed with saline or sterile water for 30 minutes. Comfort can be enhanced with a topical anesthetic. Irrigation should be continued until neutral pH is noted with litmus paper testing.

This patient is seen again 3 weeks after the injury. At that time he has 20/20 vision in the left eye and no permanent sequelae (figures 49-3 and 49-4).

Discussion

According to the Consumer Product Safety Commission, the eyeball is the most common body site injured by consumer fireworks among children in the United States, and burns are the most common type of fireworks-related injury. Pediatricians should educate parents and their children about the dangers of fireworks and counsel them to attend public displays rather than use fireworks at home. Other common causes of thermal eye burns in children may involve exposure to gas stoves or grills, and electrical outlets.

Key Points

- A pediatric ophthalmologist should be called at once if the pediatrician suspects or sees globe rupture, eyelid laceration, embedded foreign body, or chemical exposure.
- Chemical eye burns are true ocular emergencies, and the sooner the eye is copiously irrigated, the better the visual prognosis.
- Failure of the patient to improve while on therapy is another indication for a subspecialist referral.

Suggested Reading

American Academy of Pediatrics Committee on Injury and Poison Prevention. Fireworks-related injuries to children. *Pediatrics.* 2001;108(1):190–191

Danis RP, Neely D, Plager DA. Unique aspects of trauma in children. In: Kuhn F, Pieramici DJ. *Ocular Trauma: Principles and Practice.* New York, NY: Thieme Medical Publishers; 2002:307–319

Fish R, Davidson RS. Management of ocular thermal and chemical injuries, including amniotic membrane therapy. *Curr Opin Ophthalmol.* 2010;21(4):317–321

Chapter 50

Trauma, Decreased Vision, and Irregular Pupil

Tina Rutar, MD

Presentation

A 5-year-old boy is brought into the emergency department by his parents for a suspected injury to the right eye. His brother was running in the kitchen with a fork in his hand and accidentally poked him in the eye. The patient cried immediately. Since the injury 2 hours ago, he has mostly kept the right eye closed.

There is mild swelling of the right upper and lower eyelids, without lacerations. When the uninjured left eye is covered for vision examination, the child cannot read any letters on the eye chart, identify how many fingers are being held up by the examiner, or tell whether the examiner's hand is moving. He can, however, detect a bright light. His right pupil is distorted and not reactive, whereas the left pupil is normal. The conjunctiva of the right eye is bright red and bulging temporally. There is brown tissue on the temporal aspect of the corneal surface, which appears to have a laceration. The anterior chamber is flat, and the pupil is peaked toward the temporal corneal laceration.

The physician attempts to obtain a red reflex to examine the fundus but sees a dull reflex. On penlight examination, a white lens is visible in the center of the pupil.

Diagnosis

The child has sustained a traumatic penetrating injury of the right eye that involves the cornea and possibly the sclera. The iris has prolapsed out of the eye through the laceration and is temporarily "plugging" the wound. There is subconjunctival hemorrhage in the area of the injury.

The white in the center of the distorted pupil is a traumatic cataract, which occurred when the fork penetrated the anterior capsule of the lens, causing normally clear lens proteins to hydrate and opacify. Lack of pupillary reaction is not caused by damage to the retina or optic nerve, the afferent arm of the pupillary response, but by mechanical damage to the iris, the efferent arm of the pupillary response.

An open globe or full-thickness injury to the cornea, sclera, or both should be suspected when there is history of sharp trauma (eg, pencils, forks, knives), severe blunt trauma (eg, tennis ball, bungee cord, strong punch), or ballistic injury (eg, gunshot wound, fireworks) near the eye or orbit. Also, open globe should be suspected in any patient with an eyelid laceration occurring between the upper eyebrow and lower orbital rim.

Any child with a history of trauma and a severely swollen, ecchymotic (bruised) eyelid needs to have the eye examined to evaluate whether it is intact. The pediatrician should lift the upper eyelid by putting pressure on the bony rim of the orbit and not on the eye itself. If the globe is open, pressure on the eye could cause expulsion of additional intraocular contents. Sedation may be necessary to perform the examination if the child is otherwise uncooperative.

In a cooperative child, the examiner should first attempt to assess vision in the eye by covering the contralateral eye and gently elevating the swollen upper eyelid. Vision is typically severely decreased with open globe injuries, but rarely, laceration of the peripheral cornea (Figure 50-1) or sclera can allow near-normal vision. The examiner should then assess pupillary response, including an assessment for an afferent pupillary defect. A distorted pupil or any brown tissue on the surface of the cornea or under the partially transparent conjunctiva is a sign of an open globe. In a child with a history of eye trauma, a 360° subconjunctival hemorrhage may conceal scleral rupture. However, localized subconjunctival hemorrhage with a history of minor trauma and normal vision is very common and not concerning. Laceration or rupture of the cornea or limbus (junction of cornea and sclera) is often obvious on penlight examination. If unsure, the pediatrician

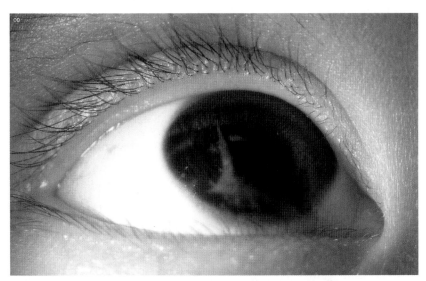

Figure 50-1. Large L-shaped corneal laceration occurred when the corner of a picture frame fell onto this 3-year-old boy's eye. He underwent repair of corneal laceration, with removal of corneal sutures 2 months later. Note the slightly pigmented corneal scar with visible suture tracts. Fortunately, the injury resulted only in additional minor trauma to the iris but no injury to the lens. The patient ultimately recovered 20/30 visual acuity. Courtesy of Tina Rutar, MD.

should compare findings to the uninjured eye. The anterior chamber, the space between the cornea and iris, can be examined by observation with a penlight from the side. Signs of a possible open globe include a shallow or flat anterior chamber or hyphema (blood in the anterior chamber), which may be layered inferiorly. A white cataract may develop after sharp or blunt trauma to the eye. Other reasons for loss of the red reflex include bleeding into the vitreous and retinal detachment.

Orbital imaging is not necessary for routine assessment of open globes. However, a noncontrast orbital computed tomography scan should be obtained if there is proptosis, suspicion of an orbital fracture, or potential intraocular or intraorbital foreign body. Do not obtain orbital magnetic resonance imaging if there is any possibility of a metallic foreign body.

Differential Diagnosis

Diagnoses besides a ruptured globe that should be considered include the following *(Note:* all of the following can coexist with an open globe injury):

Corneal Abrasion

Corneal abrasion is an injury involving only the superficial layer of the cornea. It causes severe eye pain, tearing, and mild redness (but not hemorrhage) of the conjunctiva. Vision may be decreased if the abrasion affects the central cornea. A corneal abrasion stains with fluorescein. The anterior chamber and pupil appear normal.

Conjunctival Hemorrhage

This is blood accumulating under and within the conjunctiva. It appears bright red and has a sharp border separating it from otherwise relatively white or uninflamed conjunctiva. It is painless, and visual acuity is normal.

Conjunctival Laceration

Conjunctival laceration is a laceration of the mucous membrane covering the sclera but not penetrating the sclera itself. A conjunctival hemorrhage is visible around the area of laceration, but visual acuity, the anterior chamber, and the pupillary response are normal.

Hyphema

This is blood in the anterior chamber. Vision is decreased; eye pressure may be increased causing eye pain; and the patient often experiences photophobia. The anterior chamber remains formed, not flat.

Traumatic Iritis

Traumatic iritis is inflammation involving the anterior segment of the eye due to (usually) blunt trauma. Visual acuity is mildly decreased, the conjunctiva appears red, and the pupil may be sluggishly reactive but is typically round, not peaked.

Traumatic Cataract

Traumatic cataract is white opacification of the lens of the eye (usually) caused by blunt trauma. Visual acuity is severely decreased, but the pupil is typically round, and no laceration is visible on the surface of the eye.

Vitreous Hemorrhage

Blood in the vitreous, the jelly occupying the portion of the eye between the lens and retina, is called a vitreous hemorrhage. The condition is painless. Visual acuity is decreased, and the red reflex is absent.

Traumatic Retinal Detachment or Dialysis

When the retina separates from underlying tissue called retinal pigment epithelium (detachment), or when the peripheral retinal edge peels away (dialysis), it is called traumatic retinal detachment or dialysis. These are painless but are often accompanied by flashes of light and/or floaters. Visual acuity is decreased only if the central retina is involved. Peripheral vision is decreased. An afferent pupillary defect is present.

Traumatic Optic Neuropathy

Traumatic optic neuropathy is shear injury to the optic nerve accompanying severe head trauma or actual mechanical disruption of the optic nerve from a penetrating injury. Visual acuity is decreased, and there is an afferent pupillary defect.

Orbital Hemorrhage

Blood accumulating in the soft tissues surrounding the globe leads to orbital hemorrhage. The globe is proptotic, intraocular pressure is elevated, and eye movements are limited.

When to Refer

If an open globe is suspected, the pediatrician should consult an ophthalmologist immediately. The ophthalmologist need not be a pediatric ophthalmologist; a general ophthalmologist can perform the initial management steps of open globe repair. If the pediatrician's facility does not have an ophthalmologist on call, the patient should be transferred to a tertiary care center immediately. The accepting facility must have operating room facilities and anesthesia for children.

Treatment

Management of this patient is as follows:

- Cover eye with shield and do not examine further.
- Request emergent ophthalmology consultation.
- Obtain intravenous (IV) access.
- Administer broad-spectrum IV antibiotic (eg, ampicillin with sulbactam).
- Give IV pain medication as needed.
- Inquire about tetanus prophylaxis.
- Give nothing by mouth in anticipation of surgery under general anesthesia.

While waiting for consultation with an ophthalmologist, it is important for the pediatrician and staff to keep the child calm. Sedation, pain relief, and antiemetics may be necessary to prevent the increase in intraocular pressure that occurs when a child screams or vomits. The eye should be covered with a metal shield. If one is not available, the bottom of a disposable paper or polystyrene foam cup will suffice. It is advisable to not wipe any mucus from the eye or irrigate the eye because any material on the eye could represent intraocular contents. (The exception to this is a chemical injury to the eye, which, if severe, could melt the surface of the eye and cause an open globe. In this situation, copious irrigation is the first and most important step.) Broad-spectrum IV antibiotics should be administered. The pediatrician should not administer eyedrops. Provide tetanus prophylaxis, if necessary. The child should have nothing by mouth in anticipation of surgical correction. Otherwise healthy children rarely require ancillary studies before general anesthesia, but if the pediatrician's institution requires a complete blood cell count, electrolyte measurement, chest radiograph, or electrocardiogram, these should be obtained to avoid additional delays in getting the child to the operating room.

If there are other head or systemic injuries, they should be addressed in appropriate order. If the mechanism of injury raises suspicion for child abuse, the practitioner should obtain appropriate additional examinations and consult social work and the facility's child protection team.

The ophthalmologist will confirm diagnosis of open globe and plan for additional exploration and repair in the operating room. Surgical repair is emergent if the eye and vision are to be saved. Even if the patient has no light perception, which makes recovery of any vision unlikely, the ophthalmologist will generally attempt to repair and save the eye itself.

With blunt trauma, the site of globe rupture occurs at the weakest points of the sclera: posterior to the insertions of the rectus muscles, at the limbus (Figure 50-2), and at sites of prior intraocular surgery (unlikely in children). If the site of rupture is not immediately apparent, the ophthalmologist will perform a 360° conjunctival dissection to expose the surface of the sclera and examine it, including areas behind the extraocular muscle insertions. It is acceptable for the ophthalmologist to perform open globe exploration even if clinical suspicion of

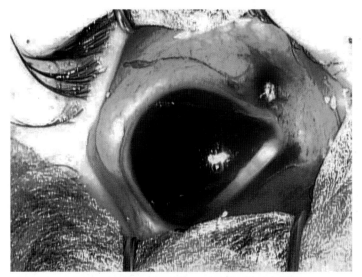

Figure 50-2. A 3-year-old boy rain into a doorknob with his eye, causing the globe to rupture. This photo was taken after the patient was under general anesthesia and prepped for eye surgery. There is extensive globe rupture along the limbus, with chemotic (swollen) and hemorrhagic conjunctiva overlying the site of rupture. The eye appears deflated, and blood fills its interior. There is no pupil visible. Brown tissue on the surface of the conjunctiva is extruding uvea. Despite repair of the globe rupture, this patient lost all vision, and the eye eventually underwent an involutional process called phthisis. Courtesy of Tina Rutar, MD.

rupture is only moderate. It is better to explore than to miss an open globe injury. Once the site of rupture or laceration is found, the site is closed with fine interrupted sutures under an operating microscope. Sometimes, cyanoacrylate glue is used to close complex corneal wounds (Figure 50-3). Very posterior scleral ruptures are not closed but allowed to heal on their own because challenging surgical access to those areas could induce additional expulsion of intraocular contents.

Certain intraocular contents—vitreous, lens material, and necrotic uvea—are excised, whereas other intraocular contents—retina and non-necrotic uvea—are reposited into the eye. If a white cataract already has developed, the ophthalmologist may remove it immediately with initial eye closure or at a later date. The ophthalmologist will likely remove an accessible intraocular foreign body. If the foreign body lies in the posterior segment (behind the lens), a retinal specialist may be

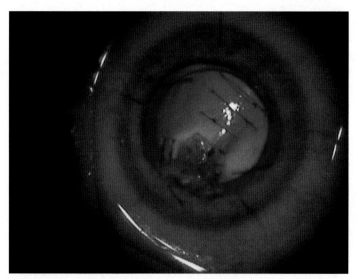

Figure 50-3. A 2-year-old boy sustained a complex stellate corneal laceration from an unobserved penetrating injury that occurred while roughhousing at the playground. Multiple corneal sutures and cyanoacrylate glue were required to close the wound. The patient also sustained a traumatic cataract, which was removed, and the native lens was replaced with an intraocular lens. Ultimately, after removal of the glue and corneal sutures and extensive amblyopia therapy, the patient recovered visual acuity of 20/40. Courtesy of Tina Rutar, MD.

called to remove it. Orbital foreign bodies made of vegetable matter or certain toxic metals are removed, whereas inert orbital foreign bodies are better left alone. Antibiotics are administered by injecting them into the eye or subconjunctival space. Often, corticosteroids are also administered via intraocular injection, subconjunctival injection, or via IV because severe intraocular inflammation can cause permanent damage to an eye.

Postoperatively, the patient generally continues IV antibiotics for 2 days and then begins oral antibiotics for a total 7-day course. Topical antibiotic, steroid, and cycloplegic drops or ointments are also administered. An eye shield is worn for approximately 2 weeks. The child requires close ophthalmologic follow-up to monitor intraocular pressure, assess for signs of severe intraocular inflammation or potential infection, remove sutures, and perform additional intraocular procedures. Occasionally, severely traumatized, painful eyes with no light perception may require replacement with a prosthesis. Traumatized eyes may develop complications such as glaucoma and retinal detachment years later. It is also important for the ophthalmologist to closely monitor the health of the fellow, nontraumatized eye because that fellow eye will likely be the patient's better-seeing eye for the duration of life, and there is a small chance of sympathetic ophthalmia in the fellow eye. Sympathetic ophthalmia is an autoimmune attack of the fellow eye because of exposure of the immune system to antigens from the traumatized eye's uveal tissues.

Because of the risk of amblyopia, children younger than 8 years should be managed in collaboration with a pediatric ophthalmologist. The risk of severe amblyopia is inversely proportional to the child's age at time of injury. Opacity in the visual axis, astigmatism (distorted shape of the eye, frequently caused by corneal sutures [Figure 50-4]), and removal of the lens contribute to amblyopia.

A child with permanently decreased vision in the traumatized eye requires full-time polycarbonate spectacle wear to protect the uninjured eye.

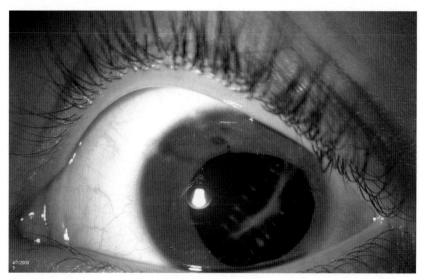

Figure 50-4. This 7-year-old girl injured her eye when a rock flew out from under a lawn mower 1 year ago. She sustained a corneal laceration, iris injury (note permanently dilated and irregular pupil), and cataract. The lens was removed at the time of corneal laceration repair. When a lens is absent, contact lens wear is necessary to correct high induced refractive error. This patient developed inward crossing of the eye because of the disruption of clear and binocular vision. Vision with spectacles is only finger counting at 2 feet in this eye. Vision may improve with a rigid contact lens to correct irregular astigmatism and with amblyopia therapy. Courtesy of Tina Rutar, MD.

Discussion

Ocular trauma is more common in boys than girls. Trauma is the leading cause of monocular blindness in children worldwide.

Many eye injuries can be prevented by close parental supervision and proper protective eyewear when children engage in potentially dangerous activities or sports, including activities with projectiles, such as paintball and baseball, and sports with close contact, such as basketball.

Key Points

- An open globe injury should be suspected when there is history of sharp trauma, blunt trauma, or ballistic injury near the eye or orbit.
- Signs of open globe include decreased vision, irregular pupil, full-thickness eyelid laceration, 360° subconjunctival hemorrhage, brown tissue on the surface of the eye, shallow or flat anterior chamber, blood in the anterior chamber (hyphema), and white pupil (white traumatic cataract).
- A suspected open globe should be managed with eye protection and medications that will keep the child calm and comfortable until an ophthalmologist can treat the patient.
- A child with a traumatized eye should maintain follow-up with an ophthalmologist to monitor for long-term complications and to routinely assess the health of the uninjured eye.
- A child who has undergone successful repair of an open globe will likely have permanently decreased vision because of associated intraocular injuries and amblyopia.
- A child with unilateral decreased vision should wear polycarbonate spectacles full-time to protect the uninjured eye.
- Many pediatric open globe injuries can be prevented by children wearing appropriate eye protection when engaging in potentially dangerous activities and sports.

Suggested Reading

American Academy of Pediatrics, American Academy of Ophthalmology. Protective eyewear for young athletes. *Pediatrics.* 2004;113(3):619–622

American Academy of Pediatrics, American Association of Certified Orthoptists, American Association for Pediatric Ophthalmology and Strabismus, American Academy of Ophthalmology. Eye examination in infants, children, and young adults by pediatricians. *Pediatrics.* 2003;111(4):902–907

Salvin JH. Systematic approach to pediatric ocular trauma. *Curr Opin Ophthalmol.* 2007;18(5):366–372

Chapter 51

Eyelid Laceration After Dog Bite

Katherine M. Whipple, MD
Don O. Kikkawa, MD
Bobby S. Korn, MD, PhD

Presentation

A 5-year-old boy well known to the pediatrician presents to the local emergency department (ED) after being bit on the right cheek by the family dog. Laceration of the right lower eyelid is noted on examination (Figure 51-1). While at the ED, the child receives a dose of intravenous antibiotics. Rabies postexposure prophylaxis is withheld because the patient's and pet's immunizations records are available and up to date. Neurologic findings are normal. Instead of suturing, the emergency

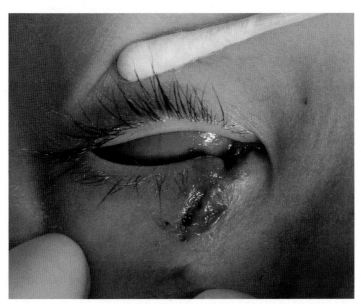

Figure 51-1. Laceration of right eyelid after dog bite. Courtesy of Bobby S. Korn, MD, PhD.

medicine physicians adhere the lacerated cheek skin with sterile strips of tape. Follow-up evaluation is scheduled at the pediatrician's office.

At the follow-up visit, the boy is his usual playful self, but his mother remarks that his right eye has been "weeping" ever since the injury. The pediatrician observes the patient continuously wiping his eye, which is not red or inflamed. Visual acuity is 20/20 in both eyes. There is no fluorescein uptake on either cornea. Pupils react equally to light with no relative afferent pupillary defect. Extra-ocular movements are full and without pain. Examination with direct ophthalmoscope reveals sharp optic nerve borders and good foveal reflexes. The pediatrician inspects the wound, noticing that the laceration extends from the lower eyelid through the medial eyelid margin. On closer inspection, the pediatrician is able to visualize torn edge of the canaliculus, which has white-appearing lumen (Figure 51-2).

On the basis of these findings, the pediatrician refers the patient to an oculoplastic surgeon because the boy likely needs surgical repair.

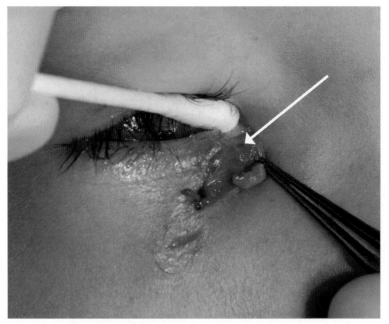

Figure 51-2. Torn edge of canaliculus has white-appearing lumen (arrow). Courtesy of Bobby S. Korn, MD, PhD.

Diagnosis

The oculoplastic surgeon agrees with the pediatrician's assessment of canalicular trauma and need for surgery.

Constant tearing (epiphora) after traumatic injury should raise suspicion of retained foreign body, corneal abrasion, increased intraocular pressure, or even ruptured globe. The first priority in evaluation of any case of periocular trauma is to rule out life-threatening conditions. Although uncommon, severe periocular trauma could result in orbital roof fracture or associated cerebral injury. The next priority is to rule out ruptured globe.

Finally, attention is directed toward the eyelid trauma. In every case of eyelid laceration, concomitant damage to the lacrimal drainage system must be ruled out. This is because the upper and lower canaliculi are located near the medial canthus. Shear force trauma, as is the case with most dog bite injuries, causes traction on the medial canthus, and resultant eyelid lacerations are often associated with canalicular tears. History of recurrent epiphora should raise suspicion of canalicular trauma.

Differential Diagnosis

Diagnoses beside canalicular laceration that should be considered for epiphora following trauma include the following:
- Ruptured globe
- Nasolacrimal duct obstruction
- Conjunctivitis
- Trichiasis
- Entropion

When to Refer

All lacerations of the eyelid should be referred to an ophthalmologist for full evaluation.

Treatment

The patient is taken promptly to the operating room for repair. A full-thickness eyelid laceration involving white lumen of the canalicular system is evident, and the proximal end of the torn canaliculus is visualized (Figure 51-3).

The first step is to intubate the lacrimal system with a silicone stent placed through the inferior punctum and the distal end into the common canaliculus (Figure 51-4). The stent is then retrieved through the nasolacrimal duct in the inferior nasal meatus.

The stent is also passed through the undamaged superior canaliculus and then tied in the nose, creating a loop. This maneuver ensures that the entire lacrimal system remains intact. Once the stent is in place, absorbable sutures are used to reapproximate pericanalicular tissues and reconstruct the eyelid margin.

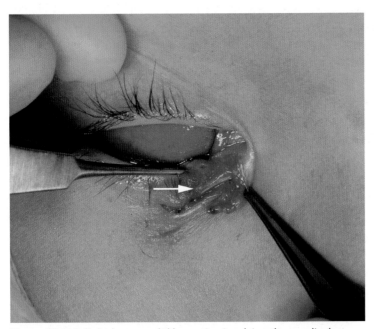

Figure 51-3. Full-thickness eyelid laceration involving the canalicular system is evident, and the proximal end of the torn canaliculus (arrow) is visualized. Courtesy of Bobby S. Korn, MD, PhD.

The silicone stent is visible passing through superior and inferior puncta. This stent allows anatomic healing of the canaliculus. The stent is well tolerated and remains in place for a minimum of 3 months. Combination steroid-antibiotic ointment is used postoperatively (Figure 51-5).

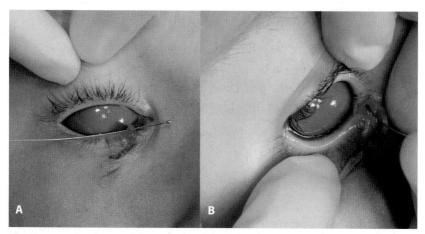

Figure 51-4. A, Silicone stent is placed through the inferior lacrimal punctum. **B,** Stent is placed through the distal end of the punctum into the common canaliculus. Courtesy of Bobby S. Korn, MD, PhD.

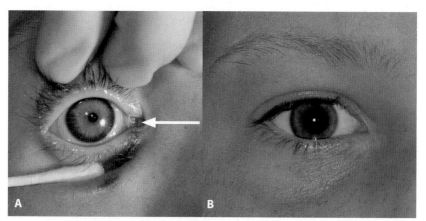

Figure 51-5. A, Silicone stent is visible passing through superior and inferior lacrimal puncta (arrow). **B,** Postoperative photograph of right eyelid laceration 2 years after repair. Courtesy of Bobby S. Korn, MD, PhD.

Discussion

Most victims of dog bites are children, and the face is the most frequently bitten area in children. Research shows that periocular dog bites involve the canaliculi more often than eyelid lacerations due to other causes. Therefore, practitioners should have a high index of suspicion for canalicular laceration when examining patients who have dog bites involving the eyelid.

Had the eyelid laceration been repaired alone and the canalicular laceration overlooked, the result could be a lifetime of tearing for this child, with the potential of impairment of vision in that eye.

To help prevent dog bites, parents should be told to supervise their children around dogs.

Key Points

- Because of the proximity of eyelid and lacrimal system anatomy, eyelid trauma is often associated with canalicular lacerations.
- A missed diagnosis of canalicular laceration can result in permanent tearing for the child.
- Constant tearing can range in severity from annoying to causing substantial vision loss.
- All lacerations of the eyelid should be referred to an ophthalmologist for full evaluation.
- Canalicular lacerations are ideally repaired less than 48 hours after the injury to prevent permanent scarring of the eyelid and canaliculus.

Suggested Reading

Kikkawa DO, Lemke BN. Orbital and eyelid anatomy. In: Dortzbach RK, ed. *Ophthalmic Plastic Surgery: Prevention and Management of Complications.* New York, NY: Raven Press; 1994:1–29

Manning SE, Rupprecht CE, Fishbein D, et al. Human rabies prevention—United States, 2008: recommendations of the Advisory Committee on Immunization Practices. *MMWR Recomm Rep.* 2008;57(RR-3):1–28

Spalton DJ, Hitchings RA, Hunter PA. *Atlas of Clinical Ophthalmology.* 3rd ed. Mosby; 2004:701–706

Chapter 52

Head Injury in an Infant

David B. Granet, MD
Alex V. Levin, MD, MHSc

Presentation

A 5-month-old girl presenting with unexplained loss of consciousness is brought to the hospital. Pregnancy and delivery were uncomplicated. The patient had no problems at her 2- and 4-month well-baby examinations. Her mother found the child unconscious and not breathing in the crib. On arrival at the hospital, the child is comatose, with seizures, fixed and dilated pupils, and bulging anterior fontanelle. Physical findings reveal no external signs of trauma and no malformations. Using a direct ophthalmoscope, the pediatrician examines the eyes and sees that retinal hemorrhages are present (Figure 52-1).

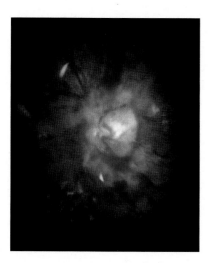

Figure 52-1. Intraretinal and preretinal hemorrhages surrounding the optic nerve (peripapillary hemorrhages). Note that there is no papilledema. This field of view is somewhat bigger than the direct ophthalmoscope allows. Courtesy of Alex V. Levin, MD, MHSc.

Computed tomography (CT) scan of the head demonstrates subdural and subarachnoid hemorrhage. Her coagulation profile and complete blood cell count are normal. Skeletal survey radiographs do not demonstrate any fractures.

Head trauma is suspected. The physician asks an ophthalmologist to perform a retinal examination.

Diagnosis

The ophthalmologist examines the patient and notes bilateral, innumerable, flame-shaped superficial intraretinal, and dot/blot deeper intraretinal hemorrhages as well as preretinal hemorrhages. The hemorrhages are seen mainly in the posterior pole but extend to the edge of the retina (ora serrata). The right eye shows perimacular retinal folds and splitting of the retinal layers with blood accumulated in the intervening space (retinoschisis). Published research, including optical coherence tomography, strongly suggests that retinal folds are caused by vitreous traction. These findings, in the absence of a history such as a fatal motor vehicle accident or a fatal crush injury of the head, are highly suggestive of abusive head trauma (AHT) characterized by repetitive acceleration-deceleration forces with or without blunt head impact (shaken baby syndrome).

When a child younger than 5 years presents with unexplained alteration of mental status, an abusive cause should be considered in the differential diagnosis. Appropriate studies include CT or magnetic resonance imaging of the brain and skeletal radiography. The constellation of fractures of the long bones, ribs, or skull; brain injury (subarachnoid or subdural hemorrhage, cerebral edema, or cerebral contusion or laceration); and retinal hemorrhage are highly suggestive of AHT.

Non-ophthalmologists should attempt direct ophthalmoscopy and can recognize the presence or absence of retinal hemorrhage. The direct ophthalmoscope offers a limited view of the retina, and it may be difficult to further characterize types of hemorrhage that are present. Any type of retinal hemorrhage (or none) can be seen in AHT. Hemorrhages that are too numerous to count, involve multiple layers, and extend to the ora serrata, beyond the view of the direct ophthalmoscope, greatly increase the likelihood that abuse has occurred. Therefore, consultation is required with an ophthalmologist who is well versed in this diagnosis and in examining children by indirect ophthalmoscopy with pharmacologic dilation of the pupils (unless they are fixed and dilated as a result of the brain injury).

Diagnosis of AHT is difficult because external injury is often lacking, and perpetrators do not often volunteer a history of the abuse. Victims of sublethal shaking may have a history of several days or weeks of lethargy, poor feeding, vomiting, and irritability. Retinal hemorrhage is an important sign for correct diagnosis. A 53% to 80% incidence of retinal hemorrhage is found in AHT, in contrast to a less than 3% incidence with most accidental head trauma.

Although retinal hemorrhage is common after birth, flame-shaped hemorrhages resolve by 1 week, and dot/blot hemorrhages resolve by 4 to 6 weeks. Retinoschisis does not occur. Some medical conditions can also cause severe hemorrhagic retinopathy (see "Differential Diagnosis" below). When AHT is suspected, coagulation abnormalities should be excluded. Confounding causes such as increased intracranial pressure and hypoxia differ in that retinal hemorrhages are almost always few in number and confined to the area around the optic nerve. Infant immunizations do not cause retinal hemorrhage. Cardiopulmonary resuscitation rarely, if ever, causes retinal hemorrhage, and when it does, just a few hemorrhages.

Differential Diagnosis

Some of the diagnoses besides AHT that should be considered include the following:

Accidental Trauma

Short falls do not cause the diffuse constellation of symptoms and physical signs described in this case.

Aneurysm

Ruptured aneurysm has been associated with widespread retinal hemorrhage in infants. This diagnosis is readily distinguished from AHT on neuroimaging.

Coagulation Defects

These conditions can be associated with mild hemorrhagic retinopathy but generally have a more central distribution. Other manifestations of bleeding sites are often present (eg, bruising). Coagulopathies can be confirmed by blood work.

Leukemia

Some forms of acute leukemia can cause severe hemorrhagic retinopathy, but this diagnosis would be readily evident on routine blood work. Patients usually also have retinal leukemic infiltrates.

Glutaric Aciduria Type 1

This metabolic disorder can mimic the subdural hemorrhage of AHT, but the brain injury is very different and shows a predisposition for the basal ganglia. Retinal hemorrhages are almost always few in number and confined to the area around the optic nerve or macular retina (posterior pole). Preexisting macrocephaly is a clinical feature in most affected children.

Meningitis or Sepsis

Retinal hemorrhages are almost always few in number and confined to the central retina. More severe retinal hemorrhages are only seen in fatal purulent meningitis.

When to Refer

Referral for pediatric ophthalmologic consultation is essential for all infants and toddlers in whom there is an unexplained alteration of mental status or other reason to suspect AHT.

Treatment

There is no treatment for the retinal hemorrhage of AHT. Retinal hemorrhage usually resolves without sequelae, although resolution rate is variable depending on the size and type of hemorrhage. Therefore, retinal hemorrhage cannot be used to date the time of injury with any specificity. The most common cause of visual loss in AHT is cortical visual impairment caused by the brain injury, followed by optic atrophy and less commonly, retinal scarring. Other associated ocular sequelae, such as amblyopia, may need treatment. Thus ophthalmologic follow-up is essential in short- and long-term management of AHT victims.

Prevention is the best treatment. Educating parents about the management of normal infant crying may be the most effective method to reduce the incidence of AHT.

Discussion

Evidence of prior child abuse may or may not be present in AHT. Outcomes in non-accidental head injury are worse than those of accidental head injury. Abusive head trauma has a high rate of morbidity and mortality.

Key Points

- When a child younger than 5 years presents with unexplained alteration of mental status, an abusive cause should be considered in the differential diagnosis.
- Diagnosis of abusive head trauma (AHT) can be difficult, particularly when presenting signs are nonspecific (eg, irritability) and there are no obvious external signs of trauma.
- Referral for pediatric ophthalmologic consultation is essential for all infants and toddlers in whom there is an unexplained alteration of mental status or other reason to suspect AHT.

Suggested Reading

Barr RG, Barr M, Fujiwara T, Conway J, Catherine N, Brant R. Do educational materials change knowledge and behaviour about crying and shaken baby syndrome? A randomized controlled trial. *CMAJ.* 2009;180(7):727–733

Levin AV. Retinal haemorrhages and child abuse. In: David TJ, ed. *Recent Advances in Paediatrics.* No. 18. London, England: Churchill Livingstone; 2000:151–219

Levin AV. Retinal hemorrhage in abusive head trauma. *Pediatrics.* 2010;126(5):961–970

Levin AV, Christian CW; American Academy of Pediatrics Committe on Child Abuse and Neglect and Section on Ophthalmology. The eye examination in the evaluation of child abuse. *Pediatrics.* 2010;126(2):376–380

McCabe CF, Donahue SP. Prognostic indicators for vision and mortality in shaken baby syndrome. *Arch Ophthalmol.* 2000;118(3):373–377

Morad Y, Kim YM, Mian M, Huyer D, Capra L, Levin AV. Nonophthalmologist accuracy in diagnosing retinal hemorrhages in the shaken baby syndrome. *J Pediatr.* 2003;142(4):431–434

Sturm V, Landau K, Menke MN. Optical coherence tomography findings in shaken baby syndrome. *Am J Ophthalmol.* 2008;146(3):363–368

Togioka BM, Arnold MA, Bathurst MA, et al. Retinal hemorrhages and shaken baby syndrome: an evidence-based review. *J Emerg Med.* 2009;37(1):98–106

Chapter 53

Black Eye

Andrea D. Molinari, MD

Presentation

An 8-year-old boy comes to the pediatrician's office after his right eye was injured with a wooden stick while he was playing with his classmates several hours earlier. No adult witnessed this accident, and it is not known how severe this injury might be or whether it involves the eye. The pediatrician can see that the child has a "black eye" and that both right eyelids are swollen. There is a small wound in the inner part of the upper eyelid (Figure 53-1).

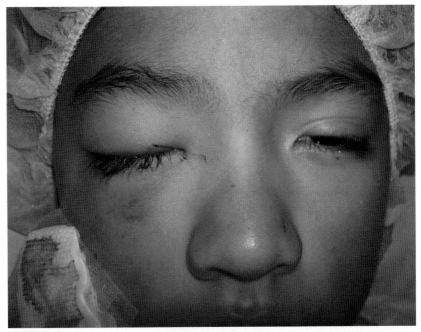

Figure 53-1. Swollen and ecchymotic right upper and lower eyelids with upper medial laceration. Courtesy of Andrea D. Molinari, MD.

Gently, the pediatrician tries to open both eyelids by resting his fingers on the bony orbital rim to assess integrity of the ocular globe. The pediatrician is mindful to not put any pressure on the eyeball itself (Figure 53-2). During examination, anesthetic eyedrops are administered to lessen eye pain and allow a better view of the injured eye. Examination of the eye reveals a wound compromising the temporal bulbar conjunctiva (Figure 53-3).

Although difficult to do, the pediatrician evaluates visual acuity in this eye, finding that the patient's vision is 20/25. This gives an idea how severely ocular function is affected as a consequence of trauma. Given the extent of injury, the pediatrician immediately sends this patient to an ophthalmologist.

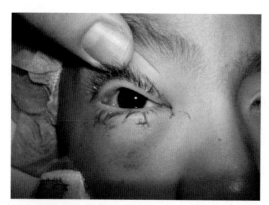

Figure 53-2. Technique to assess globe injury places gentle pressure on the orbital bones and not the globe. Courtesy of Andrea D. Molinari, MD.

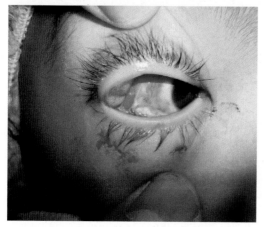

Figure 53-3. Conjunctival wound in patient with "black eye." Courtesy of Andrea D. Molinari, MD.

Diagnosis

Periorbital ecchymosis, more commonly known as a black eye, usually occurs from blunt force eye injuries that can happen in fighting, competitive sports, or at play, as in this case. If the object causing trauma is sharp enough, a wound in the eye or surrounding tissues can be seen, as in this patient.

Apparently insignificant wounds, such as the one seen in the superior eyelid of this patient, might involve important structures. In this case the superior tear duct is severed (Figure 53-4). If these tear duct lesions are not repaired immediately, permanent tearing of the eye can be seen, especially if the lower tear duct is compromised (see Chapter 51).

Swelling around the eye may hide severe injuries to the globe or facial skeleton, which if undiagnosed may lead to loss of vision, ocular motility disturbances, or facial deformity. See Chapter 50 for further information on examination and imaging of ocular injuries.

A black eye can be the external manifestation of more serious injuries, such as the following:
- Hyphema (presence of blood in anterior chamber of eye)
- Unsuspected retinal tears that can lead to retinal detachment
- Macular edema
- Orbital wall fracture causing limitation of eye movements or enophthalmos (backward displacement of eyeball into orbit) due to luxation of orbital content into the maxillary sinus (Figure 53-5)

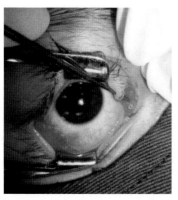

Figure 53-4. The small superior eyelid wound was compromising the superior tear duct, seen when the tear duct is probed with metal instrument and found to be noncontiguous. Courtesy of Andrea D. Molinari, MD.

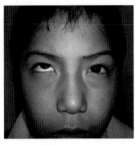
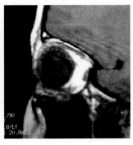

A

B

Figure 53-5. A, Limitation of elevation of left eye. **B,** Limitation is caused by entrapment of left inferior rectus muscle in an orbital floor fracture produced by blunt trauma. Courtesy of Andrea D. Molinari, MD.

A fracture deep inside the skull also can cause bilateral black eyes sometimes referred to as the raccoon sign, even though the ocular area itself was not injured.

Differential Diagnosis

Diagnoses besides traumatic periorbital ecchymosis that should be considered include the following:

Allergic Reaction

Reaction can be bilateral but might be unilateral, eg, there is no history of trauma but history of allergies and sometimes exposure to a cat or another animal. The patient complains of itching.

Orbital Cellulitis

With orbital cellulitis, there is often fever, general malaise, and a history of infection in the upper respiratory system but generally no history of trauma. See Chapter 16.

Skull Fracture

Black eye is usually bilateral and there is no history of direct trauma over the periocular area.

When to Refer

If injury in the eye or surrounding tissues is suspected or present in a child with a black eye, ensure that the patient is evaluated promptly by an ophthalmologist, ideally a pediatric ophthalmologist.

Treatment

In this case, the pediatrician patched the affected eye, gave the patient an immediate booster immunization with an anti-tetanus vaccine, covered him with general antibiotics, and referred him to the pediatric ophthalmologist. Surgery for repairing the eyelid, conjunctival wounds, and tear duct section was performed a day later under general anesthesia.

Whenever an injury in the eye or surrounding tissues is suspected, the pediatrician should initially patch the eye without applying any pressure. If there is no eye patch available, a small paper cup will suffice. Because there may be a perforating wound compromising the eye wall, antibiotic therapy should be started. Tetanus immunization should be reinforced with a booster immunization.

If no ancillary damage is noted, most black eyes heal completely and do not cause any problem to the eye. Treatment may include

- Application of cold compresses to the eye for the first 24 hours
- Warm compresses to the eye after the first 24 hours, until swelling resolves
- Keeping the child's head elevated during sleep to help decrease the amount of swelling

Discussion

Although black eyes are most often uncomplicated contusions, severe injury must always be ruled out. Blunt and penetrating trauma are major causes of visual loss. Prevent Blindness America states that about one-third of cases of eye loss in children younger than 10 years result from injury to the eye.

Key Points

- In a child with a black eye, if intraocular involvement is suspected or uncertain, ensure that the patient is evaluated promptly by a pediatric ophthalmologist.
- A black eye can be a sign of more serious ocular injury, such as hyphema, retinal tear, macular edema, or orbital wall fracture.
- Never press on an injured eye for examination or when covering with protection.

Suggested Reading

Macewen CJ. Eye injuries: a prospective survey of 5671 cases. *Br J Ophthalmol.* 1989;73(11):888–894

MacEwen CJ, Baines PS, Desai P. Eye injuries in children: the current picture. *Br J Ophthalmol.* 1999;83(8):933–936

McGwin G Jr, Xie A, Owsley C. Rate of eye injury in the United Sates. *Arch Ophthalmol.* 2005;123(7):970–976

Section 8

Abnormal Eye Movements/ Position

Chapter 54

Apparent In-turning of Eyes

Adele Marie Mediano Roa, MD
Shira L. Robbins, MD

Presentation

A young couple took their 18-month-old son to the pediatric clinic because they observed an in-turning of his eyes. The mother has seen this occasionally for close to a year and says it usually happens when the boy looks to the side. The father is not as sure. However, the grandmother, who is with them, is certain the child's eyes cross. She even brought photographs. These first-time parents claim that the child's eyes track well and he likes to look at colorful objects. The mother is Asian, and the father is white.

On entering the examination room, the pediatrician observes that both of the child's eyes seem slightly turned in and there is a wide nasal bridge and presence of an extra fold of skin on each side of the medial eyelid (Figure 54-1). The patient fixes and follows well, with full movements of each eye. The pediatrician shines a diffuse light on both eyes and sees that the corneal light reflex is symmetrically at the center of each pupil. The pediatrician alternately covers each eye while the patient looks at a toy (cover and cross-cover test), which shows eyes that are straight and stable. Further, the child is not unhappy when either eye is covered. Physical and neurologic findings as well as the medical history are all unremarkable.

Although the parents seem comfortable with the pediatrician's reassurances that the baby's eye alignment is normal, the grandmother is not. The pediatrician decides to refer them to a pediatric ophthalmologist.

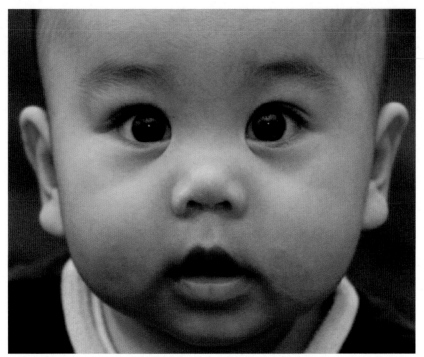

Figure 54-1. Presence of wide nasal bridge with extra fold of skin on medial side of each lid. Courtesy of Shira L. Robbins, MD, and Erika Acera, OC(C).

Diagnosis

The pediatric ophthalmologist confirms the pediatrician's conclusion. The child has a form of "fake" or pseudostrabismus; in this case, pseudoesotropia (eyes falsely appear to turn in).

Pseudoesotropia is the most common form of pseudostrabismus, which is the false appearance of strabismus despite normal eye alignment. Essentially this is an optical illusion. In pseudoesotropia there usually is a flat, wide nasal bridge and a prominent fold of skin on the medial aspect of the eyelid (epicanthal fold) covering the nasal sclera, making the eyes look in-turned. This apparent in-turning is more marked when the child looks to the side because as the eye moves nasally, it is covered under the extra fold of skin. On motility examination with the cover and cross-cover test, the eyes are straight (orthotropic), and no deviation is found. Corneal light reflexes for both eyes are at the center of each pupil. A gentle pinch and lift of the skin along the nasal bridge reveals normal alignment of the eyes because more of the nasal conjunctiva is visible.

This finding is more common in infancy and gradually improves as the child "grows a nose" and the nasal bridge narrows. A prominent epicanthal fold is a normal finding in those of Asian ancestry, but it is not abnormal in non-Asians. Pseudostrabismus is also present in those with narrow interpupillary distance and is more evident when the patient focuses at near objects.

Another form of pseudostrabismus is the presence of a positive or negative angle kappa. Angle kappa is the angle between line of sight and the corneal-pupillary axis. A negative angle kappa is found if the fovea (center of vision located on the retina) is displaced nasally. A light reflex is observed temporal to the center of the cornea, simulating an esodeviation (eyes turned in). When the fovea is temporal to the pupillary axis, corneal light reflex is seen nasally, simulating an exodeviation (eye deviated outward). This is called a positive angle kappa. It is found in retinopathy of prematurity because of cicatricial changes as the retina is pulled temporally from development of fibrovascular tissue of the anterior retina.

Differential Diagnosis

True strabismus can include eso- (inward), exo- (outward), or vertical deviations. Anatomic variations associated with pseudostrabismus (large epicanthal folds, wide nasal bridge, or close-set eyes) can also be present in cases of true strabismus, masking or augmenting the look of eye misalignment.

When to Refer

If there is any concern from parents or any doubt about diagnosis, children who appear to have strabismus despite normal results of ocular motility testing should have a complete eye examination from an ophthalmologist. A few of these patients could have true deviation of the visual axes.

Treatment

There is no real ocular deviation in pseudostrabismus, and thus no treatment is necessary other than parental reassurance.

Discussion

Although pseudostrabismus does not require treatment, it can easily be confused with true strabismus. Some forms of strabismus are intermittent and therefore not readily identified on a pediatrician's examination. These cases should be evaluated by an eye alignment specialist, with a pediatric ophthalmologist to make the call whether disease is present and treatment is needed. In cases of pseudostrabismus, reassurance by an ophthalmologist that there is no eye misalignment can be a powerful tool to counteract parent concern when they are seeing apparent eye crossing every day when they look at their child.

Key Points

- In pseudostrabismus, the eyes seem to be misaligned, but there is no real ocular deviation seen on cover and cross-cover test or Hirschberg reflex.
- Commonly found in Asians, a type of pseudostrabismus involves the presence of a wide nasal bridge and a prominent fold of skin on the medial aspect of each eyelid.
- As the child grows, this prominent epicanthal fold gradually improves and thus no treatment is necessary, but a complete ophthalmologic examination is still warranted.

Suggested Reading

American Academy of Ophthalmology. Pediatric ophthalmology and strabismus. In: *Basic and Clinical Science Course.* San Francisco, CA: American Academy of Ophthalmology; 2008

Spalton DJ, Hitchings RA, Hunter PA. *Atlas of Clinical Ophthalmology.* 3rd ed. St. Louis, MO: Mosby; 2004

Wright KW, Spiegel PH. *Pediatric Ophthalmology and Strabismus: The Requisites in Ophthalmology.* St. Louis, MO: Mosby; 1999

Chapter 55

Infant With Crossed Eyes

Shira L. Robbins, MD

Presentation

A 6-month-old girl is brought to the pediatrician's office because of an eye turning in over the past several months (Figure 55-1). Her grandmother first noticed it occurring occasionally at 1 month of age, but now it has become constant. Another pediatrician told them that the girl would "probably grow out of it." There is no family history of eye misalignment. Her health history is unremarkable.

On ocular motility testing with the cover test, the infant becomes fussy when her right eye is occluded. In-turning, or esotropia (manifest in-turning), seems about the same when she looks up, down, right, and

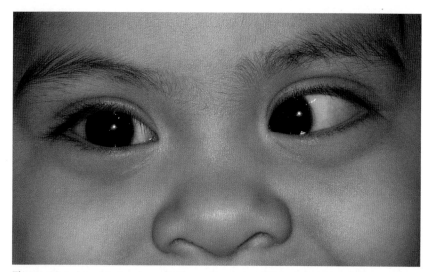

Figure 55-1. Large in-turning of left eye. Courtesy of Shira L. Robbins, MD.

left. The pediatrician tries to test her ability to abduct her eyes (move toward her ear) but finds it difficult to get her to maintain gaze on abduction. When the pediatrician covers her opposite eye, she abducts a little more, but movement is still not full. The pediatrician picks her up and spins her to see her ability to fully abduct her eyes.

Diagnosis

The pediatrician refers the patient to a pediatric ophthalmologist, who confirms the pediatrician's suspicion of unequal vision. The patient favors her right eye and therefore becomes fussy when it is covered.

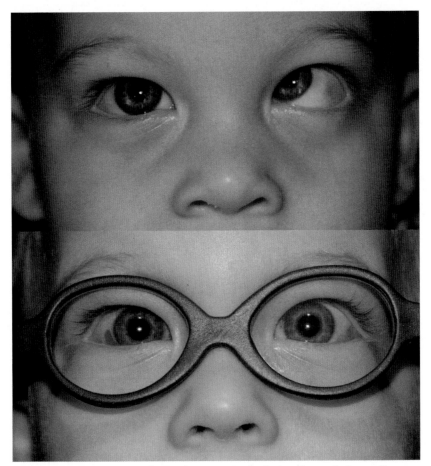

Figure 55-2. Another case of infantile esotropia displaying the vertical as well as horizontal misalignment preoperative and postoperative. Courtesy of Shira L. Robbins, MD.

Although both eyes turn inward, the left eye turns more. She also has a vertical component of her eye misalignment (Figure 55-2). She is moderately farsighted, with otherwise normal ocular anatomy.

This infant has infantile (sometimes called congenital) esotropia. This is defined as a large in-turning of the eyes before 6 months of life. Sometimes infantile esotropia does resolve on its own; however, most cases of eye in-turning that resolve during the first year of life are not this variety of esotropia. Until age 3 to 4 months, ocular alignment may be unstable due to typical neurologic and ocular development. In addition, the ciliary muscles responsible for focusing at different distances are not functioning optimally. The combination of eye movement, ciliary muscle, and visual immaturity commonly creates intermittent eye in-turning in normal infants. Another reason for an apparent esotropia that an infant grows out of is pseudoesotropia due to normal facial variations (see Chapter 54). Furthermore, the patient's left eye has amblyopia (poorer vision).

Unilateral or bilateral cranial sixth nerve paresis needs to be ruled out before making a diagnosis of infantile esotropia. Another potentially life-threatening disease, retinoblastoma, can also lead to early eye misalignment. (See "Differential Diagnosis" below.) Additional differential diagnoses are discussed in Chapter 60.

Differential Diagnosis

Diagnoses besides infantile esotropia that should be considered include the following:

Sixth Cranial Nerve Paresis

A sixth cranial nerve palsy can be caused by many diseases including an intracranial mass, raised intracranial pressure, Arnold-Chiari malformation, head trauma, and viral infection. Full abduction is demonstrated when the temporal conjunctiva is covered by the lateral canthus. This can be seen when the infant fixates on a toy or, if necessary, during the doll's head maneuver or its variation, the spin test. During the spin test, the infant's eyes should move opposite to the direction of spin. If a true abduction deficit is seen, neurologic examination and neuroimaging may be necessary.

Retinoblastoma

The esotropic type of strabismus is one of the many ways this eye tumor can be manifested. (See Chapter 24.)

Duane Syndrome

A rare strabismus syndrome caused by miswiring of the neurologic innervation of the eye muscles, Duane syndrome is the absence or hypoplasia of the abducens nucleus in combination with anomalous innervation of the lateral rectus muscle by a branch of the oculomotor nerve.

Nystagmus Blockage Syndrome

A rare condition in which the eyes wiggle (nystagmus), vision is improved when the eyes are crossed while looking in the distance. If the eyes are straightened surgically, the crossing will recur because the reason for crossing has not been changed.

When to Refer

Children older than 3 or 4 months whose eyes continue to turn in should be referred to a pediatric ophthalmologist. If a child is younger than 3 or 4 months but has a large, constant in-turning of the eyes, this patient also should be referred to a pediatric ophthalmologist because most of the cases of esotropia that resolve with age involve small angle or intermittent eye in-turning.

Treatment

Both eyes need to be looking at the same thing (straight) for good vision and depth perception to develop and be maintained in both eyes. Eyeglasses may be prescribed if the infant is severely farsighted, there is an asymmetry of refractive status, or as a temporizing treatment of alignment.

Amblyopia of the left eye is treated with an eye patch to improve vision in the amblyopic eye before eye-muscle surgery. Some surgeons may choose to realign eyes during patching treatment if the amount of esotropia is extreme. Because there are some cases of spontaneous resolution, repeated measurements of eye misalignment are necessary to establish stability before eye-muscle surgery is undertaken. Optimal timing of surgical alignment is controversial. There are an increasing number of studies that suggest the earlier the surgical procedure, the better potential for visual and depth perception outcomes, ranging from realignment by 3 to 6 to 12 months. Given the timing of anatomic ocular and neurologic maturation, referral and treatment to a pediatric ophthalmologist by the earliest time frame mentioned can be impractical. This patient underwent amblyopia patching treatment and subsequent eye muscle surgical realignment. Figure 55-3 shows her 1 month after surgery.

Discussion

Infantile esotropia can be challenging to treat. These patients can overrespond or under-respond to horizontal eye muscle surgery. This condition can also lead to vertical eye misalignment as a child grows older. This may require additional eye-muscle surgeries. Nystagmus (eye wiggling) with monocular occlusion is associated with this condition and may result in a small anomalous head position. Over an extended time, instability of the ocular motor system may again necessitate further surgery.

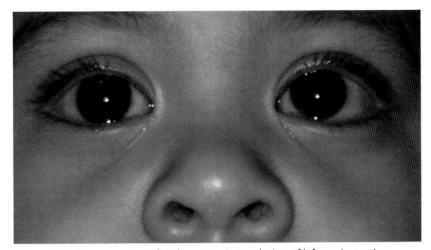

Figure 55-3. Postoperative infantile esotropia; resolution of left eye in-turning. Courtesy of Shira L. Robbins, MD.

Key Points

- Sixth cranial nerve paresis and retinoblastoma must be considered in an infant with in-turned eyes.
- By 3 to 4 months of age, infants should be able to maintain straight eyes except when looking at something very close to their face.
- If a child is younger than 3 to 4 months but has large, constant in-turning of the eyes, the child should be referred to a pediatric ophthalmologist.
- Because studies have shown that earlier surgical realignment leads to better outcomes, it is important that these infants are referred to a pediatric ophthalmologist early to start the process of diagnosis and treatment.

Suggested Reading

Birch EE, Stager DR Sr. Long-term motor and sensory outcomes after early surgery for infantile esotropia. *J AAPOS.* 2006;10(5):409–413

El-Sahn M, Robbins SL. Infantile esotropia. EyeWiki. http://eyewiki. aao.org/Infantile_Esotropia. Updated June 5, 2011. Accessed May 8, 2012

Ing MR, Okino LM. Outcome study of stereopsis in relation to duration of misalignment in congenital esotropia. *J AAPOS.* 2002;6(1):3–8

Pediatric Disease Investigator Group. Spontaneous resolution of early-onset esotropia: experience of the Congenital Esotropia Observational Study. *Am J Ophthalmol.* 2002;133(1):109–118

von Noorden GK. *Binocular Vision and Ocular Motility: Theory and Management of Strabismus.* 6th ed. St. Louis, MO: Mosby; 2002:322

Wright KW, Edelman PM, McVey JH, Terry AP, Lin M. High-grade stereo acuity after early surgery for congenital esotropia. *Arch Ophthalmol.* 1994;112(7):913–919

Chapter 56

Intermittent Cross-eye

Elysa A. Brown, MD, MS
Edward W. Brown, MD

Presentation

A 2-year-old girl is brought to the pediatrician's office by her mother who has observed her child's right eye crossing. She first noticed the crossing when her child was ill with a cold 3 weeks ago. She notices that the crossing is intermittent and is more prominent when the child looks at objects up close. The mother states that the child rubs her right eye and often becomes frustrated with visual tasks when she is tired. The only notable family history is that her father is farsighted and began wearing glasses at age 3. The girl's visual history has been unremarkable until now. She is otherwise developing normally and has been healthy except for her recent cold.

The child is given a toy to play with, and as she looks at it, her right eye crosses. When she looks at the nurse across the room, her right eye continues to cross. The pediatrician looks at her corneal light reflexes and notices that the light reflex is centered in her left eye but is displaced temporally in her right eye (Figure 56-1). As the child looks at the nurse across the room, the pediatrician occludes her right eye with a hand, and the gaze of her left eye remains fixed. While occluding the left eye, the pediatrician notices a shift of her right eye as it re-fixates on the nurse. The girl also seems a bit fussy when the pediatrician covers her left eye.

Diagnosis

Based on the findings and history, the pediatrician tells the mother that her child has esotropia, which is acquired, and also mentions the possibility of amblyopia in her right eye. A referral to a pediatric ophthalmologist for further assessment and treatment is recommended.

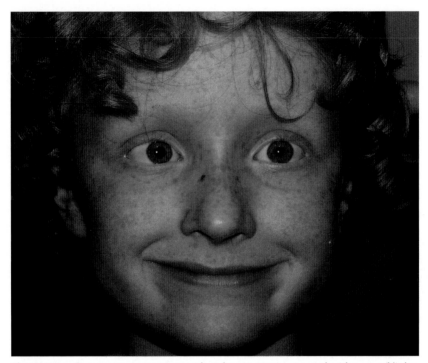

Figure 56-1. Representative patient with right eye turning inward with corneal light reflex temporal in right pupil. Courtesy of Shira L. Robbins, MD.

At the pediatric ophthalmologist's office, a comprehensive eye examination is performed on the child. Her visual acuity is checked using a picture chart with crowding bars. Visual acuity in the right eye is found to be less than that in her left eye. The magnitude of the misalignment is measured at distance and near fixation. Extraocular muscle testing shows full abduction (movement toward the ear) in each eye. A cycloplegic refraction is performed, and a large amount of hyperopia (farsightedness) is confirmed in each eye. Retinal nerves, vessels, and maculae are examined and found to be normal.

In the consultation letter to the pediatrician, the ophthalmologist explains that the child's esotropia appears to be accommodative (focusing) in nature because of the large amount of hyperopia. Amblyopia is present in the right eye. The letter explains that other common causes of esotropia were ruled out based on the findings. These include a sixth nerve palsy because her abduction functions are normal, and a sensory esotropia because the right eye is healthy.

Differential Diagnosis

Diagnoses besides accommodative esotropia that should be considered include the following:

Sixth Nerve Palsy

Abduction functions are abnormal in a sixth cranial nerve palsy but are normal in accommodative esotropia.

Sensory Non-accommodative Esotropia

In this type of esotropia, a tumor or severe ocular abnormality is present, whereas the eye is healthy in accommodative esotropia.

Non-accommodative Acquired Esotropia

In non-accommodative acquired esotropia, glasses do not control mis-alignment and surgery is needed to realign the eyes. The child is usually older and a brain tumor must be ruled out with magnetic resonance imaging.

When to Refer

Children suspected of accommodative esotropia should be referred as early as possible to a pediatric ophthalmologist for further evaluation to prevent amblyopia, restore binocular functions, and rule out more serious causes of strabismus.

Treatment

The pediatric ophthalmologist prescribes eyeglasses for full-time wear to correct the girl's hyperopia. Patching of the left eye is to be started when she can tolerate glasses. The pediatric ophthalmologist warns the mother that results may not be immediate and that a maximum result can take months to achieve. Follow-up examination to check her alignment and vision in glasses is scheduled in 2 months.

Discussion

Maintenance of ocular alignment is a balance between convergence (inward movement) and divergence (outward movement) functions. In accommodative esotropia, convergence function exceeds the weaker divergence function because of accommodative (focusing) effort. Reducing accommodative effort restores proper balance between convergence and divergence functions.

Early correction of the child's refractive error is paramount to relieve accommodative effort, stabilize ocular alignment, and reestablish binocular vision (Figure 56-2). Amblyopia, when present, is best treated with patching of the dominant eye. Follow-up examinations should be scheduled at intervals determined by the child's progress.

Glasses are typically sufficient treatment for accommodative esotropia. However, surgery may be needed in children whose eye alignment is

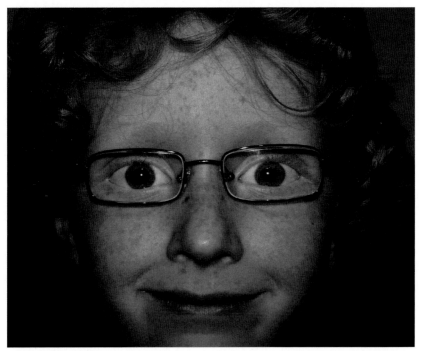

Figure 56-2. Representative patient with esotropia corrected with full farsighted eyeglasses, as seen by equal corneal light reflexes. Courtesy of Shira L. Robbins, MD.

only partially corrected initially with glasses or subsequently decompensates after wearing glasses. Bilateral medial rectus muscle recession is generally the surgical procedure of choice for correcting an in-turning ocular misalignment. In this surgery, the medial rectus muscle is removed from its original insertion point and reattached posterior to the original insertion point at a distance that is determined by preoperative measurements. The larger the deviation, the further posterior the medial rectus is attached. Despite proper muscle alignment, eyeglasses continue to be worn in most children following strabismus surgery for continued correction of existing refractive error and to prevent further crossing of the eyes.

Key Points

- Accommodative esotropia is a common form of strabismus seen in children and can usually be resolved with correction of the accompanying refractive error.
- Children suspected of accommodative esotropia should be referred as early as possible to a pediatric ophthalmologist to prevent amblyopia, restore binocular functions, and rule out more serious causes of strabismus.
- Eyeglasses are typically sufficient treatment for accommodative esotropia, but some children may need surgery.

Suggested Reading

American Academy of Ophthalmology. *Preferred Practice Pattern Guidelines: Esotropia and Exotropia.* San Francisco, CA: American Academy of Ophthalmology; 2007:3–14

Donahue SP. Clinical practice. Pediatric strabismus. *N Engl J Med.* 2007;356(10):1040–1047

Duane T, William T, Jaeger E. *Duane's Clinical Ophthalmology on DVD-ROM.* Philadelphia, PA: Lippincott Williams and Wilkins; 2011

Heidar K. Accommodative estropia. EyeWiki. http://eyewiki.aao.org/Accommodative_Esotropia. Modified June 5, 2011. Accessed June 6, 2012

Repka MX, Connett JE, Scott WE. The one-year surgical outcome after prism adaptation for the management of acquired esotropia. *Ophthalmology.* 1996;103(6):922–928

Chapter 57

Eyes Walking Away

Adele Marie Mediano Roa, MD
David B. Granet, MD
Shira L. Robbins, MD

Presentation

A man brings his 5-year-old son to the pediatrician's office because he has a persistent cough. He reports that the mother said the boy had a fever over the weekend and became worried because she saw his left eye drifting outward a couple of times. Although the father has never noticed this before, the mother told him to relay that she has seen the eye drift out in the past, just "not this much." The episodes last a few seconds and are mostly in the evening when their son is tired, day-dreaming, or simply zoning out, or when he watches television. Now that he is sick, it has been happening more often and longer than previously. The pediatrician asks the boy how his eyes feel, and he says, "My eyes are going crazy, like [they're] walking away, and I have to bring them back in."

The pediatrician does a thorough physical examination, and findings confirm an upper respiratory tract infection. Results of the neurologic examination as well as past medical history are unremarkable. There is no family history of strabismus (ocular misalignment), and the father is nearsighted. On ocular evaluation, the boy's visual acuity is 20/30 in both eyes, with full movements on all cardinal gazes. The pediatrician shines a light on both eyes and notes the corneal light reflex to be at the center of each pupil. When the pediatrician brings a pencil tip toward the boy's face, he furrows his brow but can follow it all the way in. The pediatrician covers one of the patient's eyes for a few seconds while the boy looks in the distance. When the pediatrician uncovers the eye, it is now looking off temporally (Figure 57-1).

Because of this eye alignment problem, the pediatrician decides to refer the boy to a pediatric ophthalmologist.

Diagnosis

At the ophthalmologist's office, evaluation of visual acuity, depth perception, and fusional control; eye alignment; refraction; and anatomic evaluation of the anterior and posterior (through dilation) parts of the eye are done. The boy presents with his usual good eye alignment interrupted by an episodic outward deviation of one eye occurring when he was sick, daydreaming, and tired—all characteristic of an intermittent exotropia which can be easily observed on alignment testing.

Intermittent exotropia is a type of strabismus observed as an outward drifting of an eye interspersed with periods of orthotropia (good alignment). Intermittent exotropia usually occurs early, before age 5 years, but it may be detected for the first time even later in childhood. It is often first observed by parents during periods of visual inattentiveness. The drifting becomes apparent when children are tired, sick, or drowsy from certain medications. Interestingly watching television can also bring out this deviation. Adults also manifest the deviation during these circumstances as well as during alcohol intoxication. Other

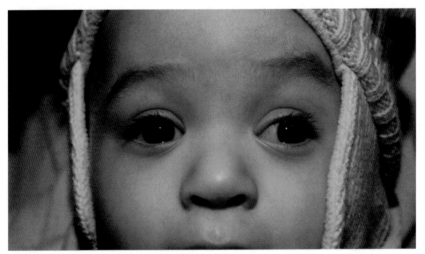

Figure 57-1. Representative photo of left eye exotropia seen after cover test. Note the different position of the corneal light reflex in the pupil/iris view. Courtesy of Shira L. Robbins, MD.

symptoms include asthenopia (eyestrain), blurring of vision, headache, difficulty with prolonged reading, and sometimes even diplopia (double vision). Squinting in bright light secondary to photophobia (light sensitivity) is commonly seen. This is thought to be a way of eliminating diplopia or confusion when exotropia is manifest.

It is an intermittent deviation because the tendency of the eye to wander is controlled by the desire to fuse the images (both eyes move nasally to fuse images into one), which keeps eyes aligned. Initially, it is a latent deviation (heterophoria) but may progress to an intermittently manifest deviation. During the latent phase, eyes are aligned most of the time, allowing them to develop good binocularity; exodeviation occurs only when there is poor fusional control in situations such as being sick and tired. The deviation may progress to become intermittently manifest and even constant, lasting for longer periods even with the slightest visual inattention. Young children with an immature visual system suppress the image of the deviated eye to eliminate double vision. Therefore, even when this occurs seemingly at a later age, lack of diplopia is reassuring that the drift is not a new phenomenon. Older children may complain of more bothersome symptoms such as asthenopia, reading difficulties, headache, blurred vision, and confusion. Amblyopia (lazy eye) is uncommon unless the exotropia progresses to constant or nearly constant exotropia at an early age or another amblyogenic factor is present.

Evaluation of control of intermittent exotropia can be done at the pediatrician's office by asking about frequency, duration, and circumstances when it occurs. Subjectively, the parent (or guardian) and physician can qualitatively assess whether alignment control is good, fair, or poor. Following are some guidelines to help with this assessment:

1. **Excellent:** Deviation is manifest uncommonly, less than 5% to 10% of waking hours, and only at distance or while daydreaming or fatigued.
2. **Good:** Deviation is manifest less than 5 times a day and only at distance.
3. **Fair:** Deviation is seen more than 5 times a day at distance, but near control of the deviation is maintained.
4. **Poor:** The patient breaks into exotropia frequently, at distance and at near, and only occasionally are the eyes straight.

The ophthalmologist can confirm good control of fusion through cover testing. Good fusional control in light of an intermittent exotropia will test as follows: when an eye is covered the eye will turn outward, and when the cover is removed the eye will resume fusion (straighten) rapidly without the need for a blink or fixation. Patients who blink or fixate to control deviation after disruption with cover testing have fair control. The patient who breaks spontaneously without any form of fusion disruption has poor control.

Differential Diagnosis

Diagnoses besides intermittent exotropia that should be considered include the following:

- Duane syndrome
- Cranial nerve palsy
- Brown syndrome
- Internuclear ophthalmoplegia
- Trauma
- Myasthenia gravis

When to Refer

For a child suspected of having an intermittent exotropia, early referral to an ophthalmologist is fundamental. Treatment depends on the child's ability to keep the eyes straight and on the level of depth perception developed.

Treatment

Treatment of exophoria (tendency to drift out) and intermittent and constant exodeviation is generally nonsurgical initially. Medical approaches may also be used to create optimal sensory conditions before surgery or when surgery must be postponed, to reinforce fusion during the waiting interval.

Large refractive errors (need for glasses), especially astigmatism and anisometropia (differences in refractive power between the eyes), should be corrected in patients with intermittent exodeviations, to create sharp retinal images, which in turn increase the stimulus to fuse (hold the eyes straight). Another way eyeglasses are used in this condition is to harness the relationship between focusing and alignment by inducing convergence to counteract the exotropia. This is done by prescribing 2 to 3 diopters of nearsighted correction in excess of what is required for good sight. This under-correction of hyperopia (farsightedness) or overcorrection of myopia (nearsightedness) can control the deviation by encouraging convergence when patients accommodate (focus at near).

Part-time monocular occlusion by patching of the dominant eye will force the patient to give attention to the image of the non-preferred eye, eliminating suppression and improving control. Alternate patching can be done when there is equal preference for both eyes.

Prisms are used to neutralize small deviations. In time, however, patients will require more prisms as they gradually develop an increasing exotropic angle. Convergence exercises like pencil push-ups or home computer exercises are used for the type of intermittent exotropia that is worse at near (convergence insufficiency).

When the deviation progresses to become manifest and constant or nearly constant, occurring more than 30% to 50% of waking hours with deteriorating control, surgical treatment may well be needed. Even now the optimal time to perform surgery is complicated. For this reason, control of the deviation is used as the guide for surgery rather than the age of the child.

Discussion

With time the deviation is likely to recur, even with surgery. This should not preclude the role of surgical realignment as it can often be effective in maintaining good visual development. Additionally, children with intermittent exotropia have recently been shown to be almost 3 times more likely to experience a psychiatric disorder later in life than youngsters without this diagnosis. Pediatricians should keep these risks in mind.

Key Points

- Intermittent exotropia is drifting out of an eye interspersed with periods of good alignment; the exotropia typically is apparent during visual inattentiveness.
- This condition can progress from latent deviation to become intermittent, then constant.
- Early referral to an ophthalmologist is fundamental because management depends on the child's ability to keep the eyes straight and the level of depth perception developed.
- Initial treatment is nonsurgical; however, it is not unusual for the condition to worsen despite medical treatment, necessitating surgical intervention.

Suggested Reading

American Academy of Ophthalmology. Pediatric ophthalmology and strabismus. In: *Basic and Clinical Science Course.* San Francisco, CA: American Academy of Ophthalmology; 2008

Rosenbaum AL. *Clinical Strabismus Management: Principles and Surgical Technique.* Philadelphia, PA: Saunders; 1999

Taylor D, Hoyt C, eds. *Pediatric Ophthalmology and Strabismus.* 3rd ed. Edinburgh, United Kingdom: Elsevier Saunders; 2005

von Noorden GK. *Binocular Vision and Ocular Motility: Theory and Management of Strabismus.* St. Louis, MO: Mosby; 2002

Wright KW, Spiegel PH. *Pediatric Ophthalmology and Strabismus.* 2nd ed. New York, NY: Springer-Verlag; 2003

Chapter 58

Smaller Turned-out Eye

Adele Marie Mediano Roa, MD
Shira L. Robbins, MD

Presentation

A 3-month-old infant is brought to the pediatric clinic because the parents noticed that the "left eye looks smaller than the right, and it turns out a bit." They originally noted this when the baby was 3 days of age. Prenatal history was unremarkable, but there was a forceps delivery. No pertinent unusual medical or family history is provided by the parents. Developmental milestones are on target for age. Results of a thorough (non-ocular) physical and neurologic examination are normal.

The pediatrician observes that the left upper eyelid is droopy, rather than the eyeball being small. When looking straight ahead, the left eye looks lower and turned out, with the upper eyelid covering most of the eye. The right upper eyelid rests slightly below the superior border of the cornea. The pediatrician checks vision by having the baby fixate and follow an object as the pediatrician moves it slowly. The baby is fussy, so examination is difficult. However, a preference for the right eye is noted because the left eye is constantly turned out and the right eye maintains intermittent fixation on the target. The pediatrician observes the patient's eye movements by lifting up the left upper eyelid and finding that the left eye has limitations in moving nasally, superiorly, and inferiorly (Figure 58-1). The right eye has full ocular movements. Pupil examination with use of a penlight shows a larger left pupil with an afferent pupillary defect.

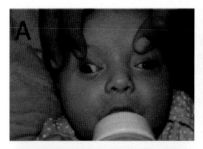
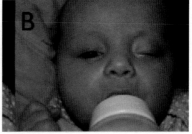
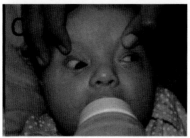

Figure 58-1. Representative photo. A, In attempted right gaze, left eye unable to adduct or look towards nose. B, Complete eyelid ptosis of left upper eyelid when patient looking straight ahead. C, Left gaze, left eye able to abduct (move temporally). Courtesy of Shira L. Robbins, MD.

Diagnosis

The pediatrician suspects a cranial nerve (CN) palsy, possibly congenital in origin, and emergently refers the newborn to a pediatric ophthalmologist and neurologist. The infant has presented with a droopy upper eyelid (blepharoptosis); an eye that is lower and turned out with limitations in adduction (moving nasally), supraduction (elevation), and infraduction (depression); and a larger pupil with an afferent papillary defect characteristic of a third CN (oculomotor) palsy. Some third CN palsies present without eyelid or pupil involvement. Onset was during the child's first year of life, and a history of traumatic birth is present. There are no associated neurologic deficits such as hemiparesis, seizures, or difficulty of speech, and non-ocular physical findings are normal, signifying that this condition could be congenital.

At the pediatric ophthalmology clinic, a thorough eye examination is performed. Examination includes tests of visual acuity, fixation preference, stereopsis, alignment, and ocular rotations, as well as dilated retinal examination, cycloplegic refraction, evaluation for amblyopia, and pupil examination. Severity of the ptosis, and therefore the extent of occlusion of the visual axis, is also assessed because the amblyopia process can begin quickly in children.

A third CN palsy can be partial or complete. It is easy to identify a complete third CN palsy by the presence of a closed eyelid, nonreactive dilated pupil, and down-and-out position of the eye caused by peripheral involvement. A central complete third CN palsy spares the pupil. Pupil involvement is a red flag for presence of a cerebral aneurysm; however, cerebral aneurysm should not be excluded as an underlying cause for pupil-sparing third CN palsies.

Partial third CN palsy is a diagnostic challenge because it can present with many associated signs. Numerous patterns can therefore arise, and oculomotor nerve palsies, such as abducens (sixth CN) and trochlear nerve (fourth CN) palsies, must be distinguished from myasthenia gravis and mechanical restrictions. Ocular fibrosis and monocular elevation defects may also look like third CN palsies. Clinical correlation of the history and physical and neurologic findings will help guide the physician to the appropriate evaluation. Neurologic deficits almost always accompany a complete third CN palsy.

A congenital third CN palsy is usually an isolated, incomplete, and unilateral form of palsy. Still, a thorough physical and neurologic examination should be performed. Presence of neurologic signs warrants neuroimaging.

An acquired third CN palsy must be fully evaluated with neuroimaging. When a third CN palsy acquired in childhood cannot be explained on the basis of clinical findings or noninvasive neuroimaging, cerebrospinal fluid should be evaluated and angiography performed.

Differential Diagnosis

Diagnoses besides third CN palsy that should be considered include the following:

- Juvenile myasthenia gravis
- Mechanical restriction
- Ocular fibrosis
- Monocular elevation defect

When to Refer

Children with pupil-involving third CN palsy accompanied by neurologic signs require a complete neurologic evaluation and should be referred to a pediatric neurologist. Referral for neuroimaging of the brain is necessary in all cases of suspected acquired childhood third CN palsy.

Treatment

Treatment of the underlying cause should be addressed (see "Discussion" below for causes). Ptosis, eye misalignment, and loss of accommodation (focusing at near) of the affected eye may prevent development of binocular vision and stereopsis. This can lead to amblyopia as well. In children who have onset of third CN palsy before visual maturity, attainment of good visual acuity may be adversely influenced by development of strabismus and deprivation amblyopia as well as inability to accommodate. This should be addressed through patching of the good eye once the affected eyelid is high enough to clear the pupil.

There is no definite treatment of the loss of nerve function. Thus, the physician must observe the patient for any recovery of third CN function and stabilization of the deviation for 6 to 12 months before any surgical intervention. Surgical intervention, through repair of ptosis to clear the visual axis and realignment of the eye through strabismus surgery, may be performed if needed. The greater the loss of function, the less likely the patient is to achieve normal eye movements or binocular vision despite surgical intervention.

Discussion

Third CN palsy in childhood is uncommon. However, the most common type is congenital (40% to 50%), followed by trauma, inflammation, viral infection, migraine, and infrequently, neoplastic lesions. Factors causing congenital palsy include difficult delivery, neonatal hypoxia, or absence of the nerve itself. Major head trauma with or without skull injury is a common cause of third CN palsy in children. Inflammatory causes include meningitis and encephalitis accompanied by systemic signs of illness. A third CN palsy associated with migraine is transient, and nerve function recovers within a few months without permanent damage. Other causes of third CN palsy include vascular disorders such as aneurysms and diabetes mellitus, but these are more commonly found in adults.

The oculomotor nerve innervates most of the extraocular muscles, including the medial rectus, superior rectus, inferior rectus, and inferior oblique muscles, as well as the musculus levator palpebrae superioris (levator muscle of the upper eyelid), pupillary sphincter muscles, and ciliary body inside the eye. Improper function of these muscles is responsible for the limitation of ocular rotations, eyelid ptosis, pupil dilation, and focusing inability. The eye is in a characteristic down-and-out position because the lateral rectus muscle (innervation by sixth CN) and superior oblique muscle (fourth CN) are unopposed.

Key Points

- Third cranial nerve (CN) palsy in children is uncommon and usually has a congenital cause.
- A down-and-out position of the eye with limitations in adduction, supraduction, and infraduction; eyelid ptosis; and pupil dilation are characteristic of this CN palsy.
- Pupil-involving third CN palsy is always accompanied by neurologic signs. Thus, a complete neurologic evaluation should be done, and findings may warrant the need for further neuroimaging.
- Routine or emergency neuroimaging, such as contrast-enhanced computed tomography or magnetic resonance imaging of the brain, is necessary in all cases of acquired childhood third CN palsy and may be considered in other cases.
- Amblyopia and loss of stereopsis are important sequelae that should be managed by occlusion therapy, strabismus surgery, and ptosis repair.
- Recovery of nerve function may take 6 to 12 months, which makes observation before surgical intervention a wise choice.

Suggested Reading

American Academy of Ophthalmology. Pediatric ophthalmology and strabismus. In: *Basic and Clinical Science Course.* San Francisco, CA: American Academy of Ophthalmology; 2008

Schumacher-Feero LA, Yoo KW, Solari FM, Biglan AW. Third cranial nerve palsy in children. *Am J Ophthalmol.* 1999;128(2):216–221

Wright KW, Spiegel PH. *Pediatric Ophthalmology and Strabismus: The Requisites in Ophthalmology.* 2nd ed. St Louis, MO: Mosby; 1995

Wright KW, Spiegel PH. *Pediatric Ophthalmology and Strabismus.* 2nd ed. New York, NY: Springer; 2003

Chapter 59

Head Tilt and Eye Misalignment

Adele Marie Mediano Roa, MD
Shira L. Robbins, MD

Presentation

Parents of a 6-year-old boy have observed over the past few months
that the child's head is slightly tilted to the right. The pediatrician
observes the head position and agrees that there is a tilt to the right. In
addition to this, the pediatrician notices a slight facial asymmetry—a
shortened right side of the face compared with the left. The pediatrician
asks the parents for old photographs of the child and sees that the head
tilt was present as early as late infancy, signifying the possibility that it
could be congenital. There is no history of head trauma or any family
history of eye misalignment. The pediatrician asks the parents if they
ever notice any eye misalignment. The parents state they occasionally
see the left eye go up and in toward the side of the nose.

The pediatrician performs a thorough physical and neurologic examination and finds nothing abnormal. Testing of visual acuity demonstrates 20/20 in both eyes. The child has good visual fixation and tracks
objects well. When his head is held totally centered and he is looking
straight ahead, his left eye is higher than the right. This is more obvious
when the pediatrician shines a penlight on the eyes and sees an unequal
corneal light reflex. When the child closes one eye, the pediatrician
observes that the head tilt improves. Then the pediatrician moves the
patient's head from side to side while the boy's eyes are closed and
notes normal neck range of motion. The pediatrician suspects an
ocular cause of this patient's torticollis and refers him to a pediatric
ophthalmologist.

Diagnosis

The child has presented with an anomalous head posture that improves spontaneously when one eye is closed. Range of motion of the neck is normal, and facial asymmetry is present. Thus, ocular-caused torticollis is suspected.

At the ophthalmology office, a pediatric ophthalmologist performs a complete eye examination. Examination includes testing of visual acuity, depth perception, eye alignment, dilated retinal examination, cycloplegic refraction, and evaluation for presence of amblyopia. The patient's visual acuity is good. Results of the ocular motility examination show that the left eye is higher (hypertropia) than the right when looking straight ahead. Hypertropia worsens on gaze to the right as well as when the head is tilted toward the left shoulder. A marked in-turning of the left eye is noted when the boy looks up slightly to the right (over-action of the left inferior oblique muscle). All these findings confirm a palsy of the fourth cranial nerve (trochlear nerve) that normally inner-vates the superior oblique (SO) muscle of the left eye.

Typically, the SO muscle intorts (superior part of the eye rotates nasally) the eye when it is abducted (eye moved temporally) and depresses the eye when it is adducted (eye moved nasally). Thus, when this muscle is weakened, the affected eye is hyper-deviated (higher than unaffected eye), with the hyper-deviation worse in down-gaze and gaze toward the nose. Therefore, these patients are most often symptomatic while reading.

A distinction needs to be made between unilateral and bilateral SO palsies. In unilateral SO palsy, the patient manifests hypertropia (eye deviates superiorly) increasing on gaze to the contralateral side (Figure 59-1) and an abnormal head posture with the head tilted away from the affected eye. There is an under-action of the SO muscle and a resulting overaction of the antagonist, inferior oblique muscle, seen best when the eye goes up and in. Therefore, a left SO palsy shows a left hypertropia that worsens on gaze to the right and adopts a compensatory head tilt to the right (away from the affected eye).

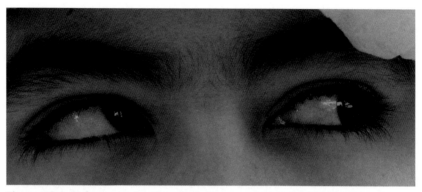

Figure 59-1. Right eye higher than the left eye on gaze to the left. Courtesy of Shira L. Robbins, MD.

Bilateral SO palsy manifests as hyper-deviation on gaze to either side that reverses on head tilt. This reversing head tilt shows the left eye higher on head tilt to the left and the right eye higher on head tilt to the right. It is associated with bilateral under-action of the SO muscle and bilateral overaction of the inferior oblique muscle.

Abnormal head posture is a common sign of SO palsy, as it is a compensatory mechanism. When the head is tilted, the eyes align, fusing what is seen into one image and therefore avoiding bothersome double vision. Presence of facial asymmetry with shallowing of midface region between the lateral canthus and edge of the mouth is characteristic of congenital SO palsy (Figure 59-2).

The most common cause of unilateral fourth nerve palsy is congenital. It has been observed in congenital SO palsy that the tendon is usually lax, long, and posteriorly inserted, or even may be absent. Because facial asymmetry in SO palsy is very strong evidence that torticollis dates to infancy, its presence may preclude the need for an expensive and unnecessary neurologic evaluation. Other symptoms that can be associated with this palsy are diplopia (double vision), asthenopia (eye strain), and amblyopia (lazy eye) of the hyper-deviated eye.

Acquired fourth nerve palsy has a number of causes, the most common of which is trauma secondary to a closed head injury. Other acquired causes include increased intracranial pressure, intracranial neoplasm, meningitis, mastoiditis, arteriovenous malformation, vascular disease,

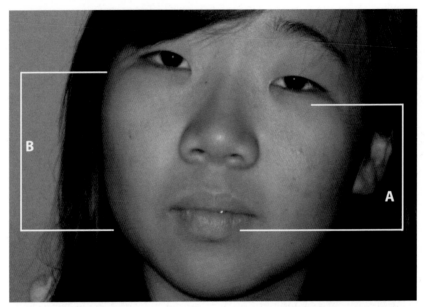

Figure 59-2. Representative image of patient with head tilt. Shows head tilt to the left, with alignment of both eyes (A) and shallowing of midfacial region of the left side as compared with the right (B). Courtesy of David B. Granet, MD.

demyelinating disease, herpes zoster ophthalmicus, diabetes mellitus, and iatrogenesis.

There are several other causes of torticollis (discussed in Chapter 86), and differentiating between an ocular and a neuromuscular torticollis is important. One way is to ask the patient to close one or both eyes and observe if head tilt improves (straightens). If it does improve, an ocular cause is more likely. Another method of differentiation is to have the patient close his or her eyes and move the neck from side to side to check for its range of motions. If range of motion is full, it reduces the likelihood of a neuromuscular cause.

Differential Diagnosis

Diagnoses besides congenital fourth cranial nerve palsy that should be considered include the following:

Congenital Neuromuscular Torticollis

Torticollis is likely to be neuromuscular if the head tilt persists when either eye is closed or covered and when the examiner is unable to passively tilt the head in the opposite direction.

Juvenile Cerebral Palsy, Juvenile Onset Wilson Disease, Juvenile Onset Huntington Disease, Severe Gastroesophogeal Reflux, Tonsillar/Retropharyngeal Abscess

All of these generally have other physical signs and symptoms associated with them.

When to Refer

If an ocular torticollis is suspected, referral to a pediatric ophthalmologist should follow. A referral might also be needed to an orthopedist, physical therapist, gastroenterologist, or other specialists depending the clinical suspicion.

Treatment

Neutralization of refractive errors (with eyeglasses) and treatment of amblyopia should be addressed appropriately before any intervention of the SO palsy. A patient with small hypertropia, a tolerable head tilt, and no bothersome symptoms may not need any treatment. In acquired-type SO palsy, the patient is observed for 6 months before strabismus surgery is considered to allow for recovery and stabilization of the deviation. For patients complaining of double vision, relief can be achieved through the use of prisms or monocular occlusion. However, prolonged occlusion can create amblyopia.

Strabismic surgical intervention is indicated in the presence of any of the following: a large deviation associated with diplopia, a worsening or unacceptable head tilt, marked facial asymmetry, and contraction of neck muscles. Physical therapy to alter the habitual head position may be required.

Discussion

Most isolated fourth nerve palsies are congenital. Thus, a review of old family photographs showing long-standing head tilt (sometimes called a "family album tomography" [FAT] scan) or simply eliciting a history of symptoms of many years' duration is sufficient to rule out an acute acquired process. Neurologic evaluation and imaging may be indicated when the palsy is associated with additional neurologic deficits; otherwise, diagnosis and management can be based solely on clinical findings.

Key Points

- Presence of a head tilt and facial asymmetry are signs to consider a diagnosis of superior oblique (SO) muscle palsy.
- Differentiation between ocular torticollis and neuromuscular abnormality of the neck should be established. Once an ocular torticollis is considered, referral to a pediatric ophthalmologist should follow.
- The most common cause of SO palsy is congenital. In these cases extensive neurologic evaluation may not be required, and diagnosis may be achieved clinically.
- An isolated SO palsy with a tolerable head tilt may not need surgical treatment, but routine ophthalmologic follow-up is needed to identify early signs of decreased vision and amblyopia.

Suggested Reading

American Academy of Ophthalmology. Pediatric ophthalmology and strabismus. In: *Basic and Clinical Science Course*. San Francisco, CA: American Academy of Ophthalmology; 2008

Rosenbaum AL. *Clinical Strabismus Management: Principles and Surgical Technique*. Philadelphia, PA: Saunders; 1999

Taylor D, Hoyt CS, eds. *Pediatric Ophthalmology and Strabismus*. 3rd ed. Edinburgh, United Kingdom: Elsevier Saunders; 2005

Wright KW, Spiegel PH. *Pediatric Ophthalmology and Strabismus*. 2nd ed. New York, NY: Springer-Verlag; 2003

Chapter 60

Acute Head Turn

Benjamin H. Ticho, MD

Presentation

A 4-year-old girl comes to the pediatrician's office because her parents noted that over the past 3 days, she has begun to turn her head to the left (Figure 60-1). She had no previous medical problems or head trauma but did have a cold earlier in the week. She is currently afebrile. She does not complain of diplopia (double vision).

Visual assessment reveals that she can fix and follow toy targets in each eye. She does not object to having her right eye covered as long as she can adopt her left head turn (of about 40 degrees). She has briskly reactive pupils with no afferent pupillary defect. Examination of the anterior

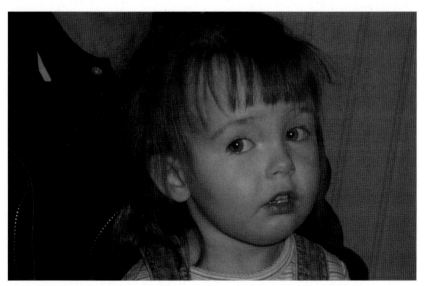

Figure 60-1. Girl with acute head turn. Courtesy of Benjamin H. Ticho, MD.

and posterior ocular segments, including optic discs, yields normal findings. Results of the non-ocular neurologic assessment are unremarkable.

With her head in its adopted leftward-turned position, she is able to demonstrate normal binocular vision (depth perception). When her head is forcibly straightened (Figure 60-2), her binocularity disappears, and a moderately sized left esotropia (eye drifting inward toward the nose) becomes apparent.

When her head is turned to the right (Figure 60-3) or when she looks to her left, an even larger left esotropia is noted.

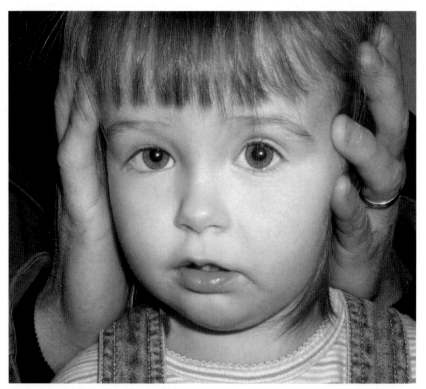

Figure 60-2. When the child looks straight ahead, she shows left esotropia. Note asymmetric corneal light reflex, with left corneal light reflex more lateral in the pupil than the right. Courtesy of Benjamin H. Ticho, MD.

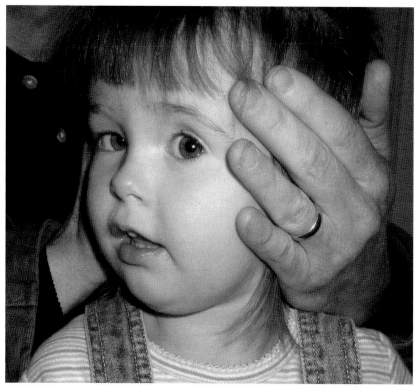

Figure 60-3. When the girl's head is turned to the right, an even larger left esotropia is noted. Courtesy of Benjamin H. Ticho, MD.

Diagnosis

Isolated inability to abduct the left eye suggests a problem with the left lateral rectus muscle, which is innervated by the sixth cranial (abducens) nerve. Given the absence of supportive data for alternative diagnoses, the most likely diagnosis is sixth cranial nerve palsy.

Alternatively, the left medial rectus muscle could be abnormally tight, restricting movement of the eye to the left. Tight medial rectus muscles may be seen in Graves ophthalmopathy, orbital abscesses from ethmoid sinusitis extension, and occasionally following medial orbital trauma (blowout fracture), as described in "Differential Diagnosis" on pages 412 and 413.

The etiology of sixth cranial nerve palsy includes the following:

- Viral infection or immunization
- Brain tumor
- Decompensated esophoria (preexisting tendency for eyes to cross inward)
- Increased intracranial pressure
- Arnold-Chiari malformation
- "Benign" sixth cranial nerve palsy—no recognizable illness or intracranial process
- Head trauma

Isolated acquired unilateral sixth cranial nerve palsy is relatively common in children. Although most such cases are postinfectious or idiopathic in this setting, the possibility of compressive lesions and elevated intracranial pressure must be considered. Bilaterality, optic disc swelling, nystagmus (involuntary rhythmic movements of the eyeball), involvement of other cranial nerves or other neurologic abnormalities, and failure to improve within 4 to 6 weeks should increase suspicion of more worrisome causes.

When a typical viral prodrome is known, and in the absence of any confounding features, observation alone is reasonable. Of course, when the words *brain tumor* are mentioned as a potential cause in discussions with parents, neuroimaging may be indicated to allay their concerns. Certainly, neuroimaging should be performed if spontaneous improvement does not occur within 4 to 12 weeks of onset or in the presence of any of the other worrisome features already mentioned.

Differential Diagnosis

Diagnoses besides sixth cranial nerve palsy that should be considered include the following:

Graves Ophthalmopathy (Thyroid Eye Disease)

Graves disease is uncommon in children. Most adult patients with thyroid eye disease have exophthalmos, or protrusion, of one or both eyeballs. This corneal exposure can lead to dry, irritated eyes. The most common presentation of pediatric thyroid eye disease is lid retraction (without proptosis or strabismus).

Orbital Abscess From Ethmoid Sinusitis Extension

Extension of ethmoid sinus infection into the orbit may create enough localized swelling to affect medial rectus function. While infection-associated orbital inflammation and edema may induce ocular misalignment, this would typically be associated with prominent eyelid swelling and edema.

Medial Orbital Trauma (Blowout Fracture)

Blunt orbital trauma (eg, from a fist or baseball) may generate enough force to cause wall fractures, typically inferiorly or medially. The medial rectus muscle may become entrapped in the fracture, leading to a restrictive esotropia that may increase in abduction. Clinically this may closely resemble abducens palsy; aside from a history of trauma, a restrictive etiology may be distinguished from neurogenic causes by forced duction test. In this test, the globe is grasped and forcibly abducted; resistance to forced duction is found in restrictive but not neurogenic strabismus.

Duane Syndrome

Duane syndrome is frequently missed during early childhood and later misdiagnosed as acquired sixth cranial nerve palsy. Duane syndrome is a congenital condition in which absence or hypoplasia of the abducens nucleus is combined with anomalous innervation of the lateral rectus muscle by a branch of the oculomotor nerve. It can be distinguished from sixth cranial nerve palsy by usual impairment to some degree of ipsilateral adduction, and by widening of the palpebral fissure in attempted abduction and narrowing with adduction.

When to Refer

Referral to an ophthalmologist is recommended in any case of acquired strabismus, particularly during early childhood, when amblyopia may develop relatively rapidly. Urgent referral of suspected abducens palsy is appropriate to confirm diagnosis and absence of complicating factors.

Treatment

In this patient, spontaneous improvement occurred within 3 weeks, with complete restoration of left abduction over an additional 3 months of observation (figures 60-4 and 60-5).

Initial approach to isolated sixth cranial nerve palsy is appropriately aimed at prevention of amblyopia (lazy eye) and preservation of binocularity. Presence of a head turn is a positive indicator of intact binocularity. On the other hand, loss of this compensatory head posture (despite persistent incomitant esotropia) is an ominous sign suggesting loss of fusion and possible development of amblyopia.

Surgical treatment of esotropia is usually reserved for stable deviations that persist for at least 4 to 6 months. Injection of botulinal toxin to the

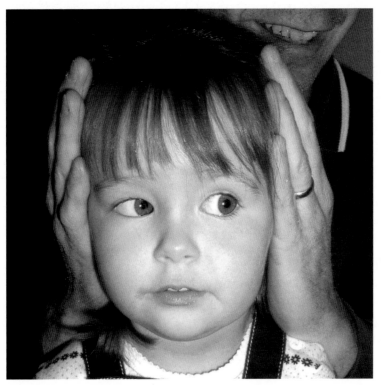

Figure 60-4. There is incomplete restoration of left abduction. Courtesy of Benjamin H. Ticho, MD.

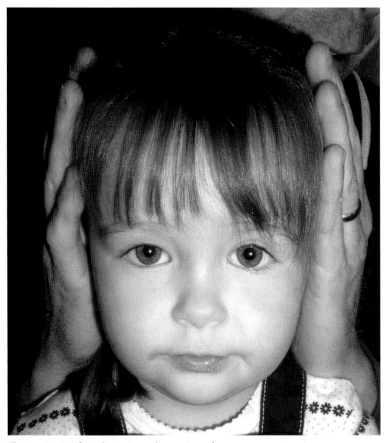

Figure 60-5. After about 3 weeks, patient shows spontaneous improvement of esotropia when looking straight ahead. Courtesy of Benjamin H. Ticho, MD.

ipsilateral medial rectus has been advocated to reduce development of muscle contracture. However, prospective multicenter studies reported in 2001 suggest that administration of botulinum toxin to the yoke (ipsilateral) medial rectus muscle within 3 months of injury does not significantly alter long-term strabismus prognosis in a mixed-age population.

Discussion

Most pediatric isolated sixth cranial nerve palsies resolve completely or nearly so. However, subtotal resolution and recurrence (weeks to years following the initial episode) are not uncommon. Sixth cranial nerve palsies occurring after head trauma spontaneously recover within 6 months of injury about 70% of the time. Poorer prognosis for recovery is suggested by complete or bilateral sixth cranial nerve palsy.

Key Points

- An inability to abduct an eye suggests a problem with the left lateral rectus muscle or abnormal tightness of the medial rectus muscle.
- Although most cases of acquired unilateral sixth cranial nerve palsy are postinfectious and idiopathic in this setting, the possibility of compressive lesions and elevated intracranial pressure must be considered.
- Bilateral sixth cranial nerve palsy, optic disc swelling, nystagmus, involvement of other cranial nerves or other neurologic abnormalities, and failure to improve within 6 weeks should increase suspicion of more worrisome causes.
- Initial approach to isolated sixth cranial nerve palsy is aimed at prevention of amblyopia and preservation of binocularity.

Suggested Reading

Holmes JM, Beck RW, Kip KE, Droste PJ, Leske DA; Pediatric Eye Disease Investigator Group. Predictors of nonrecovery in acute traumatic sixth nerve palsy and paresis. *Ophthalmology.* 2001;108(8):1457–1460

Werner DB, Savino PJ, Schatz NJ. Benign recurrent sixth nerve palsies in childhood. Secondary to immunization or viral illness. *Arch Ophthalmol.* 1983;101(4):607–608

Chapter 61

Shaking Eyes and Head

Richard W. Hertle, MD

Presentation

A 2-year-old hypopigmented girl visits the pediatrician for her 2-year well-child examination. The parents report that they have noticed both eyes wiggle since birth, and the child is now tilting and shaking her head when interested in distance objects. She is the product of a full-term, uncomplicated pregnancy with normal birth, delivery, growth, and development. They also notice some problems related to depth perception, "going up and down stairs, and judging objects coming at her."

The results of her 2-year well visit examination are otherwise normal, specifically including a general age-appropriate neurologic examination (Figure 61-1).

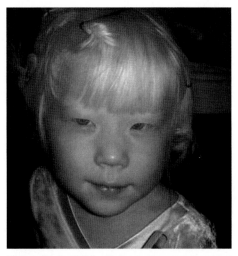

Figure 61-1. Child with hypopigmentation and nystagmus. Courtesy of Richard W. Hertle, MD.

Diagnosis

This child has nystagmus associated with albinism. Diagnosis of nystagmus is usually accomplished with a combination of history, thorough ocular examination, occasionally neuroimaging, and, most importantly, eye movement recordings (Figure 61-2), which are diagnostic of the type of nystagmus.

The most common ocular oscillations in children are typically not associated with structural disease of the brain but are commonly associated with diseases of the visual system. These eye diseases include albinism

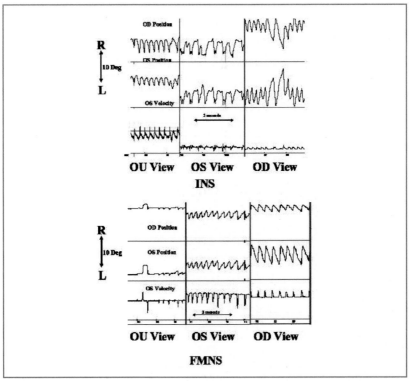

Figure 61-2. Eye movement recording showing the difference between infantile nystagmus syndrome (INS) and fusion maldevelopment nystagmus syndrome (FMNS). OD, right eye; OS, left eye; OU, both eyes. The slow phases of the oscillation have an increasing exponential waveform in INS and a decreasing exponential slow phase in FMNS. Courtesy of Richard W. Hertle, MD.

(as in this child; see Figure 61-1), optic nerve hypoplasia, congenital cataracts, and retinal dystrophies. Ocular oscillations include infantile nystagmus syndrome (previously called congenital nystagmus), which is a conjugate, principally jerk nystagmus that appears after the first few months of life, often associated with a position of gaze where the nystagmus is less intense (a null zone) and therefore vision is best. This results in head and face posturing to allow the eyes to stay in the gaze position that affords the child's best vision. These patients often have an associated head oscillation (due to the same anomalous central motor signal causing the eye oscillation also affecting the neck muscles), as well as strabismus and refractive errors.

The second most common type of ocular oscillation in children is fusion maldevelopment nystagmus syndrome (previously called latent nystagmus). This horizontal, conjugate, jerk nystagmus is always associated with strabismus and is increased or worsened by occlusion of one eye.

The last and most rare type is spasmus nutans syndrome (SNS). It is defined by the triad of anomalous head posture, asymmetric high-frequency nystagmus, and head bobbing, which spontaneously disappears by 2 to 3 years of age. Rarely, SNS is associated with hypothalamic or chiasmatic glioma or subacute necrotizing encephalomyopathy. If unilateral nystagmus is detected, SNS, internuclear ophthalmoplegia, amblyopia, blindness, brain-stem disease, and superior oblique myokymia (a uniocular torsional micro-tremor) should be considered.

Physiologic forms of nystagmus are endpoint nystagmus, which is a jerk nystagmus of fine amplitude that occurs on extreme lateral gaze; vestibular nystagmus, also a jerk nystagmus that can be evoked by altering equilibrium of the endolymph in semicircular canals; optokinetic nystagmus, which is an induced jerk nystagmus elicited by moving a repetitive stimulus across the visual field; and voluntary nystagmus. The latter (sometimes a party trick) is usually very rapid and horizontal, often associated with convergence of the eyes and pupillary constriction, and is rarely able to be sustained for more than 30 seconds at a time.

Nystagmus in infancy and childhood may also be due to structural disease of the brain stem and cerebellum, much the same as nystagmus in adulthood. Types of nystagmus associated with localizing neurologic disorders are shown in Table 61-1.

Table 61-1. Types of Nystagmus Associated With Localizing Neurologic Disorders

Nystagmus	Manifestations	Cause/Association
Convergence-retraction	Convergence on attempted upward gaze	Possible midbrain disorder
Seesaw	Pendular oscillation in which one eye rises and intorts while the other falls and extorts	Usually parasellar tumors
Periodic alternating	Horizontal nystagmus that rhythmically changes direction and intensity every 90 to 120 seconds	Cerebellar or caudal medullary disorders
Downbeat	Rapid downward nystagmus	Structural lesions at the cervicomedullary junction; neurotoxins
Upbeat	Rapid upward nystagmus	Lesions of the cerebellar vermis or medulla
Gaze paretic	Similar to endpoint nystagmus, except continuous in lateral gaze	Parieto-occipital, cerebellar, and brain-stem lesions
Central vestibular	Horizontal and torsional jerk on lateral gaze, with vertigo, tinnitus, or deafness	Usually demyelinating disease, stroke, encephalitis, or tumor
Peripheral vestibular	Usually torsional on lateral gaze opposite side of the lesion	Lesions of labyrinth or eighth cranial nerve

Differential Diagnosis

Diagnoses besides nystagmus that should be considered include

- Roving eye movements (slow, disorganized, searching eye movements seen in patients with very poor vision)
- Opsoclonus (rapid, involuntary, nonrhythmic, multidirectional eye movements usually associated with brain pathology)

When to Refer

A referral to a pediatric ophthalmologist is warranted when there is a family history of a significant childhood eye disease, a visual system abnormality is noted by a health care professional, or the child fails a vision screening evaluation.

Treatment

Numerous treatments have been described, and many are in use for nystagmus in infancy and childhood. These include dietary manipulation, medications, contact lenses, prisms, biofeedback, intermittent photic stimulation, acupuncture, injection of botulinum toxin, and a variety of surgical procedures on extraocular muscles. Except those treatments that directly improve visual acuity (spectacle and contact lens correction of refractive errors), all these treatments have a common desired effect of reducing or favorably changing nystagmus intensity directly or indirectly, allowing for an increase in visual acuity.

Discussion

Although not needed for routine pediatric care, some background helps with understanding nystagmus. Involuntary ocular oscillations have been classified in many ways, resulting in some confusion and disagreement among clinicians, physiologists, psychologists, and biomedical scientists. The National Eye Institute Workshop on Classification of Eye Movement Abnormalities and Strabismus in 2001 attempted to resolve some of these issues.

> ## Key Points
>
> - Diseases of the visual system or brain can cause nystagmus.
> - Adoption of an anomalous head position can be an involuntary accommodation in a patient with nystagmus.
> - The pattern of nystagmus on physical examination, eye movement recordings, and occasional neuroimaging is the mainstay of diagnosis.

Suggested Reading

Abadi RV, Bjerre A. Motor and sensory characteristics of infantile nystagmus. *Br J Ophthalmol.* 2002;86(10):1152–1160

Hertle RW, Dell'Osso LF. Clinical and ocular motor analysis of congenital nystagmus in infancy. *J AAPOS.* 1999;3(2):70–79

Hertle RW, Yang D. Clinical and electrophysiological effects of extraocular muscle surgery on patients with infantile nystagmus syndrome (INS). *Semin Ophthalmol.* 2006;21(2):103–110

Leigh RJ, Khanna S. What can acquired nystagmus tell us about congenital forms of nystagmus? *Semin Ophthalmol.* 2006;21(2):83–86

National Eye Institute. A Classification of Eye Movement Abnormalities and Strabismus (CEMAS). http://www.nei.nih.gov/news/statements/cemas.pdf. Accessed May 14, 2012

Chapter 62

Odd Eye Movement

Chantal Boisvert, OD, MD

Presentation

An 8-year-old boy comes to the pediatrician's office for an annual checkup. He just moved from another city and was followed by a single pediatrician since his birth. He was born at term by a spontaneous vaginal delivery and is healthy and fully immunized for his age. He does not have any eye complaints.

Physical examination yields normal results. Visual acuity is normal in both eyes (20/20). The eyes look aligned when the patient looks directly ahead in the primary position of gaze (Figure 62-1). However, the pediatrician notices that when the child looks up and to the left, his right eye does not fully move in that position (Figure 62-2). In other gaze positions the eyes move normally. The pediatrician asks the mother about this finding. She tells the pediatrician that her child has always had this "funny eye movement." She denies that he has had any ocular surgery or trauma.

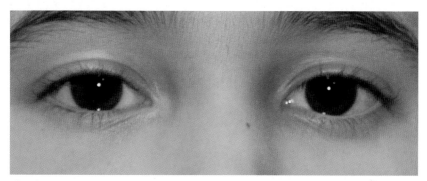

Figure 62-1. An example of a patient with straight eyes when looking straight ahead. Courtesy of Faruk H. Örge, MD.

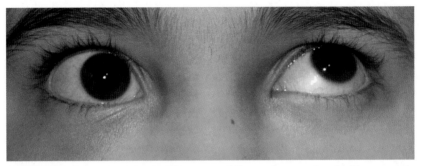

Figure 62-2. The same patient's right eye not fully moving up when looking up and to the left. Courtesy of Faruk H. Örge, MD.

Diagnosis

This child has an elevation deficiency with the right eye in adduction—looking up and in. Several conditions should be considered in the differential diagnosis. However, deficient elevation in adduction that improves with abduction is a well-recognized clinical feature of Brown syndrome (or superior oblique tendon sheath syndrome), which is the diagnosis in this patient. Brown syndrome may be present at birth (congenital) or begin later. It may be constant or intermittent. Acquired Brown syndrome is uncommon but may be seen following surgery (eg, eyelid, frontal sinus, ocular, teeth), following orbital trauma, or in association with inflammatory diseases (eg, sinusitis, lupus, juvenile or adult rheumatoid arthritis, scleroderma).

In the primary position of gaze, many patients with Brown syndrome are orthophoric (the eyes are straight), but in severe cases, hypotropia (the involved eye is lower) may develop (Figure 62-3), with a compensatory face turn toward the opposite side and a head tilt on the same side as the affected eye. This chronic tilt will cause facial asymmetry (Figure 62-4). Forced duction testing in these patients, using forceps to move the eye in the upward position, indicates restriction. The cause of this restriction is a problem of the superior oblique tendon.

No laboratory tests are specifically required in the evaluation of patients with congenital Brown syndrome. In acquired cases, tests to exclude autoimmune diseases and magnetic resonance imaging of the orbit may need to be ordered.

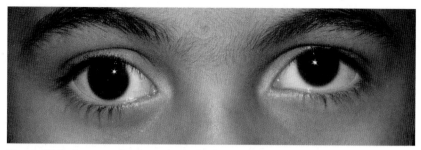

Figure 62-3. An example of a patient with severe Brown syndrome and right hypotropia in primary position of gaze. Courtesy of Irene Anteby, MD.

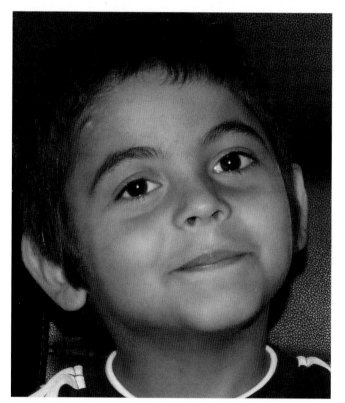

Figure 62-4. Same patient as in Figure 62-3 with compensatory face turn toward the opposite side with a pronounced head tilt toward the affected eye. Note facial asymmetry consistent with a long-standing head tilt. Courtesy of Irene Anteby, MD.

Differential Diagnosis

Diagnoses besides Brown syndrome that should be considered include the following:

Congenital Fibrosis of the Inferior Rectus Muscle

Fibrosis entrapping the inferior rectus muscle can produce a restrictive elevation deficiency. However, the deficiency is usually more marked in abduction than in adduction.

Inferior Orbital Blowout Fracture

Inferior orbital blowout fracture can produce a restrictive elevation deficiency if the inferior rectus muscle is entrapped. However, the deficiency is usually more marked in abduction than in adduction, and there is usually a history of ocular trauma.

Inferior Oblique Palsy

Inferior oblique palsy is rare and is characterized by hypotropia of the affected eye that increases in adduction and on contralateral head tilt. Unlike Brown syndrome, there is a superior oblique overaction, and forced duction test results are negative (without restriction).

When to Refer

A pediatric ophthalmologist should evaluate children with suspected Brown syndrome to determine if further treatment is needed.

Treatment

Observation (by the pediatric ophthalmologist) alone remains the most common form of management for congenital and acquired Brown syndrome and was the choice for this patient. In selected patients, range-of-motion eye exercises, oral corticosteroids, and corticosteroids injected near the trochlea have produced improvement.

In cases of acquired Brown syndrome associated with systemic inflammatory diseases, resolution may occur as systemic treatment brings the underlying disease into remission. Comanagement with a rheumatologist may be helpful.

Surgical treatment is indicated when there is large misalignment of the eyes while looking straight ahead, significant double vision, an abnormal head position, or constant eye misalignment causing amblyopia (lazy eye) and threatening binocularity. More than one surgery may be needed for optimal management.

Discussion

This syndrome can be congenital (more common) or acquired. Acquired Brown syndrome is more likely to be intermittent and resolve spontaneously. It has been attributed to a variety of causes, including superior oblique surgery, scleral buckling bands in retinal detachment surgery, trauma, sinus surgery, and inflammation in the trochlear region due to systemic causes. In some acquired cases, the patients may feel or hear a click on attempted elevation in adduction, and there may be a palpable mass or tenderness in the trochlear region. These patients may well experience diplopia (double vision) when elevating the involved eye in adduction but will learn to avoid this position of gaze. An identical motility pattern can be acquired by patients with juvenile or adult rheumatoid arthritis (stenosing tenosynovitis). Surgery can be difficult and should be reserved for specialists with experience in this disorder.

Key Points

- Brown syndrome is defined as an inability to elevate the eye in adduction actively and passively on testing.
- Most cases are congenital and do not necessitate any intervention unless they are leading to abnormal visual or binocular development.
- Acquired cases may respond to anti-inflammatory treatment.
- A pediatric ophthalmologist should evaluate children with suspected Brown syndrome to determine if further treatment is needed.

Suggested Reading

Wilson ME, Eustis HS Jr, Parks MM. Brown's syndrome. *Surv Ophthalmol.* 1989;34(3):153–172

Wright KW. Brown's syndrome: diagnosis and management. *Trans Am Ophthalmol Soc.* 1999;97:1023–1109

Chapter 63

Crossing and Limited Outward Rotation of Both Eyes

Federico G. Velez, MD
Arthur L. Rosenbaum, MD

Presentation

An 8-month-old boy is brought to the pediatric clinic by his parents, who have noted since early infancy that both eyes turn in and have limited outward rotation. They also have noted a mild right head tilt. There is a family history of strabismus in one parent. The infant was born full term with a birth weight of 8 pounds, 1 ounce, and has been in excellent medical health. The parents deny any trauma.

On ocular examination, the patient can fixate well on objects with each eye when looking straight ahead. However, he cannot follow objects with either eye to the side. He seems to prefer his left eye but can occasionally use his right. He also has esotropia (cross-eyes). The pediatrician is not sure if this is routine infantile esotropia, but clearly the child needs evaluation by a pediatric ophthalmologist.

The pediatric ophthalmologist also notes crossing of the eyes (Figure 63-1). Ocular rotations reveal severe inability to abduct either

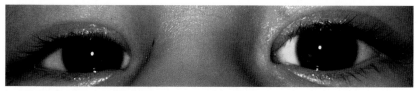

Figure 63-1. Right eye esotropia, corneal light reflex displaced temporally. Courtesy of Federico G. Velez, MD.

eye (look temporally). The eyes are noted to pull back in the orbit (globe retraction; figures 63-2 and 63-3). There is mild over-elevation of the left eye in adduction (looking in toward the nose; Figure 63-3). Each pupil measures 4.0 mm in size and reacts well to light and accommodation. The rest of the eye examination shows normal findings.

Diagnosis

The pediatric ophthalmologist finds that this infant has Duane syndrome, a congenital ocular motility disorder. This patient has type 1 Duane syndrome.

Duane syndrome is classically divided into 3 types. Type 1, the most common, is characterized by limitation of abduction with minimal to no limitation of adduction. Type 2 is characterized by limitation of adduction with minimal to no limitation of abduction. Type 3 is characterized by limitation of abduction and adduction.

Differential diagnosis of a child with esotropia and limitation of abduction is discussed on the next page. The constellation of small angle of

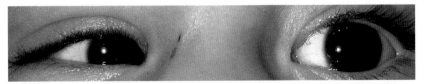

Figure 63-2. Decreased abduction of left eye on left gaze with associated widening of eyelid fissure. The right eye demonstrates narrowing of right eyelid fissure and globe retraction. Courtesy of Federico G. Velez, MD.

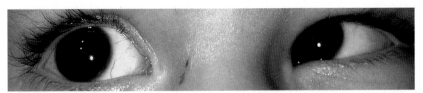

Figure 63-3. Decreased abduction of right eye on right gaze with associated widening of eyelid fissures. The left eye demonstrates narrowing of left eyelid fissures and globe retraction with mild vertical elevation on adduction. Courtesy of Federico G. Velez, MD.

deviation in the primary position, presence of globe retraction, narrowing of palpebral fissure in adduction, and mild limitation of abduction are characteristics of Duane syndrome and not other causes of esotropia. Other associated manifestations in patients with Duane syndrome include horizontal strabismus, mild vertical strabismus on adduction, anomalous head posture, amblyopia, and refractive errors. Approximately 10% of patients have associated ocular abnormalities, including eyelid ptosis, nystagmus, dermoids, cataracts, microphthalmos, optic nerve hypoplasia, and nasolacrimal duct obstruction.

Systemic associations are found in approximately 5% of patients. They include crocodile tears, hearing loss, muscle and skeletal abnormalities, pectus carinatum, meningocele, Klippel-Feil anomaly, Goldenhar syndrome (oculoauriculovertebral spectrum), Holt-Oram syndrome, and atrial septal defects. The triad of Duane syndrome, Klippel-Feil anomaly, and hypoacusis is known as Wildervanck syndrome. Every patient with Duane syndrome requires a complete physical examination to determine presence of associated systemic abnormalities.

Differential Diagnosis

Diagnoses that should be considered besides Duane syndrome include the following:

Paralysis of Sixth Cranial Nerve

Congenital sixth nerve palsy is extremely rare. It occurs in Moebius syndrome, which also compromises cranial nerves 6 and 7. History of sickness, fever, trauma, or vaccination is important in suspected acquired sixth nerve palsy.

Infantile Esotropia

In infantile esotropia, onset of deviation occurs by 3 to 4 months of age. It is characterized by large-angle esotropia while looking directly ahead, alternating crossed fixation with fixing eye closer to the nose, mild limitation of abduction, latent nystagmus, and asymmetric pursuit movements.

Fibrosis of Extraocular Muscles

Fibrosis of extraocular muscles is a congenital cranial anomolous innervation syndrome characterized by eyelid ptosis and a mechanical restriction in all gaze directions, especially elevation.

Myositis

Myositis is characterized by orbital tenderness and pain during attempted ocular rotations, proptosis (abnormal protrusion of eyeball), and conjunctival injection.

When to Refer

Children with signs of Duane syndrome (limitation of horizontal ocular rotations, especially abduction, and anomalous head posture) should be referred to a pediatric ophthalmologist. A complete ophthalmologic examination is necessary in patients with Duane syndrome to determine presence of strabismus, amblyopia, and associated ocular abnormalities, and to perform a cycloplegic refraction. Additionally, a genetic evaluation may be considered in presence of multiple associated conditions or in patients with a family history of Duane syndrome.

Treatment

When required, early therapeutic intervention is recommended to improve eye alignment, anomalous head posture, and ocular rotations as well as to decrease effects of co-contraction. This patient underwent extraocular muscle surgery to realign his eye and recover binocular vision. Patients must be checked for eyeglasses during their first eye examination. Small angles of esotropia and anomalous head posture may sometimes be corrected with the proper eyeglass prescription.

Indications for surgery include strabismus in the primary position of gaze, diplopia, anomalous head posture, and anomalous vertical movements. Surgical goals include achieving binocular single vision while looking straight ahead, expanding and centering size of the diplopia-free field, improving ocular rotations, and decreasing effects of simultaneous contraction. The surgical approach to Duane syndrome is complex and requires the expertise of a surgeon well versed in strabismus repair. Approximately 80% of patients undergoing extraocular muscle surgery for this condition regain ocular alignment in primary position and improve anomalous head posture.

Patients with Duane syndrome need ophthalmologic follow-up every 3 to 6 months for approximately the first 8 years of life. It is important to determine the presence of amblyopia and any residual ocular misalignment and anomalous head posture requiring further correction.

Discussion

Duane syndrome is an ocular motility disorder caused by anomalous innervation of the lateral rectus muscle. This is caused by absence or hypoplasia of the sixth cranial nerve (abducens nerve) resulting in abduction deficiency. Fibers of the ipsilateral third cranial nerve (oculomotor nerve) are abnormally directed to the lateral rectus muscle, resulting in contraction of the lateral rectus muscle when the medial rectus muscle is contracting. Simultaneous contraction of both horizontal rectus muscles results in globe retraction, palpebral fissure narrowing, and limitation of abduction.

Duane syndrome accounts for up to 5% of all forms of strabismus. Incidence in the general population is 0.1%. It is typically sporadic and unilateral, with the tendency to affect females and the left eye more frequently. Bilateral involvement occurs in 15% of the cases.

Although most cases are sporadic, autosomal-dominant and autosomal-recessive inherited cases have been reported. Deletions in chromosome 8q13 *(DURS1* locus) have been found in sporadic cases. Some autosomal-dominant cases have been mapped to the *DURS2* locus on chromosome 2q31 and are associated with higher incidence of bilateral disease and abnormal vertical movements. Duane syndrome is classified within congenital cranial anomolous syndromes because of mutations in genes associated with development of ocular motoneurons such as *PHOX2A, KIF21A, ROBO3, CHN1,* and *HOXA1.*

Key Points

- Duane syndrome may be associated with other ocular and systemic abnormalities.
- Limitation of horizontal ocular rotations, especially abduction, and anomalous head posture are the most important clinical manifestations.
- Differential diagnosis from sixth nerve palsy avoids unnecessary evaluation.
- When required, early therapeutic intervention is recommended to improve eye alignment, anomalous head posture, and ocular rotations and to decrease effects of co-contraction.

Suggested Reading

DeRespinis PA, Caputo AR, Wagner RS, Guo S. Duane's retraction syndrome. *Surv Ophthalmol.* 1993;38(3):257–288

Engle EC. The genetic basis of complex strabismus. *Pediatr Res.* 2006;59(3):343–348

Jampolsky A. Duane syndrome. In: Rosenbaum AL, Santiago AP, eds. *Clinical Strabismus Management.* Philadelphia, PA: Saunders; 1999:325–346

Mohan K, Sharma A, Pandav SS. Differences in epidemiological and clinical characteristics between various types of Duane retraction syndrome in 331 patients. *J AAPOS.* 2008;12(6):576–580

Velez FG, Foster RS, Rosenbaum AL. Vertical rectus muscle augmented transposition in Duane syndrome. *J AAPOS.* 2001;5(2):105–113

Section 9
Decreased Vision

Chapter 64

Floaters and Blurred Vision

Igor Kozak, MD, PhD

Presentation

A 17-year-old boy comes to the pediatrician's office with complaints of floaters and cloudy vision in both eyes for the last couple of weeks. Although the patient says he never needed glasses, his visual acuity is decreased to 20/50 in both eyes. He has no history of a similar event in the past, and nobody in his family has an eye problem. He denies history of any trauma. His health history is unremarkable. The teenager does not complain of ocular pain.

On examination ocular surface redness is not evident. There is no increased tearing, discharge, or crusting of the eyelids. Ocular motility is full in both eyes. On penlight examination the pupils constrict, and there is no photophobia.

Because this patient needs an intraocular examination, the pediatrician refers him to an ophthalmologist. At the ophthalmology office, intraocular pressures are normal bilaterally. Eye examination with slit-lamp microscope shows trace inflammatory cells in the anterior chamber. Peripheral retinal examination with scleral indentation is performed. Dilated fundus examination in one eye is shown in Figure 64-1. A wide-angle view of the retina shows optic nerve and retinal vessels superiorly and dense vitreous inflammation (vitritis) inferiorly. Next, the patient undergoes intravenous fluorescein angiography (Figure 64-2) and optical coherence tomography (real-time, noncontact, cross-sectional imaging of the retinal layers) (Figure 64-3).

Diagnosis

This patient has idiopathic intermediate uveitis.

Vitritis (inflammation of the vitreous) is a defining sign of intermediate uveitis. Other critical signs of intermediate uveitis include white exudative material over the inferior ora serrata and pars plana ("snowbank") and cellular aggregates floating in the vitreous ("snowballs"), commonly termed pars planitis. Peripheral vascular sheathing, mild anterior chamber inflammation, and cystoid macular edema are frequently present. What often delays diagnosis is the insidious course of the disease; it presents in an externally white and "quiet" eye.

Up to 50% of cases of intermediate uveitis are idiopathic. The remaining cases are most commonly associated with systemic disease (see "Differential Diagnosis" on page 440). Therefore, the patient should be questioned about systemic diseases and any prior episodes of eye inflammation. Additionally, evaluation should include chest radiography, purified protein derivative (tuberculin) skin test, serum angiotensin-converting enzyme level, rapid plasma reagin,

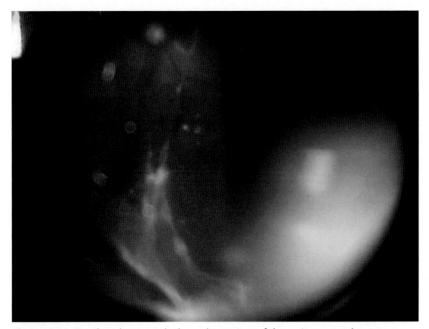

Figure 64-1. Fundus photograph shows hazy view of the retina secondary to vitreous inflammation. Superior in the image is the optic nerve with inferior whitish inflammation involving the retina. Courtesy of Igor Kozak, MD, PhD.

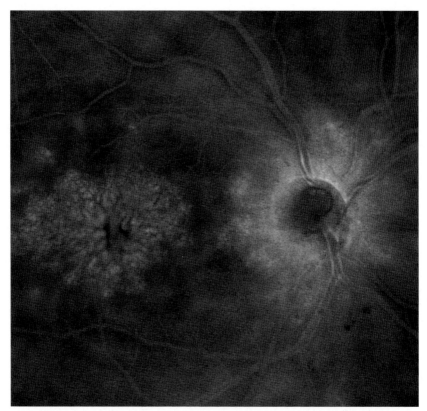

Figure 64-2. Fluorescein angiography shows leakage of fluorescein from the optic nerve (right) and cystoid macular edema (left). Courtesy of Igor Kozak, MD, PhD.

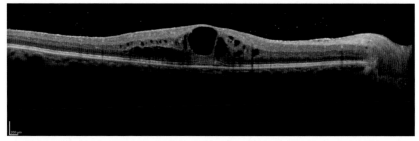

Figure 64-3. Spectral domain optical coherence tomography (cross section of retinal layers) shows cystic spaces in the retina filled with fluid. Courtesy of Igor Kozak, MD, PhD.

fluorescent treponemal antibody absorption test, enzyme-linked immunosorbent assay for Lyme disease, and serologic assay for toxoplasma and *Toxocara*. A review of focal neurologic deficits also should be performed to rule out multiple sclerosis (MS).

Differential Diagnosis

Diagnoses besides intermediate uveitis that should be considered include the following:

Sarcoidosis

Laboratory tests and biopsy establish diagnosis of sarcoidosis. Sarcoid uveitis is more common in infants than school-aged children and adolescents. Typically, older children with sarcoidosis have mainly lung involvement, without the rash and arthritis usually seen in infantile sarcoidosis. Uveitis is more often anterior and granulomatous in sarcoidosis, although intermediate uveitis can occur.

Multiple Sclerosis

Multiple sclerosis has been associated with pars planitis, which usually has a milder course than other types of intermediate uveitis. It typically affects women who are young and white. Onset of pars planitis may precede MS in up to 25% of patients, and it may precede MS by 5 to 10 years. Neurologic examination and magnetic resonance imaging scan of the brain are diagnostic.

Lyme Disease

Intermediate uveitis is one of the most common intraocular presentations of Lyme disease. Cranial nerve involvement and systemic skin and joint disease are common. Diagnosis is clinical with supportive serology.

Juvenile Inflammatory (Rheumatoid) Arthritis

Juvenile inflammatory arthritis is associated with chronic uveitis. Involvement is more pronounced in the anterior segment (iridocyclitis) with the presence of keratic precipitates, band keratopathy, posterior synechiae, and cataracts.

Syphilis

Ocular manifestations of syphilis are numerous and can masquerade as any other type of uveitis. The posterior pole is more affected than in intermediate uveitis with findings such as (necrotizing) chorioretinitis, serous retinal detachment, or optic neuropathies. Diagnosis is clinical with serologic evidence of treponemal antibodies.

Tuberculosis

Tuberculosis also presents with varied clinical findings predominantly in the posterior segment of the eye including vitritis, chorioretinitis, optic nerve involvement, or vitreous hemorrhage. Systemic disease and skin test with chest radiograph can narrow diagnosis.

Inflammatory Bowel Disease and Whipple Disease

Ulcerative colitis and Crohn disease are associated with acute uveitis. These patients tend to be HLA-B27 positive. Uveitis is more often anterior with spillover to the back of the eye. Whipple disease, a cause of malabsorption, has been associated with intermediate uveitis.

Intraocular Lymphoma

Lymphomas, usually non-Hodgkin B-lymphocyte type, can present with vitritis and mild anterior chamber reaction. They also have retinal lesions with creamy yellow subretinal infiltrates. Vitreous biopsy confirms diagnosis.

Toxocara

A peripheral *Toxocara* granuloma can present with cloudy vitreous with cyclitic membrane and can mimic pars plana snowbank in a child. Unlike intermediate uveitis, it is rarely bilateral.

Toxoplasma

Toxoplasma is characterized by dense vitritis behind which an area of retinitis can be found (often described as a "headlight in the fog"). It is commonly a unilateral disease. Serologic tests and ocular fluid polymerase chain reaction help with diagnosis.

When to Refer

If intermediate uveitis is not diagnosed early and treated promptly, loss of vision may occur. Patients with floaters and blurred vision, even in the absence of eye pain and redness, should be referred to an ophthalmologist for intraocular examination. Patients who experience chronic intermediate uveitis should see a uveitis specialist.

Treatment

The patient received a periocular injection of methylprednisolone acetate 40 mg (1 mL volume) in both eyes. His visual acuity improved to 20/25 in his right eye and 20/32 in his left eye over 6 months. It is imperative to exclude an underlying infectious disease or malignancy and decide whether treatment is really indicated. Therapy may not be needed in quiescent cases with good visual acuity.

Topical 1% prednisolone acetate every 2 hours is administered if there is anterior chamber reaction with reduced visual acuity. For treatment of pars planitis (a form of intermediate uveitis), periocular or sub-Tenon capsule injections of triamcinolone acetate or methylprednisolone acetate are repeated until the vitritis subsides, cystoid macular edema clears, and visual acuity improves. Intravitreal dexamethasone implants with releasing time up to 6 months are available. Patients with acute cases follow up every 2 weeks, and those with chronic cases follow up every 2 to 6 months based on clinical status.

In patients who do not respond to local corticosteroid therapy, systemic therapy with 0.5 to 1 mg/kg of prednisolone (or cyclosporine 2.5 mg/kg, the first-line steroid-sparing agent) is administered. Cryopexy (freezing therapy) of the pars plana or vitrectomy surgery is reserved for refractory cases.

Discussion

Intermediate uveitis accounts for up to 15% of all uveitis cases. It primarily affects children and young adults and is usually bilateral. The course is chronic, with flare-ups and remissions, in 40% to 60% of patients.

Visual outcome depends on clarity of optical media as well as presence and severity of macular edema. A good visual outcome requires aggressive treatment of active inflammation.

Key Points

- Intermediate uveitis can present with any or none of the following symptoms: sustained floaters, vision loss, white or red eye, and occasionally eye pain.
- Diagnosis of intermediate uveitis in children can be delayed if the child does not complain of symptoms.
- If this type of uveitis is not diagnosed early and treated promptly, visual loss may develop.
- Possible vision-reducing sequelae of intermediate uveitis are amblyopia, posterior subcapsular cataract, secondary glaucoma, and chronic cystoid macular edema.
- If amblyopia is suspected it should be treated concurrently.
- Cataracts can develop as a result of ocular inflammation and corticosteroid therapy.
- Underlying systemic disease may be present and must be considered, particularly multiple sclerosis.

Suggested Reading

Donaldson MJ, Pulido JS, Herman DC, Diehl N, Hodge D. Pars planitis: a 20-year study of incidence, clinical features, and outcomes. *Am J Ophthalmol.* 2007;144(6):812–817

Nussenblatt RB, Whitcup SM. *Uveitis: Fundamentals and Clinical Practice.* 4th ed. Philadelphia, PA: Elsevier; 2010

Chapter 65

Decreased Vision and a "Normal" Eye

Richard W. Hertle, MD

Presentation

An otherwise healthy 5-year-old girl is found to have unilateral loss of vision in the right eye when tested in the pediatrician's office as part of vision screening. Her eyes are straight and move together, and she has no structural disease of the ocular surface or media opacity that the pediatrician can detect in the office with direct ophthalmoscope. On obtaining further family history, the pediatrician finds that there are several family members who had a "lazy eye" as children (asymmetric vision).

Diagnosis

This child has amblyopia in the right eye, often erroneously called lazy eye. Amblyopia is a decrease in vision and visual functions in one eye, or less often, both eyes, resulting from abnormal or unequal visual input during development in infancy and early childhood. Vision loss ranges from mild (worse than 20/25) to severe (20/200 to hand motion). Confusingly, the ocular anatomy looks otherwise normal.

If central visual pathways are not properly stimulated by equally clear images during development of the visual cortex, amblyogenesis results. Several conditions in childhood are amblyogenic, including suppression of one eye associated with strabismus (eye misalignment), uncorrected refractive errors (farsightedness, nearsightedness, astigmatism), or image deprivation (most often due to cataract but can be caused by eyelid, corneal, lens, vitrous, or retinal disease). These conditions result in 3 major types of amblyopia: strabismic, anisometropic, and deprivation, respectively.

The diagnosis of vision loss due to amblyopia occurs when an amblyogenic factor is detected and other eye disease is excluded. Complete ocular and family history is obtained. Vision is measured in preverbal children using fixation behavior or visual matching tasks. A reliable and valid test of vision in children up to 7 years of age is the single-surrounded HOTV optotype test (Figure 65-1).

Direct ophthalmoscope to detect the presence of equal and symmetric red reflexes in the pupils as well as corneal light reflexes can be used to check for ocular media opacities, refractive errors, and ocular alignment (Figure 65-2). Red reflex should be equally present, diffuse, and luminous. Location of the small white corneal light reflection from both eyes (typically slightly nasal to the center of the pupil) should be symmetric. Irritability in a content and cooperative child while one eye is covered suggests vision loss in an eye.

Differential Diagnosis

Diagnoses besides amblyopia that should be considered when there is vision loss in normal-appearing eyes include the following:
- Cortical vision loss
- Seizures
- Visual conversion reaction

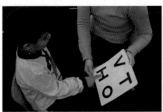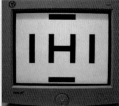

Figure 65-1. Single surrounded HOTV optotype vision testing. Courtesy of Richard W. Hertle, MD.

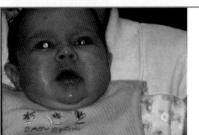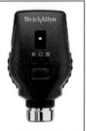

A B

Figure 65-2. Red reflex test (A) using direct ophthalmoscope (B). Courtesy of Richard W. Hertle, MD.

When to Refer

Prompt referral of a child with amblyopia to an ophthalmologist is crucial to prevent permanent loss of vision. Any child with visual acuity in either eye of 20/40 or worse from ages 3 to 5 years, 20/30 or worse at 6 years and older, or a 2-line difference in acuity between eyes should be referred for further evaluation.

Treatment

This patient was given full optical correction (glasses) and patching of the good eye 2 hours a day, to which she responded with improved vision in 3 months. Treatment is individualized depending on the cause of amblyopia. Although treatment after age 10 years was previously thought to offer little benefit, results from recent studies suggest that treatment even in adolescence results in sustained improvement in visual acuity. Duration of therapy depends on degree of vision loss and rate at which the child regains vision.

Treatment of amblyopia is a 3-step process. First, structural abnormalities of the eye are treated if present (eg, cataract removal). Second, refractive error is corrected by prescribing spectacles. Third, penalization of the better eye is initiated. The most common method of penalization is placement of an adhesive patch over the better-seeing eye (Figure 65-3). Patching regimens vary depending on severity of vision loss, ranging from 2 hours a day to all waking hours (full time). Additional options include wearing opaque contact lenses, placement of a cloth occluder over glasses, and adjustment of prescription glass in the preferred eye to blur vision.

Another alternative type of penalization therapy uses atropine eyedrops. A single drop of atropine (0.5% or 1% solution) will blur the good eye for 2 to 7 days. This paralyzes accommodation, thus blurring near

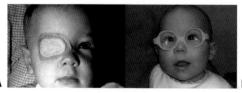

Figure 65-3. Amblyopia treatment: patching (A) and penalization spectacles (B). Courtesy of Richard W. Hertle, MD.

A   B

vision and encouraging use of the amblyopic eye at near. Atropine may be especially useful in children who cannot comply with occlusive patch therapy. Multiple studies have shown that patching and atropine are effective therapies. Atropine is well tolerated and cost-effective. Local skin irritation is the most common adverse reaction with patching. Topical atropine use is associated with greater incidence of light sensitivity, mild eye irritation, flushing of the skin, and headache, although these side effects rarely necessitate discontinuation of therapy. Parents should be advised to keep atropine eyedrops in a locked cabinet; if eyedrops are swallowed, there can be a serious effect on heart rate.

While using a patch or atropine, the child should engage in active nearvision therapy, such as writing or drawing. Such activities require the child to concentrate on fine visual detail.

Surgery for associated strabismus is usually accomplished after amblyopia therapy is completed. Surgery for those conditions causally related to amblyopia (ie, cataracts, glaucoma, and ptosis) is completed at the same time or prior to initiation of optical penalization therapy.

An amblyogenic condition beginning at birth needs to be treated within 12 to 17 weeks after birth to prevent irreversible loss in vision; this is often called the critical period.

The success of amblyopia therapy is highly dependent on compliance. It is paramount to educate parents and families about the nature of vision loss and consequences of noncompliance.

Visual acuity can be improved to 20/32 or better in at least 75% of patients. However, amblyopia may recur months or years after successful therapy, which has prompted a common practice of maintenance patching (usually a few hours per week) after a visual plateau is reached. If amblyopia recurs, patching and penalization may be resumed until the amblyopic eye has reached its maximum vision. A risk associated with untreated amblyopia is that damage to the healthy eye may lead to bilateral vision loss.

Discussion

Amblyopia is a major public health problem, with a prevalence of 1% to 4%. It is the most common cause of monocular vision loss in children and young adults.

Early recognition of amblyopia is important to help prevent permanent visual loss. Despite multiple organizations, including the American Academy of Pediatrics, endorsing screening children for visual abnormalities, only about 20% of school-aged children have routine vision screening examinations. Age-appropriate vision screenings should be a part of all well-child examinations.

Key Points

- Amblyopia is a treatable disease only if diagnosed and treated during childhood.
- Eyeglasses, patching, and atropine eyedrops are all commonly used treatments.
- Compliance with amblyopia treatment is the key to successfully treating this disease.
- The American Academy of Pediatrics has guidelines for screening vision of all children between 3 and 4 years of age, which can lead to identification of children who have or are at risk of amblyopia.

Suggested Reading

American Academy of Pediatrics Committee on Practice and Ambulatory Medicine and Section on Ophthalmology, American Association of Certified Orthoptists, American Association for Pediatric Ophthalmology and Strabismus, American Academy of Ophthalmology. Eye examination in infants, children, and young adults by pediatricians. *Pediatrics*. 2003;111(4):902–907

Hertle RW, Scheiman MM, Beck RW, et al. Stability of visual acuity improvement following discontinuation of amblyopia treatment in children aged 7 to 12 years. *Arch Ophthalmol*. 2007;125(5):655–659

Kemper AR, Clark SJ. Preschool vision screening by family physicians. *J Pediatr Ophthalmol Strabismus*. 2007;44(1):24–27

Repka MX, Wallace DK, Beck RW, et al. Two-year follow-up of a 6-month randomized trial of atropine vs patching for treatment of moderate amblyopia in children. *Arch Ophthalmol.* 2005;123(2):149–157

Scheiman MM, Hertle RW, Beck RW, et al. Randomized trial of treatment of amblyopia in children aged 7 to 17 years. *Arch Ophthalmol.* 2005;123(4):437–447

Wu C, Hunter DG. Amblyopia: diagnostic and therapeutic options. *Am J Ophthalmol.* 2006;141(1):175–184

Chapter 66

An Infant Who Seems Not to See

Avery H. Weiss, MD

Presentation

During a routine visit to the pediatrician, the parents of a healthy, full-term, 3-month-old girl raise concerns about her vision. They state that she often stares and does not appear to fixate or follow objects in her environment. Otherwise, she is thriving and reaching age-appropriate milestones.

At first the pediatrician agrees with the parents' concern, but on further observation the pediatrician discovers that the baby intermittently makes eye contact and fixates on targets. Eye alignment is normal, gaze-holding is steady, and her eyes seem to move in all directions normally. Pupils respond briskly to light. Red reflex is normal and symmetric between eyes. The parents deny a family history of ocular disorders associated with reduced vision.

Diagnosis

Having confirmed that neurodevelopment and results of the eye examination are normal, the pediatrician reassures the parents that the observed behavior represents visual inattention, a transient immaturity in vision. This delay in attentional maturation should resolve by 4 months of age, and almost certainly by 6 months.

As a developmental specialist, the pediatrician is aware that visual acuity is immature at birth and undergoes considerable development after birth. Infants can normally select and acquire objects of interest between 2 and 4 months of age. Infants with visual inattention demonstrate normal visual-orienting behaviors when placed in an uncrowded room where multiple objects do not compete for their attention.

Visual inattention should be distinguished from delayed visual maturation. The latter refers to delay in visual acuity development that occurs in the context of cerebral visual impairment (CVI) or infantile nystagmus associated with visual sensory disorders. Cerebral visual impairment refers to visual disabilities caused by abnormalities of visual cortical function. Children with CVI frequently have superimposed deficits of visual attention and delayed visual maturation that contribute to their subnormal visual behaviors. Visual acuity in children with CVI commonly improves over time, taking months to years, but seldom reaches normal levels. Children with CVI are uniformly delayed, have abnormal neurologic findings (especially microcephaly, hypotonia, and seizures), and generally demonstrate abnormalities on brain imaging studies. In comparison, infants with visual inattention are normal developmentally and neurologically.

Evaluation of CVI should include referral to an ophthalmologist to quantify visual acuity and exclude ocular disorders. Presence of age-appropriate visual acuity can be confirmed by behavioral measures such as the Teller preverbal visual acuity test or visual evoked potential (VEP) techniques. Diagnosis of CVI and assessment of severity are most reliably documented by VEP (electrophysiologic) testing. Because visual cortex immaturity is reflected in VEP testing for the first 6 months of life, this testing is most reliable when performed in patients after 6 months of age.

If there are developmental delays and neurologic findings, brain imaging studies should be considered.

Differential Diagnosis

Diagnoses that should be considered in a visually inattentive infant include the following:

- Delayed visual maturation as part of cortical visual impairment is excluded by the infant meeting developmental milestones and normal neurologic examination.
- Absence of normal visual-orienting behaviors because of anatomic abnormalities (eg, cataract, optic nerve hypoplasia, coloboma) and

functional abnormalities (eg, congenital nystagmus, retinal dystrophy) are excluded by the presence of normal visual acuity and normal eye examination.

When to Refer

Infants older than 6 months with persistent inability to fix and follow targets should be referred to an ophthalmologist for an eye examination to quantify visual acuity and exclude ocular disorders. Younger infants with subnormal visual-orienting behaviors should be referred for an eye examination if they have a systemic disorder with global developmental delays, suggesting the possibility of CVI.

Treatment

Because the patient's visual inattention is transient, no treatment is recommended. Persistence of visual or developmental concerns after 4 months, and certainly 6 months, should prompt reevaluation.

Discussion

Postnatal visual improvements are primarily related to maturation of the macula and optic nerve, along with refinements in visual abilities at lower and higher cortical levels. Visual processing is initiated by decomposition of objects into essential bits of information, such as form, color, and motion, followed by cortical reconstitution of the viewed object. The task of selecting one object over another depends on the infant's ability to make decisions about importance of the object and to allocate attention to the selected object (Figure 66-1). Once the decision process is completed, the infant must disengage from the current object of interest and transform relevant visual information into a gaze shift to the selected object. It is a complicated process we all take for granted.

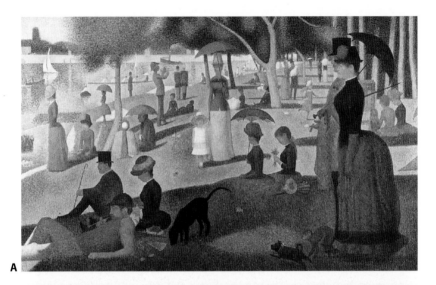

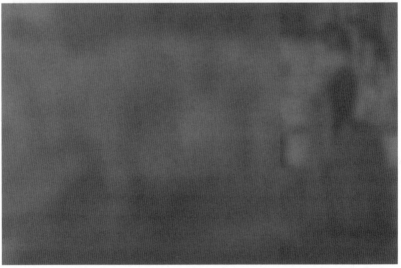

Figure 66-1. Infant vision testing is based on the concept of preferential looking. **A,** a complex scene matched to the acuity of an older child with 20/20 vision. (From: Georges Seurat French, 1859–1891, A Sunday on La Grande Jatte – 1884, 1884–86, Oil on canvas. 81¾ x 121¼ in. [207.5 x 308.1 cm], Helen Birch Bartlett Memorial Collection, 1926.224, The Art Institute Chicago.) **B,** matched to the acuity level of an infant, depicts selective attention to the female figure and emphasizes the relative blur of unattended objects in the scene.

Key Points

- Visual inattention typically gets better in an infant with normal development and a normal eye examination.
- Infants older than 6 months with persistent subnormal visual-orienting behaviors should be referred to an ophthalmologist.
- Cerebral visual impairment usually is accompanied by systemic issues or global delay.

Suggested Reading

Hunnius S. The early development of visual attention and its implications for social and cognitive development. *Prog Brain Res.* 2007;164:187–209

Johnson MH. Brain and cognitive development in infancy. *Curr Opin Neurobiol.* 1994;4(2):218–225

Weiss AH, Kelly JP, Phillips JO. The infant who is visually unresponsive on a cortical basis. *Ophthalmology.* 2001;108(11):2076–2087

Chapter 67

Decreased Visual Acuity in Both Eyes

Chantal Boisvert, OD, MD

Presentation

A 5-year-old boy comes to the pediatrician's office for a preschool medical evaluation. According to his mother, he has always been healthy and does not complain of any vision problems. Visual acuity was measured by the pediatric nurse and was 20/50 in the right eye and 20/40 in the left eye. There is no familial history of eye diseases. Previous vision examinations were normal. The mother has worn glasses for correction of myopia (nearsightedness) and astigmatism (irregular corneal curvature) since she was 13 years old.

The pediatrician shines a light in front of the patient's eyes and finds that both reflexes are centered. No abnormal eye movement is evident, and the anterior segment of the eye seems grossly normal. The pediatrician repeats the visual acuity test with a pinhole occluder. Visual acuity is now 20/25 in both eyes. The mother is surprised by this finding and asks the pediatrician's opinion about the boy's seemingly concerning vision loss.

Diagnosis

Lowered visual acuity is a worry for family and physician. As in most of medicine, this sign can have ominous and innocuous causes. Reduced visual acuity may indicate that this child needs corrective lenses to obtain normal vision, or indicate a pathologic eye condition. Pinhole visual acuity is a quick method to distinguish between these. By the patient looking through a pinhole (Figure 67-1), the refractive errors of the peripheral cornea and lens are greatly reduced or eliminated, and acuity simulates that with proper glasses in place. Going back to optics, a central ray is unaffected by passage through a lens. Thus, the pinhole duplicates a corrective lens by creating a beam of light not influenced

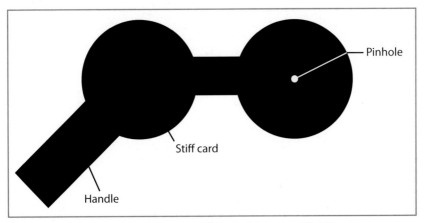

Figure 67-1. Pinhole aperture. Courtesy of Chantal Boisvert, OD, MD.

by refractive error. In this child, there is an improvement in visual acuity with the pinhole. The pediatrician is now more confident about a diagnosis of refractive error.

The pediatrician refers this child to an eye specialist for a complete ocular examination, including cycloplegic refraction. Use of eyedrops to relax and paralyze the lens (cycloplegic retinoscopy) remains the best method of determining a child's refraction. The eye examination is normal; only vision is slightly off. The eye specialist diagnoses mild myopia (nearsightedness) and astigmatism in both eyes.

On rare occasions the pediatrician will find improved vision with a pinhole occluder that will not improve with glasses. These cases are all caused by medical conditions; lenticular opacities (cataract), corneal opacities or scarring, keratoconus, and Marfan syndrome are some examples.

In children, there are 4 types of refractive errors, or ametropia.

1. **Myopia** (nearsightedness): Distant objects appear blurred because their images are focused in front of the retina rather than on it (the eyeball is too long or the optics too strong). Childhood myopia falls into 2 groups, congenital (usually high) and developmental (generally manifesting itself between 7 and 10 years). In general, the earlier the onset of myopia, the greater the progression (Figure 67-2).

2. **Hyperopia** (farsightedness): Images are focused behind the retina when accommodation is completely relaxed. Vision is better for distant objects than near objects (Figure 67-3). Hyperopia is the normal refractive state of the eye in childhood. Uncorrected hyperopia forces the patient to accommodate (put effort into focusing the lens of the eye) to sharpen the retinal image, thus leading to increasing convergence and sometimes to strabismus (eye misalignment) and amblyopia (lazy eye).

3. **Astigmatism:** Abnormal curvature, usually of the cornea (much like a football), can cause 2 focal points to fall in 2 different locations, making objects up close and at a distance appear blurry (Figure 67-4).

4. **Anisometropia:** A condition in which eyes have unequal refractive power.

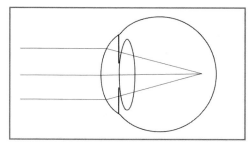

Figure 67-2. Myopia. The myopic (nearsighted) eye has excess power or the eye is too long, resulting in parallel light rays being focused in front of the retina, producing a blurred image on the retina. Courtesy of Chantal Boisvert, OD, MD.

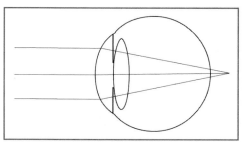

Figure 67-3. Hyperopia. The hyperopic (farsighted) eye has insufficient focusing power (is too short) to bring parallel light rays to a point of focus on the retina. Courtesy of Chantal Boisvert, OD, MD.

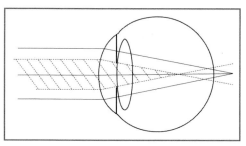

Figure 67-4. Astigmatism. A defect in the eye caused by a deviation from spherical curvature prevents light rays from meeting at a common focus, resulting in distorted images. Courtesy of Chantal Boisvert, OD, MD.

Most of the time, refractive errors are easy to correct and do not induce amblyopia. Anisometropic amblyopia develops when unequal refractive error in the eyes causes the image on one retina to be chronically defocused. A bilateral reduction in acuity (isometric amblyopia) can result from large, approximately equal, uncorrected refractive errors in both eyes of a young child. High hyperopia, high myopia, and high astigmatism in both eyes carry a greater risk of inducing bilateral amblyopia.

Differential Diagnosis

Any pathologic eye condition can lead to decreased visual acuity in a child. Diagnoses besides refractive error that should be kept in mind include the following:

Amblyopia

Amblyopia (lazy eye) is the reason for more vision loss in children than all other causes put together. Amblyopia is a decrease in the child's vision that can happen even when the eye structure is perfectly normal. It can be caused by refractive error, strabismus (eye misalignment), or vision deprivation (cataract, eyelid ptosis). If it is not treated, it can cause permanent loss of vision.

Cortical Visual Impairment

Cortical visual impairment (CVI) is bilateral decreased visual response caused by an abnormality affecting the part of the brain responsible for sight. It is one of the most frequent causes of visual impairment in children from developed countries. Infants with CVI demonstrate varying degrees of visual attentiveness and usually have some level of vision which can improve over time.

Infantile/Juvenile Cataract

Pediatric cataracts are responsible for nearly 10% of all vision loss in children worldwide. It is estimated that 1 in 250 newborns has some form of cataract. The evaluation of red reflexes by the child's health provider is the best screening test possible when looking for leukocoria.

Albinism

Albinism is an inherited condition characterized by reduced or lack of pigment that normally gives color to the skin, hair, and eyes. Vision can range from normal to legal blindness (vision less than 20/200) or worse. Generally, those who have the least amount of pigment have the poorest vision. Iris transillumination (iris has little to no pigment) and nystagmus (shaking of the eyes) are usually present.

Optic Nerve Hypoplasia

Optic nerve hypoplasia (ONH) is a congenital condition in which the optic nerve is underdeveloped (too small). The diagnosis of ONH is typically made by the appearance of a small, pale optic nerve on ophthalmoscopic examination of the eye. Magnetic resonance imaging is sometimes used to confirm the diagnosis and rule out septo-optic dysplasia. Endocrine disorders are commonly associated with this condition. Vision impairment from ONH ranges from mild to severe and may affect one or both eyes. Nystagmus may also be noted.

Retinal Disorders

Most disorders of the retina involve a disruption in the transmission of information from photoreceptors to the brain. Symptoms of a retinal disorder vary widely from patient to patient, depending on the type of disorder, where in the retina it originates, and whether it affects rod or cone cells, or both. About 10% of cases of congenital blindness or severely reduced vision are caused by Leber congenital amaurosis. Retinopathy of prematurity is a potentially blinding disease caused by abnormal development of retina blood vessels in premature newborns.

When to Refer

A child with visual loss should be referred to an eye specialist for a complete ocular examination, including cycloplegic refraction.

Treatment

This child simply needs glasses to correct his decreased vision. Prescribing visual correction for children often has 2 goals: first and most commonly, to provide a focused retinal image, and secondly, achieving the optimal balance between accommodation and convergence (in case of strabismus).

Relatively low myopic corrections (if vision without glasses is better than 20/30–20/40) should be worn for school but may be optional at other times.

The correction of hyperopic refractive error is dependent on the patient's ability to accommodate (change the focus of the internal crystalline lens) and the presence of amblyopia or strabismus. Most of the time, mild hyperopia does not need to be corrected and is considered normal.

High astigmatic error and unilateral ametropia (or when there is a large asymmetry between the eyes) should be corrected to prevent the development of amblyopia. Anisometropic (unequal refractive power between the eyes) and isometropic amblyopia may improve considerably with refractive correction alone over several months. Occlusion therapy of the good eye may sometimes be necessary.

Although many attempts have been made to arrest the development of school-aged myopia, these treatments are generally not well tolerated and yield only modest changes in myopic growth at best. These include use of bifocals and atropine eyedrops. Use of contact lenses to change refractive error by warping the eye overnight (orthokeratology) is of limited effectiveness in permanently eliminating refractive error. This technique may be used for those in whom wearing spectacles or glasses during the day is a serious problem but is not recommended because of the increased risk of bacterial corneal ulcers. Newer work has demonstrated that time spent outside may be more valuable as an environmental effect to slow myopia progression.

Daily use of contact lenses can be considered for psychosocial purposes or functional reasons (like sports) when the child is motivated to insert the lenses and responsible enough to care for them properly. Typically, this is early in middle school for most children.

Despite common belief, prescription glasses properly prescribed have not been demonstrated to worsen refraction of the eye.

Discussion

Refractive errors are thought to occur because of a combination of genetic and environmental factors. The prevalence of refractive error among ethnic groups differs greatly. The natural history of refractive error has been the subject of numerous investigations. Most babies are born hyperopic and shift toward emmetropia (no refractive error) by 6 to 8 years of age. This process is called emmetropization, meaning that small to modest refractive errors generally disappear with development. In premature newborns less than 36 weeks of gestational age, there is a higher incidence of myopia than in full-term infants.

Key Points

- Low hyperopia is the most common refractive error of childhood and generally does not need to be corrected with eyeglasses.
- In the United States, refractive error that requires correction affects 25% of the population by the age of 15 years.
- Myopia is the most common refractive error requiring correction encountered in children.
- All types of refractive errors can affect global school performance.
- In most cases, refractive error is easily remedied by corrective eyeglasses.
- Wearing corrective glasses does not speed the progression of refractive disorder.

Suggested Reading

Fulton AB, Dobson V, Salem D, Mar C, Petersen RA, Hansen RM. Cycloplegic refractions in infants and young children. *Am J Ophthalmol.* 1980;90(2):239–247

Saw SM, Gazzard G, Au Eong KG, Tan DT. Myopia: attempts to arrest progression. *Br J Ophthalmol.* 2002;86(11):1306–1311

Chapter 68

Normal Vision in a Patient With Poor Blood Glucose Control

Ruben Carmona, BS
Janet Lee, BS
Daniel Kasuga, MD
Xiaolei Wang, MD
Kang Zhang, MD, PhD

Presentation

A 17-year-old girl, whom the pediatrician has known for years, has type 1 diabetes mellitus. Despite much parental guidance and patient education, she has poor blood glucose control. Diabetes was diagnosed at the age of 12 years, and the girl was immediately placed on an insulin therapy regimen. Her daily injection dose is 0.80 U/kg. Her blood pressure is 120/71 mm Hg. Her fasting blood glucose level is 118 mg/dL, and her hemoglobin A_{1c} (HbA$_{1c}$) test result is 8.0%. She has a healthy weight for her height, with a body mass index of 21.3 kg/m². Her visual acuity is 20/20 when tested in the pediatrician's office.

Because current guidelines from the American Academy of Pediatrics recommend an initial retinopathy screening 3 to 5 years after diagnosis of type 1 diabetes in children older than 9 years, the pediatrician correctly refers her for evaluation by a pediatric ophthalmologist. Being well versed in eye examinations, the pediatrician takes a look with direct ophthalmoscope and notices that there are no abnormal-appearing blood vessels growing from the retina into the vitreous gel that fills the eye. This lack of neovascularization rules out the more advanced stage of diabetic retinopathy, proliferative diabetic retinopathy (PDR). The patient is referred for a full ophthalmologic examination.

Diagnosis

The pediatric ophthalmologist performs a dilated funduscopic examination on this patient. A few capillary microaneurysms are noted in her retinas due to weakened capillary walls that have allowed a bulging outward of the endothelial lining of the vessels (Figure 68-1). This could be diabetic retinopathy, but at what stage? There is no swelling, macular edema, or presence of exudates. Furthermore, the retinal tissue looks healthy and does not have the appearance of decreased blood flow (ischemia). This effectively rules out severe non-proliferative diabetic retinopathy (NPDR). However, the patient does display an initial sign of NPDR—microaneurysms.

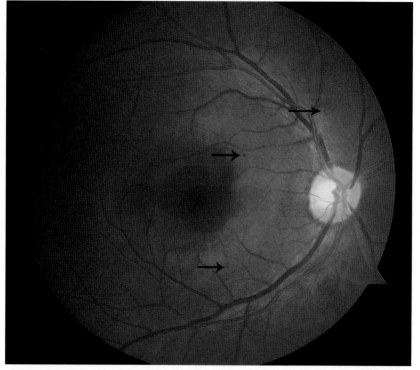

Figure 68-1. Fundus image of the girl's right eye reveals a few small microaneurysms (arrows), which are indicative of mild non-proliferative diabetic retinopathy. Courtesy of Kang Zhang, MD, PhD.

Major diagnostic clues in this case are the child's medical history, lifestyle and daily habits, funduscopic findings, and fasting blood glucose and HbA$_{1c}$ levels. Hemoglobin A$_{1c}$ measures serum glycosylated hemoglobin, which is an indicator for average level of serum glucose for 3 preceding months. Glycemic control, along with duration of diabetes, have been found to correlate closely with development of diabetic retinopathy.

Diabetic retinopathy refers to all abnormalities of retinal blood vessels caused by diabetes. Usually in young patients with type 1 diabetes, no clinically significant retinopathy can be seen in the first 5 years after initial diagnosis of diabetes is made. However, substantial retinopathy may become apparent shortly thereafter at 6 to 7 years after onset of the disease.

Diabetic retinopathy progresses from non-proliferative to proliferative and can normally be divided into 4 stages (Table 68-1). In NPDR, vision is usually normal, but blood vessels in the retina may become weak and begin to bulge. These vessels eventually leak, forming small hemorrhages. If the condition worsens, neovascularization will occur and can leak blood into the center of the eye, thereby blurring vision. This stage is called PDR.

Table 68-1. Stages of Diabetic Retinopathy

Mild Non-proliferative
• Microaneurysms

Moderate Non-proliferative
• Microaneurysms, intraretinal hemorrhages, venous beading • Hard exudates, cotton-wool spots

Severe Non-proliferative

• One or more of the following (4-2-1 rule):
  – Microaneurysms or hemorrhage in 4 or more quadrants
  – Venous beading in 2 or more quadrants
  – Intraretinal microvascular abnormalities in 1 or more quadrants

Proliferative
• Neovascularization of optic disc, retina, or iris • Vitreous hemorrhage

Differential Diagnosis

Diagnoses besides diabetic retinopathy that should be considered include the following:

Hypertensive Retinopathy

This is associated with arteriolar narrowing and nicking of the veins.

Radiation Retinopathy

There is history of radiation therapy to the eye or nearby tissue.

Sickle Cell Retinopathy

Clinical findings include salmon patch hemorrhages, black sunburst lesions, and sea-fan neovascularization.

Coats Disease

This disease usually affects young males. Fundus examination shows telangiectatic and aneurysmal retinal vessels and subretinal exudates.

Central Retinal Vein Occlusion

Clinical findings include diffuse retinal hemorrhages, tortuous veins, and optic disc swelling. Patients often complain of sudden painless loss of vision in one eye.

Branch Retinal Vein Occlusion

Clinical findings include superficial hemorrhages along a retinal vein that do not cross midline. Patients often complain of sudden painless decrease of vision in one eye.

When to Refer

Children with type 1 diabetes mellitus who are older than 9 years should receive initial retinopathy screening 3 to 5 years after diagnosis with subsequent annual examinations.

Treatment

No treatment is needed in the eyes during the earliest stages of diabetic retinopathy, but patients should be closely followed by an ophthalmologist. To prevent a child's progression of diabetic retinopathy, it is important for patients to control their levels of blood glucose, blood pressure, and blood cholesterol. The Diabetic Control and Complications Trial demonstrated that tight glucose control reduced incidence and progression of diabetic retinopathy in patients with type 1 diabetes mellitus. The American Diabetes Association recommends that HbA_{1c} levels of less than 7.5% should be the aim in adolescents 13 to 19 years old. A lower goal of less than 7% may be reasonable if it can be achieved without excessive hypoglycemia. In this case, the girl should also make a follow-up appointment for approximately 6 months to detect risk of disease progression.

Patients exhibiting PDR with neovascularization require timely treatment to prevent potentially severe loss of vision. Panretinal photocoagulation is the mainstay of treatment. If vitreous hemorrhage or retinal detachment occurs because of neovascularization, patients may require vitrectomy surgery in addition to photocoagulation therapy (laser).

Discussion

The leading cause of vision loss in young adults is diabetic retinopathy. Children younger than 10 years with type 1 diabetes mellitus are at minimal risk of developing diabetic retinopathy. However, prevalence of the disease rises steadily following puberty. Risk of visual loss from diabetic retinopathy can be reduced with early identification and treatment.

Key Points

- In initial stages of diabetic retinopathy, patients are generally asymptomatic.
- Families need to be proactive about seeking fundamental diabetes education and practicing effective diabetes management.
- A healthy lifestyle and good control of blood glucose levels will likely help protect vision in young diabetic patients.
- Intensive diabetes treatment delays onset and slows progression of diabetic retinopathy. However, therapy must be tailored to the patient to avoid hypoglycemic events.

Suggested Reading

The effects of intensive diabetes treatment on the progression of diabetic retinopathy in insulin-dependent diabetes mellitus. The Diabetes Control and Complications Trial. *Arch Ophthalmol.* 1995;113(1): 36–51

Klein R, Klein BE, Moss SE, Davis MD, DeMets DL. The Wisconsin epidemiologic study of diabetic retinopathy. II. Prevalence and risk of diabetic retinopathy when age at diagnosis is less than 30 years. *Arch Ophthalmol.* 1984;102(4):520–526

Lueder GT, Silverstein J, American Academy of Pediatrics Section on Ophthalmology and Section on Endocrinology. Screening for retinopathy in the pediatric patient with type 1 diabetes mellitus. *Pediatrics.* 2005;116(1):270–273

The relationship of glycemic exposure (HbA1c) to the risk of development and progression of retinopathy in the diabetes control and complications trial. *Diabetes.* 1995;44(8):968–983

Retinopathy and nephropathy in patients with type 1 diabetes four years after a trial of intensive therapy. The Diabetes Control and Complications Trial/Epidemiology of Diabetes Interventions and Complications Research Group. *N Engl J Med.* 2000;342(6):381–389

Silverstein J, Klingensmith G, Copeland K, et al. Care of children and adolescents with type 1 diabetes: a statement of the American Diabetes Association. *Diabetes Care.* 2005;28(1):186–212

Chapter 69

White Mass on the Eye

Salma Khayali, MD
Shira L. Robbins, MD
Bobby S. Korn, MD, PhD
Don O. Kikkawa, MD

Presentation

A new patient, a 5-month-old boy, presents to the pediatric clinic for routine care. He is reported to be otherwise healthy, according to his parents.

Complete physical examination reveals preauricular skin tags, partially formed ears, mandibular hypoplasia, and cleft palate. Ocular examination reveals an elevated dome-shaped white lesion at the edge of the cornea inferotemporally of the left eye (Figure 69-1). The infant reacts to light in both eyes and appears to have normal pupillary responses and grossly full ocular motility. No other eyelid or anterior segment abnormalities are noted, and red reflex is equal in both eyes. Further examination reveals a cardiac murmur.

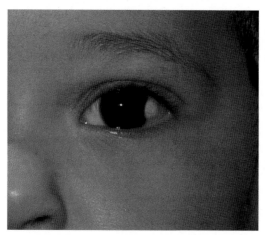

Figure 69-1. White raised lesion covering part of the lateral conjunctiva and cornea. Courtesy of Don O. Kikkawa, MD.

Diagnosis

This patient has findings consistent with facioauriculovertebral (FAV) spectrum, also termed Goldenhar syndrome or oculoauriculovertebral (OAV) dysplasia. Therefore, the pediatrician refers the infant to a pediatric ophthalmologist to perform a full eye examination.

The pediatric ophthalmologist performs a penlight examination (often sufficient) to identify a limbal dermoid (a dermoid at the limbus, the edge of the cornea) and possible eyelid abnormalities. The ophthalmologist also tests for eye preference, strabismus (eye misalignment), and anterior and posterior segment abnormalities, including iris and choroidal colobomas. This infant's findings are consistent with FAV; he has a limbal dermoid and a preauricular skin tag.

Facioauriculovertebral spectrum is the most common craniofacial malformation. The FAV spectrum is present at birth and occurs sporadically in most cases. It is a spectrum of findings that results from disruption of development of the first and second branchial arches during fetal development. The disorder is characterized by a wide spectrum of findings that vary in severity. The most common characteristics include
- Epibulbar dermoid
- Microtia
- Microstomia
- Mandibular hypoplasia
- Preauricular skin tag and inner ear anomaly
- Vertebral anomaly

Other ocular findings that have been documented with FAV spectrum include eyelid defects and iris and choroidal colobomas. Other, less common findings include microphthalmia (small eye), lacrimal duct stenosis, and strabismus, including Duane syndrome (see Chapter 63).

In FAV, the ocular dermoid is present from birth but can enlarge with age. It is typically found in the inferotemporal quadrant of the globe. The dermoid is bilateral in about 25% of cases. A subconjunctival lipodermoid or dermolipoma (lipoma covered by keratinized or nonkeratinized epithelium with hair on the surface) is found in the superotemporal quadrant in about 50% of cases. A coloboma (or notch) of the upper eyelid is present at the junction of the middle and inner third of the eyelid in about 25% of cases. Vision is often affected, as the dermoid can distort the normal corneal surface, resulting in irregular astigmatism. Ocular dermoids can lead to amblyopia (lazy eye) in 1 of 2 ways. The dermoid may cause astigmatism or refractive changes that result in unequal focusing power between the eyes (anisometropic amblyopia) or, if obstructing the visual axis, the dermoid may cause deprivation-type amblyopia.

Auricular anomalies, typically on the same side as the ocular dermoid, include periauricular appendages, posteriorly displaced ears, and stenosis of the external auditory meatus (Figure 69-2). Sensorineural or conductive hearing loss has been reported to occur in 50% of patients. The cause of hearing loss varies and can be the result of outer ear malformations, narrow or missing ear canals, or abnormal skin cartilage on or in front of the ears.

Vertebral anomalies occur in two-thirds of patients, including fused cervical vertebrae, hemivertebrae, spina bifida, and occipitalization of the atlas. Failure of segmentation is the most common abnormality

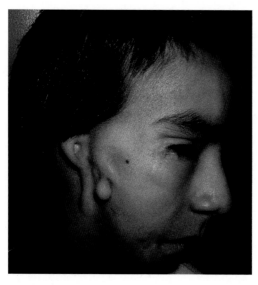

Figure 69-2. Facioauriculovertebral patient with auricular abnormalities, including preauricular appendage. Courtesy of Shira L. Robbins, MD, and the Rady Children's Hospital Craniofacial Clinic.

present in the neck region, and failure of formation most frequently occurs in the upper thoracic spine.

Cardiac disease is also seen in high frequency in patients with FAV spectrum. Especially common are ventricular septal defect, atrial septal defect, patent ductus arteriosus, tetralogy of Fallot, and coarctation of the aorta.

A high incidence of structural abnormalities of the pharynx and larynx has been associated with this syndrome. This is an important implication for any general anesthesia that is to be administered throughout the patient's lifetime. Renal, genitourinary, and gastrointestinal defects are also known associations with FAV spectrum and should be screened for routinely.

Differential Diagnosis

Diagnoses besides FAV spectrum that should be considered include the following:

Treacher Collins Syndrome

These patients can have some of the same features as FAV spectrum. These include abnormalities of the ear in which the outer part of the ear may be missing or partially formed. They may also have micrognathia, cleft palate, flat cheekbones, and hypoplasia of the facial bones. Mandibular hypoplasia may cause airway obstruction. Ocular abnormalities include colobomas of the eyelid, aplasia of the lid lashes, and down-slanting palpebral fissures. Ocular dermoids are not a typical feature of Treacher Collins syndrome.

Hallermann-Streiff Syndrome

This is a rare condition that can also have some similar features to FAV spectrum. These patients also may have mandibular hypoplasia; however, they often have distinctive, characteristic birdlike facies including a prominent thin pointed nose, extreme thinness of the skin, and severe dental abnormalities. They also have hypotrichosis. They do not typically have auricular abnormalities. Ocular findings include congenital cataracts, microphthalmos, and eyelid abnormalities.

When to Refer

Patients with findings consistent with FAV spectrum require a thorough screening examination for possible systemic associations as well as referral to a pediatric ophthalmologist for a complete eye examination.

Treatment

The patient had a complete ophthalmic examination and was noted to have a significant degree of astigmatism in the eye with the limbal dermoid. He was prescribed glasses to correct for the astigmatism and his vision was noted to be equal in both eyes on subsequent examinations. He did not require amblyopia therapy or surgical intervention. Limbal dermoids are often difficult to surgically remove, as the lesion may extend into deeper structures of the eye. Because of this, conservative treatment is usually attempted initially as long as visual development is not adversely affected. For patients with astigmatism, glasses with or without patching may be prescribed to stave off amblyopia. If the dermoid has encroached on the visual axis, dilating eyedrops may be prescribed to enlarge the visual axis. If amblyopia does develop, more intense patching treatment and dilating drops may be used.

Limbal dermoids may also require periodic removal of irritating cilia or topical lubrication to prevent foreign body sensation. Excision is considered only after amblyopia treatment fails and when the risks of scar formation or surgical complications are outweighed by the likelihood of improving the patient's vision or cosmesis.

The procedure of choice for removal of a dermoid is a superficial sclerokeratectomy (removing the involved sclera and cornea) performed flush with the globe. The exposed sclera is then covered by the conjunctiva or donor scleral tissue. Any uncovered or exposed areas can result in scarring of the conjunctiva and cornea to the eyelids (Figure 69-3).

Other associated ocular findings are evaluated and treated as needed, including possible nasolacrimal duct probing for obstruction, strabismus surgery for eye misalignment, and at least one dilated eye examination for evaluation of posterior colobomas.

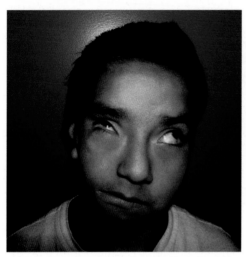

Figure 69-3. Same patient as in Figure 69-2 with history of surgery to remove dermoid; note the eyelid scarring to the conjunctiva with resultant abnormal eyelid shape on upgaze. Courtesy of Shira L. Robbins, MD, and the Rady Children's Hospital Craniofacial Clinic.

Discussion

Craniofacial malformations are rare conditions that can present in multiple patterns and varying degrees of severity. There are several common ophthalmic abnormalities related to craniofacial malformations, such as telecanthus, hypertelorism, eyelid malposition, and nasolacrimal duct obstruction.

The classification of craniofacial malformations is difficult to standardize because of the large variation of the disease. They can be divided into 2 broad categories, facial cleft syndromes and craniosynostosis.

Common facial cleft syndromes include FAV spectrum, Treacher Collins syndrome, and Hallermann-Streiff syndrome (see "Differential Diagnosis" on page 476).

Craniosynostoses are the result of premature fusion of a single or multiple cranial sutures. They are usually present at birth. Early closure of cranial sutures can cause facial deformities, increased intracranial pressure, visual loss from papilledema in severe cases, and developmental delay.

The most common craniosynostoses are Crouzon disease and Apert and Pfeiffer syndromes (Figure 69-4). These disease/syndromes are the result of bilateral coronal suture synostosis and lead to an abnormal shape of the skull called brachycephaly. The skull has a characteristic shortened anteroposterior diameter, with a flat forehead and corresponding enlargement of the bitemporal and biparietal diameters. Because of changes in orbital anatomy, most commonly shallow orbits, the eyes are pushed forward. This can result in visual loss from optic atrophy due to narrowing of the optic canal or stretching of the optic nerve. Because of abnormal suture development, these patients may develop papilledema and resultant optic nerve swelling. Patients with craniosynostoses are also at risk of corneal exposure, as the globe is anteriorly positioned in the shallow orbit. Patients should be screened for the development of these ocular complications.

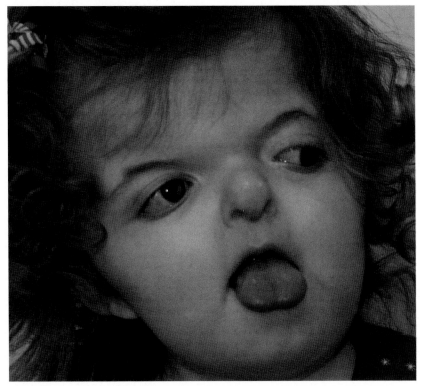

Figure 69-4. Patient with Apert syndrome and typical facial features. Courtesy of Shira L. Robbins, MD.

These syndromes share common clinical characteristic features. Observed extracranial abnormalities include varying degrees of midfacial hypoplasia, hypertelorism, and proptosis (abnormal protrusion of the eyeball) secondary to shallow orbits. Proptosis is usually more prominent in Crouzon disease than Apert syndrome. Apert syndrome is typically characterized by a varying degree of strabismus with down-slanting of the palpebral fissures. Syndactyly of hands and feet is common in Apert syndrome (Figure 69-5). Pfeiffer syndrome also has digital anomalies of broadening of the thumb and great toe. Intellectual capacity is usually normal in patients with Crouzon disease or Pfeiffer syndrome, whereas hydrocephalus and developmental delay are more frequent in Apert syndrome. An autosomal-dominant pattern of inheritance occurs in most cases of Crouzon disease. Sporadic transmission is more common in Apert and Pfeiffer syndromes.

Ophthalmic manifestations of craniofacial malformations can affect the orbit, eyelids, and lacrimal system.

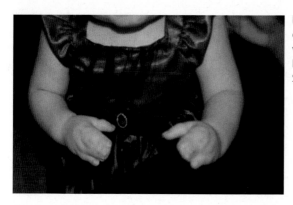

Figure 69-5. Syndactyly of the hands in the patient with Apert syndrome from Figure 69-4. Courtesy of Shira L. Robbins, MD.

Key Points

- The facioauriculovertebral (FAV) spectrum is the most common craniofacial malformation, with limbal dermoids as its most prevalent ocular finding.
- An estimated 30% of patients with dermoids have associated systemic abnormalities, including FAV spectrum.
- Patients suspected of having FAV spectrum should undergo thorough examination for possible systemic associations, including hearing loss, spinal malformations, and cardiac disease.
- Initial epibulbar dermoid treatment is conservative and may include glasses, dilating eyedrops, and patching.
- Craniosynostoses require long-term follow-up for development of papilledema and strabismus.

Suggested Reading

Gorlin RJ, Pindborg JJ. Oculoauriculovertebral dysplasia. In: *Syndromes of the Head and Neck.* New York, NY: McGraw-Hill; 1964:546–552

Kaufman A, Medow N, Phillips R, Zaidman G. Treatment of epibulbar limbal dermoids. *J Pediatr Ophthalmol Strabismus.* 1999;36(3): 136–140

Mader TH, Stulting D. Technique for the removal of limbal dermoids. *Cornea.* 1998;17(1):66–67

Nelson L, Olitsky S. *Harley's Pediatric Ophthalmology.* 5th ed. Lippincott Williams & Wilkins; 2005:233–234

Nesi FA, Lisman RD, Levine MR. *Smith's Ophthalmic Plastic and Reconstructive Surgery.* 2nd ed. Mosby; 1998

Chapter 70

Droopy Eyelid and Eyelid Nodule

Edel M. Cosgrave, FRCOphth
Anthony J. Vivian, FRCS, FRCOphth

Presentation

A mother brings her 3-year-old son to see the pediatrician for a second opinion on swelling of his left upper and lower eyelids (Figure 70-1). The child has completed a 1-week course of antibiotics to treat an eyelid infection. Eyelid swelling has almost fully resolved except for a slight ptosis and a small nodule in the lower lid. The mother tells the pediatrician that her son's left lid has always been a little droopy, but she is concerned about the nodular swelling.

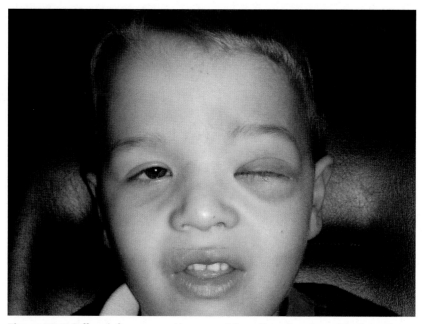

Figure 70-1. Diffuse left upper and lower eyelid swelling. Courtesy of Anthony J. Vivian, FRCS, FRCOphth.

While palpating for lymphadenopathy, the pediatrician notices that the patient has a café au lait spot on his neck. When the pediatrician asks the parent about any other birthmarks, she removes the boy's T-shirt to reveal several more café au lait spots on his back and 2 small neurofibromas on his shoulder (Figure 70-2).

Because of these findings in conjunction with the eyelid nodule, the pediatrician becomes suspicious and sends the patient with his parents to see an ophthalmologist.

The ophthalmologist carries out a slit-lamp microscopic examination of the boy's eyes and notes a number of Lisch nodules on the irises (Figure 70-3). Both parents' eyes are also examined, but they do not have any Lisch nodules. The ophthalmologist is also concerned that the boy has a mild degree of proptosis (bulging forward of the globe) and a pale optic nerve on the left side. Therefore, the ophthalmologist arranges for a biopsy of the eyelid nodule and a computed tomography (CT) scan of the orbits (Figure 70-4).

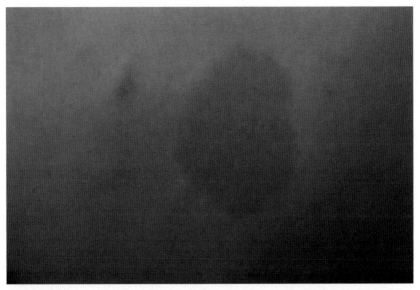

Figure 70-2. Classic café au lait spot on child's back. Courtesy of Anthony J. Vivian, FRCS, FRCOphth.

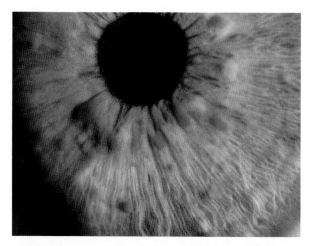

Figure 70-3. Iris Lisch nodules, benign pigmented lesion. Courtesy of Anthony J. Vivian, FRCS, FRCOphth.

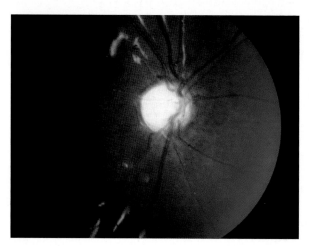

Figure 70-4. Severe pallor of the optic nerve with pathologic large optic cup. Courtesy of Anthony J. Vivian, FRCS, FRCOphth.

Diagnosis

The biopsy is reported as consistent with plexiform neurofibroma. The CT scan shows a left optic nerve glioma with no evidence of sphenoid bone dysplasia. The diagnosis is neurofibromatosis type 1 (NF1). Arrangements are made for regular ophthalmic assessments to monitor visual function. The family is referred to the medical center's genetics department, where gene testing of the family and genetic counseling are commenced.

Eight subtypes of neurofibromatosis have been described to date, but the National Institutes of Health defined 2 distinct types. Neurofibromatosis type 1 (formerly called von Recklinghausen disease) affects 90% of patients, and neurofibromatosis type 2 (NF2, or bilateral acoustic neuromas and schwannomas) affects 10%. Whereas NF1 most often is diagnosed in early childhood, NF2 usually presents in the teen years or adulthood.

The clinical diagnosis of NF1 requires 2 or more of the following:
- Six or more café au lait spots larger than 5 mm in diameter in prepubertal children and larger than 15 mm in postpubertal children
- A plexiform neurofibroma (or 2 or more neurofibromas of any type)
- Crowe sign (multiple freckles in the axillary or inguinal region)
- A first-degree relative with confirmed NF1
- Optic nerve glioma
- Two or more Lisch nodules
- Sphenoid dysplasia, cortical thinning in long bones, or other distinctive osseous lesion

Lisch nodules of the irises are the ocular hallmark of NF1 but do not affect vision. The prevalence of Lisch nodules increases with age, occurring in 40% of children aged 3 to 4 years and 100% of those older than 20 years. The number of Lisch nodules does not correlate with clinical severity of NF1.

Neurofibromas may affect any organ in the body. Cutaneous neurofibromas occur infrequently before puberty. A plexiform neurofibroma is a diffuse elongated fibroma that frequently involves the trigeminal or upper cervical nerves. Development of a plexiform neurofibroma in the eyelid can cause a classic S-shaped ptosis in the pediatric patient. It often appears within the first 2 years of life and can be associated with overlying hyperpigmentation. Plexiform neurofibromas can induce refractive errors (astigmatism), and if the visual axis is compromised, amblyopia (lazy eye) and strabismus (eye misalignment) can develop. Rarely, plexiform neurofibromas can undergo malignant transformation (about 10%) to become malignant peripheral nerve sheath tumors.

The child with NF1 is also at risk of glaucoma, typically in the eye on the side of the plexiform neurofibroma. Iris ectropion (visible, darkly pigmented underside of the iris) also indicates a risk of glaucoma.

Optic nerve gliomas occur in 12% to 15% of patients with NF1, most occurring in the first decade of life and tending to be nonprogressive. Thirty percent are bilateral, and up to 40% have involvement of the optic chiasm. They appear as fusiform enlargement of the optic nerve and its sheath on CT scan and are noncalcified.

Rapid enlargement of a glioma can present with visual loss, proptosis, and ocular motility problems. The optic disc can appear swollen or atrophic, sometimes showing an optociliary shunt vessel. Visual evoked potentials are a useful way of determining optic nerve function, detecting chiasmatic involvement, and monitoring progression or regression of chiasmatic gliomas.

Differential Diagnosis

It is mainly the cutaneous features of NF1 that are shared with other conditions. Multiple café au lait spots may occur with no other features of NF1 inherited in an autosomal-dominant fashion. They are also a feature of Albright syndrome (in association with polyostotic fibrous dysplasia) and LEOPARD syndrome (in association with hypertelorism, deafness, and congenital heart disease).

Multiple skin nodules occur in multiple endocrine neoplasia type 2b (with neuromas of the conjunctiva and oral mucosa and pheochromocytoma), multiple lipomatosis, congenital generalized fibromatosis, and Proteus syndrome (with regional overgrowth and multiple lipomas.

Skin lesions and Lisch nodules may rarely be a feature of NF2 (associated with cranial nerve neuromas, especially acoustic neuromas).

When to Refer

Children with NF1 should be referred routinely to a pediatric ophthalmologist. Yearly review is suggested to detect progressive optic nerve or chiasmatic involvement. However, if there is a significant occlusion of an eye by ptosis or eyelid lesion or the eye itself looks abnormal, particularly in a young child, referral should be made urgently.

Treatment

This patient has undergone a number of debulking operations of his plexiform neuroma as it progresses. He has required occlusion treatment of his better eye to limit the development of amblyopia in his affected eye.

Blepharoptosis surgery is indicated if the visual axis is compromised by a plexiform neurofibroma. Postoperatively this type of neurofibroma may recur and require further surgery. Ptosis surgery performed to improve appearance is best delayed until after the age of 18 years.

Optic nerve gliomas are treated with expectant observation unless serial imaging studies detect aggressive growth. Progressive disease interfering with vision may require surgical excision, chemotherapy, or less often, radiation therapy.

Pediatricians should provide health supervision to children with NF1 according to American Academy of Pediatrics policy. Children with neurofibromatosis also often need multidisciplinary care. Management of children with NF1 includes an annual eye examination by a pediatric ophthalmologist or an ophthalmologist familiar with the disorder.

Discussion

Neurofibromatosis type 1 is an autosomal-dominant disorder with an incidence of 1 case per 3,000 to 4,000 people. Genetic defect is found on chromosome 17, causing a mutation in the neurofibromin gene. Fifty percent of cases are new mutations. In familial cases, expressivity of the disorder is variable, but penetrance is 100%.

Most children with NF1 are mildly affected. However, they have an increased risk of morbidity and life-threatening problems, which does not correlate with their findings in childhood.

Key Points

- Ophthalmic assessment of a child suspected of having neurofibromatosis type 1 can reveal much more than the presence of Lisch nodules.
- Lisch nodules appear over time. Therefore, normal eye examination results at an early age do not rule out diagnosis of neurofibromatosis.
- Be aware of the possibility of glaucoma on the side of an eyelid plexiform neurofibroma.
- In children with neurofibromatosis, visual loss can result from optic nerve gliomas, glaucoma, blockage of the visual axis because of eyelid neurofibromas, astigmatism, and amblyopia.

Suggested Reading

Hersch JM, American Academy of Pediatrics Committee on Genetics. Health supervision for children with neurofibromatosis. *Pediatrics.* 2008;121(3):633–642. http://aappolicy.aappublications.org/cgi/content/full/pediatrics;121/3/633. Accessed May 22, 2012

Jett K, Friedman JM. Clinical and genetic aspects of neurofibromatosis 1. *Genet Med.* 2010;12(1):1–11

Zeid JL, Charrow J, Sandu M, Goldman S, Listernick R. Orbital optic nerve gliomas in children with neurofibromatosis type 1. *J AAPOS.* 2006;10(6):534–539

Chapter 71

Absence of Tearing

Ronald Antonio N. Reyna, MD

Presentation

An 8-month-old girl is brought to the pediatric clinic because she has absence of tearing as well as feeding difficulties. Her previous pediatrician is contemplating performing blood tests and genetic testing, but the parents prefer getting a second opinion from another pediatrician before proceeding with the tests. Unfortunately, previous health records are not available. The mother claims that the infant was born at term with no known labor complications and with an unremarkable prenatal history. However, she informs the pediatrician that her daughter has been hospitalized twice for treatment of pneumonia, which was treated with unrecalled antibiotics.

The pediatric nurse gives the pediatrician the weight and length of the baby and on plotting the data, the pediatrician finds that the baby is below the 50th percentile for weight and height. The pediatrician then asks about feeding problems. The mother claims that the baby does not tolerate solid foods and that she usually vomits after liquid feedings. The mother also claims that the infant does not produce tears when she cries. The pediatrician goes through past medical and social history and finds out that the family recent emigrated from Europe and are of Eastern European Jewish descent. No one in the family has had similar problems.

On examination, the pediatrician notices that the patient's skin generally appears blotchy, and the girl has several scratch marks on her arms and cheeks. When the pediatrician questions the mother, she answers that the scratches occur frequently whenever she forgets to cut her daughter's nails. The pediatrician then shines a light from a direct ophthalmoscope and discovers some mild horizontal opacities along the inferior border of the cornea of both eyes. As the family mentioned, the pediatrician sees an absence of tearing. The infant does not seem to be having ocular discomfort.

Routine examination of corneal opacities requires staining the eyes with fluorescein dye to check for uptake of the dye by the de-epithelialized cornea. The pediatrician has a bottle of fluorescein solution mixed with anesthetic but because of the concerning absence of symptoms, the pediatrician pauses. Why is this child not in pain? The pediatrician decides to check for corneal sensitivity. With a wisp of cotton, the pediatrician gently touches the cornea from the temporal side to avoid visually inducing a blink reaction. Unsurprisingly, the patient does not blink on contact. The pediatrician places a drop of fluorescein dye on both eyes and on shining a blue light from the direct ophthalmoscope, notes the presence of yellow-green uptake of dye along opacified areas. Otherwise, the patient has a bright red-orange reflex coming from within the pupil of both eyes.

Diagnosis

Given the history, physical findings, and ancestry of the patient, the pediatrician's primary consideration is familial dysautonomia, also called Riley-Day syndrome. The pediatrician gives the infant artificial tears and refers the patient to an ophthalmologist.

Differential Diagnosis

- Congenital causes of alacrima can be seen in patients with maldeveloped eyes.
- In cryptophthalmos, the skin grows over the eyeball without separation of the eyelids with associated maldevelopment of other ocular tissues.
- With anophthalmia, there is complete failure of eye development resulting in absence of eye tissues.
- Acquired causes of alacrima may be secondary to scarring from previous ocular infection, chemical burns, Stevens-Johnson syndrome, vitamin A deficiency, or Mikulicz syndrome.

- With familial dysautonomia, eye structures are fully developed. The absence of preexisting conditions such as trauma, rash, or infection and presence of autonomic and sensory dysfunction support diagnosis of familial dysautonomia.

When to Refer

A patient with possible familial dysautonomia should be referred to an ophthalmologist to test for tear production and to check for corneal damage using slit-lamp biomicroscopy.

Treatment

Treatment is supportive only. Medications may be given to help control abnormal blood pressure, nausea, and vomiting. Artificial tears can be helpful, and appropriate topical antibiotics may be given in the presence of secondary bacterial infection. Safety goggles or the use of glasses over contact lenses is advised to protect eyes from environmental damage or fingernail-induced corneal abrasions. Special consideration should be given in choosing protective eyewear in patients with dysautonomia. Improperly fitted glasses or frames with sharp edges should be avoided because some frames have been known to cause skin abrasions along areas of contact such as the nasal bridge, temple, and just above the ears.

Lastly, genetic counseling can be helpful in educating parents about their potential genetic risk if they are contemplating having more children. Prenatal testing for the *IKBKAP* gene is now possible and can be offered to people at risk of carrying this gene.

Discussion

Alacrima is a condition characterized by the absence of or markedly reduced tear production. This may be present from birth in conditions where conjunctivae and the eye failed to develop, or in patients with autonomic dysfunctions. Familial dysautonomia is a rare autosomal-recessive genetic disorder that almost exclusively affects people of Eastern European (Ashkenazi) Jewish descent. It is estimated that 1 in 27 people of this population is a carrier of the familial dysautonomia gene identified as *IKBKAP.* Dysfunction is a result of incomplete development and progressive degeneration of the neurons affecting the autonomic and sensory nervous systems. The autonomic nervous system is responsible for tear production, breathing, digestion, and regulation of blood pressure and body temperature. The sensory nervous system is responsible for protective response to pain, perception of hot and cold, and taste. A definitive diagnosis of familial dysautonomia can be made with a blood test that will show mutations in the *IKBKAP* gene in an affected individual.

Ocular health is highly dependent on adequate lubrication as provided by our tears. The surface of the eye is also supplied by nerve endings that stimulate tear production and blinking whenever the eye gets irritated or when basic tear production is inadequate. Diminished or lack of sensation on the ocular surface may lead to inadequate tear production or lack of reflex tearing, and a diminished blink reflex.

Affected individuals become susceptible to having frequent corneal abrasions and exposure keratopathies, both of which manifest clinically as areas of opacity frequently involving the inferior part of the cornea (Figure 71-1). Secondary bacterial infections of damaged corneas may lead to corneal ulcerations and, if left untreated, extension of the infection to intraocular tissues, with subsequent blindness.

Prognosis used to be poor with life expectancy averaging up to 5 years old, with chronic pulmonary failure and aspiration as common causes of death. However, reports of mild to moderate vision loss secondary to optic atrophy usually after the first decade of life are increasing as advances in treatment have increased life expectancy of patients.

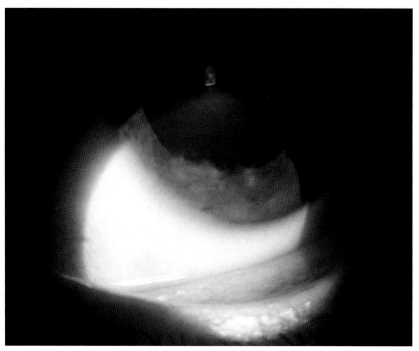

Figure 71-1. Inferior cloudiness on cornea. Courtesy of Ronald Antonio N. Reyna, MD.

Key Points

- Familial dysautonomia is a rare autosomal-recessive genetic disorder that affects almost exclusively people of Ashkenazi Jewish descent.
- Because most patients with familial dysautonomia are asymptomatic, regular pediatric and ophthalmologic evaluations are needed to detect problems that are otherwise unknown to the affected individuals.
- Families of children with familial dysautonomia are advised to seek professional help as soon as possible for dysautonomic crisis, or when there are signs of possible corneal involvement such as whitish opacities and presence of ocular discharge or redness.

Suggested Reading

Axelrod FB. Familial dysautonomia: a review of the current pharmaco-
logical treatments. *Expert Opin Pharmacother.* 2005;6(4):561–567

Mondino BJ, Brown SI. Hereditary congenital alacrima. *Arch Ophthalmol.* 1976;94(9):1478–1484

Chapter 72

Pale, Shaking Eyes

Ronald Antonio N. Reyna, MD

Presentation

An infant boy comes to the pediatrician's office for his 2-month well-baby visit. The pediatrician has known this infant since birth. On interviewing the parents, their main concern is that 2 weeks ago, the child was noted to have "wiggly" eyes. The parents are not sure how long this has been going on, only that it is getting more noticeable. The infant is also noted to be squinting his eyes in brightly lit conditions. Otherwise, he is healthy and growing normally for his age. He was born full term with no complications. He is the product of light-skinned white parents and has a slightly lighter complexion than his parents.

On examination, the pediatrician notes that the patient's eyes do wiggle from side to side. The patient tends to avoid the light from a direct ophthalmoscope by squinting. The pediatrician asks the parents if anyone in the family has the same condition. The mother says that one of her uncles had wiggly eyes.

The patient has a bluish to green iris. Light reflex is centered on both eyes, and pupils look round and reactive to light. The pediatrician looks through the direct ophthalmoscope to check for presence of cataracts or any other ocular disorders that may block the visual axis. Blood vessels appear prominent, but there is an indistinct fovea, the small area in the retina that affords acute vision (Figure 72-1). Normally, if the pediatrician shines a light through the iris, it is reflected back within the pupil through the direct ophthalmoscope. The pediatrician shines a light and manages to get a bright red reflex coming from within the pupil but also diffusely through the iris of each eye. This effect is more obvious when the room lights are turned off and is called iris transillumination (Figure 72-2).

Finally, the pediatrician wonders about the inheritance of this disease and examines the mother. The pediatrician closely examines her iris and notes that it is hazel to light brown in color with absence of transillumination defects. Using the direct ophthalmoscope, the pediatrician looks at her fundus and notes no pigmentary abnormalities. The pediatrician then refers the family to an ophthalmologist for further management and to check whether the mother is a carrier.

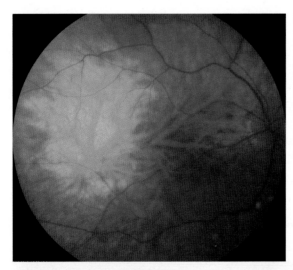

Figure 72-1. Retina of patient; note the prominent choroidal vessels easily seen because of lack of retinal pigmentation. There is also foveal hypoplasia (lack of pigment), which leads to decreased vision. Courtesy of Ronald Antonio N. Reyna, MD.

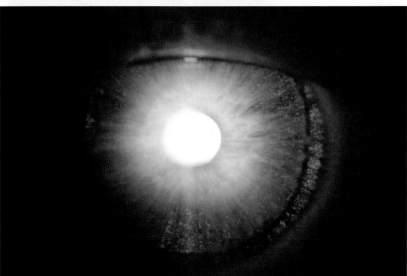

Figure 72-2. Iris transillumination defects seen as orange color due to lack of iris pigment. Natural lens edge is revealed as curvilinear line usually hidden by iris pigment. Courtesy of David B. Granet, MD.

Diagnosis

Light from a direct ophthalmoscope can be seen through areas of defect in the iris of patients with albinism because of lack of pigment. Given the transillumination defects of the iris as well as the presentation, family history, and presence of nystagmus (rapid involuntary movement of the eyes as a result of instability in the sensory motor system of the eyes), the pediatrician's primary consideration is ocular albinism.

Differential Diagnosis

Patients with tyrosinase-negative oculocutaneous albinism are easier to diagnose because they have no skin, hair, or ocular pigments. Diagnosis may be difficult in cases with ocular albinism or tyrosinase-positive oculocutaneous albinism because the reduced amount of pigmentation may not be as obvious.

Presence of nystagmus during the first few months of life should prompt the physician to look for different causes of severe vision loss. Evaluation and comparison of red reflex using a direct ophthalmoscope is invaluable in assessing anterior segment anomalies such as corneal opacities, colobomas, and congenital cataracts. Aniridia is a congenital disorder also characterized by poor vision and foveal hypoplasia. It can easily be distinguished from albinism by the absence of much of the iris tissue in patients with aniridia.

In patients with a normal-appearing anterior segment and in the absence of an iris transillumination defect, as is often the case if the examination is limited by use of a direct ophthalmoscope, a dilated fundus examination is needed to identify posterior pathologies such as retinal detachment, retinopathy of prematurity, hemorrhages, exudates, tumors, infections, and scars. Optic nerves should be evaluated as well for color and size because an abnormal-appearing optic nerve is usually indicative of a central nervous system abnormality and may necessitate a neurologic workup.

In some patients with retinal photoreceptor dysfunction, the anterior segment as well as the fundus may appear normal, and diagnosis is confirmed with electrophysiologic testing such as electroretinogram. Among those presenting with severe vision loss and nystagmus include Leber congenital amaurosis, congenital stationary night blindness, and achromatopsia. Normal funduscopic appearance is in contrast with lack of pigment, prominence of choroidal vessels, as well as presence of macular hypoplasia in patients with albinism.

When to Refer

A child with an ocular abnormality, such as nystagmus, should be referred to an ophthalmologist experienced in the care of children. When albinism is suspected, slit-lamp examination and funduscopy should be performed on the patient as well as the carrier mother to help confirm diagnosis. A thorough ophthalmologic examination on the patient may also help identify other associated ocular abnormalities that have been associated with albinism, such as anterior segment dysgenesis, glaucoma, strabismus, and high refractive errors.

A referral for neurologic workup is advised in cases in which onset of nystagmus is after 6 months of age or there is history of severe prematurity, complicated labor, coexisting genetic or developmental disease, presence of other neurologic signs, or history of exposure to drugs or toxins.

Treatment

Patients with high refractive errors are given optical correction in the form of glasses, contact lenses, or low-vision aids. Soft contact lenses may be a better option because they have been shown to dampen nystagmus and avoid eyeglass-induced distortion with ocular movement. Patching may be needed to prevent amblyopia (lazy eye). Surgery may be performed to correct strabismus, slow nystagmus, restore a more typical appearance, and improve self-image.

Treatment also includes limitation of exposure to sunlight and use of tinted glasses, hats, and sunblock because patients are more prone to ultraviolet damage and skin cancer.

Another important aspect to treatment is attention to emotional and social adjustment to this condition. Support groups are available to help deal with the emotional stress as well as to provide more information to the families involved. Referral to a geneticist for counseling may provide additional information to families if they are contemplating having more children.

Discussion

Nystagmus is often associated with multifactorial visual impairment such as albinism, aniridia, achromatopsia, congenital cataracts, retinopathy of prematurity, or optic nerve hypoplasia. It is often a first sign that a child has vision loss.

Albinism refers to a group of hereditary disorders that involve an abnormality of melanin synthesis or distribution. Clinically it presents as a pigmentation abnormality of the skin, hair, eyes, or all of these. It can be divided into 2 broad categories: oculocutaneous and ocular. Oculocutaneous albinism is primarily an autosomal-recessive disorder that involves the skin and eyes. Ocular albinism is X-linked in most cases and affects mainly the eyes, with minimal to no skin involvement. Both forms of albinism have similar ocular symptoms and signs, which include iris transillumination defects, high refractive errors, photophobia (light sensitivity), nystagmus, strabismus (eye misalignment), and decreased central visual acuity. Severity of visual acuity defect tends to be proportionate to the degree of hypopigmentation. Another common problem in patients with albinism is abnormal decussation of optic nerve fibers. Normally, temporal retinal nerve fibers go to the same side of the brain, whereas nasal fibers cross to the opposite side. From the eye with ocular albinism, more of the nerve fibers cross to the other side. This results in patients being unable to fuse images, manifesting clinically with difficulty in depth perception.

The main problem with the eye in patients with albinism is in the fovea. The fovea does not develop completely, presumably because melanin pigment is needed for its development. Therefore, the eye cannot process a sharp image no matter how well focused with glasses. Normally, light entering the eye is absorbed by the pigment of the retinal pigment epithelium (RPE). Because of lack of pigment, the patient with albinism has a "blonde fundus" with prominence of the underlying choroidal vessels (Figure 72-1). The RPE normally acts to absorb light entering the pupil. With abnormal RPE, illumination scatters freely within the eye, resulting in photophobia.

Visual difficulties in these patients are multifactorial, including light being focused on an underdeveloped fovea, stray unfocused light entering through iris defects, nystagmus, and nerve signals following an unusual route to the brain. Hence, it is not surprising to see patients with visual acuity ranging around 20/100 to 20/200, although acuities as good as 20/40 or better have been reported.

Lastly, some forms of albinism are not limited to the skin and eyes. Chédiak-Higashi syndrome is a tyrosinase-positive form of albinism characterized by the patient's susceptibility to infection, as well as tendency to develop lympho-follicular malignancy. Hermansky-Pudlak syndrome is characterized by bleeding tendencies or prolonged bleeding time as a result of platelet dysfunction. Sensorineural deafness has also been known to occur in patients with albinism.

Key Points

- Nystagmus can herald many eye diseases.
- Ocular albinism can occur even when there is some iris pigment present and the patient's skin is not affected.
- Vision loss in albinism is multifactorial and can require multiple treatments, including low-vision aids, sunglasses, and eye muscle surgery.

Suggested Reading

Riordan-Eva P, Cunningham ET Jr, eds. *Vaughan & Asbury's General Ophthalmology.* 18th ed. New York, NY: McGraw-Hill; 2011

Taylor D, Hoyt CS, eds. *Pediatric Ophthalmology and Strabismus.* 3rd ed. Edinburgh, United Kingdom: Elsevier Saunders; 2005

Wright KW, Spiegel PH, eds. *Pediatric Ophthalmology and Strabismus.* 2nd ed. New York, NY: Springer-Verlag; 2003

Chapter 73

Slanted Eyelid Fissures and Poor Vision

Lance M. Siegel, MD

Presentation

A pleasant 4-year-old boy presents to a new pediatrician. The boy is small for his age and developmentally delayed, and appears to have problems seeing. His mother reports that he has a genetic syndrome that required heart surgery as an infant. He is the only 1 of 3 children to be affected. The parents are apparently healthy and in their late 40s. The child has had no formal eye examinations after the initial check in the newborn nursery, when the mother was told everything was fine.

The pediatrician notices an atypical slant to the eyelids and focal paleness in the patient's peripheral irises (Figure 73-1). The child seems to fixate and follow objects with each eye but prefers the right eye, which is demonstrated by a left esotropia (inward eye turning). The patient has good red reflexes.

Diagnosis

History and physical findings suggest Down syndrome. A genetic karyotype would be confirmatory and may have been performed in association with this patient's cardiac evaluation as an infant. On eye examination, the pediatrician finds esotropia and likely amblyopia in the deviated eye. Because of these findings, the pediatrician refers the child to a pediatric ophthalmologist for dilated retinoscopy.

An equal and symmetrical red reflex, as seen in this boy, is important to help exclude cataracts, which are much more prevalent in individuals with Down syndrome than the rest of the population. Hypopigmented areas on the boy's peripheral iris are Brushfield spots and are present in 60% of patients with Down syndrome.

It is estimated that more than 80% of patients with Down syndrome have some clinically significant ocular pathology. Such conditions include refractive error requiring glasses (50%–70%), strabismus (40%),

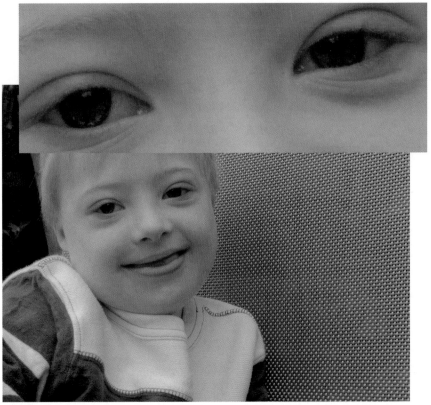

Figure 73-1. Patient with atypical slant of eyelids with the lateral canthi slightly higher than the medial canthi. Inset shows pale spots in the peripheral iris called Brushfield spots. Courtesy of the Hank family, cofounders, DS Action.

and nystagmus (30%). Blepharitis is very common in children with Down syndrome (80%; see Chapter 6). Nasolacrimal duct obstruction (see Chapter 14), exacerbated by small midface and poor blink, occurs frequently as well (20%). Eyelid ptosis (see Chapter 18), visually significant cataracts, optic neuropathy, and glaucoma also occur in increased frequency in patients with Down syndrome. Fine lens opacities that are not visually significant may present in up to 60% of patients with Down syndrome. Children with Down syndrome are also predisposed to eye rubbing and keratoconus (progressive, large, abnormal corneal curvature). This conical change in the cornea can lead to visually significant astigmatism and refractive error that cannot be corrected with glasses. Many patients with Down syndrome have nystagmus (see Chapter 61).

This rapid, rhythmic eye movement can be present at birth due to obvious or occult central nervous system abnormalities (congenital), or develop later, as in this case, from severe sensory deprivation.

Differential Diagnosis

Many of the constellation of findings in Down syndrome patients, which may include hypotonia, strabismus, cardiac problems, developmental delay, hyper-flexibility of joints, anomalous auricles, gastrointestinal and genitourinary abnormalities, and short fingers or clinodactyly, can be found in many other syndromes and require consideration in differential diagnosis.

Other diagnoses to consider include trisomy 18, Zellweger syndrome, peroxisomal disorders, and higher order multiple X chromosomes.

When to Refer

A child with Down syndrome should be examined by a pediatric ophthalmologist or an ophthalmologist who has experience with children with special needs. A special dilated retinoscopy examination is needed to determine if the child needs glasses. This technique gives refractive data without requiring subjective information, making it ideal for nonverbal patients.

Treatment

Eyeglasses compliance is often difficult and may require behavioral modification and reinforcement techniques. Blepharitis often responds to eyelid hygiene with or without antibiotics (see Chapter 6).

Many of the ocular conditions noted in patients with Down syndrome—eyelid ptosis, nasolacrimal duct obstruction, strabismus, cataracts, and glaucoma—may require surgery.

Discussion

While most patients do not achieve 20/20 vision due to many factors (eg, neurologic, developmental, and refractive abnormalities), most can be expected to have functional vision. Those who wear eyeglasses from an early age have a better prognosis from refractive amblyopia. Surgical correction for strabismus and ptosis has a success rate similar to the rest of the population. Nasolacrimal duct surgery (because of small anatomy) and cataract surgery (because of complex irregularities of the lens) often have lower surgical success than the rest of the population.

In addition to having increased risk of ocular problems, children with Down syndrome are at high risk of hearing loss and otitis media. They should be examined by an otolaryngologist or audiologist following the schedule recommended in the American Academy of Pediatrics (AAP) clinical report, "Health Supervision for Children With Down Syndrome" (see "Suggested Reading" below). Additionally, these children should be evaluated for the other medical problems common to patients with Down syndrome, including congenital heart defects and obstructive sleep apnea. Age-specific anticipatory guidance should conform to the AAP guidelines.

Key Points

- There is high prevalence of ocular comorbidities in patients with Down syndrome.
- Some of the major associated ocular findings in Down syndrome are iris Brushfield spots, need for eyeglasses (refractive error), blepharitis, nasolacrimal duct obstruction, eyelid ptosis, strabismus, cataracts, glaucoma, and optic neuropathy.
- Pediatricians are often the first to notice cataracts on red reflex test and should specifically look for them when Down syndrome is suspected.
- Because most patients with Down syndrome are not fully verbal, it is necessary for a pediatric eye care specialist who is familiar with objective examination techniques and the medical aspects of this disease to evaluate these children.

Suggested Reading

Bull MJ, American Academy of Pediatrics Committee on Genetics. Health supervision of children with Down syndrome. *Pediatrics.* 2011;128(2):393–406

Creavin AL, Brown RD. Ophthalmic abnormalities in children with Down syndrome. *J Pediatr Ophthalmol Strabismus.* 2009;46(2): 76–82

Chapter 74

Eye Misalignment, Eyelid Ptosis, and Shaking Eyes

Sri Thyagarajan, MRCOphth, BSc
Anthony J. Vivian, FRCS, FRCOphth

Presentation

An 18-month-old girl is referred from a community general physician to a pediatrician for evaluation of abnormal eye movements and delayed motor development. She was born following normal delivery at full term. She was found to have profound bilateral sensorineural deafness and fitted with hearing aids at 1 year of age. The parents report that she has never fed well and has always been a bit "floppy" (generalized lack of muscle tone.)

The girl reacts to lights and follows faces, but the pediatrician notes that she holds toys quite close to her face. She has unusually shaped ears and bilateral eyelid ptosis (drooping). Eye examination reveals a mild alternating divergent strabismus (exotropia) as well as vertical nystagmus when she looks up, but otherwise she has full eye movements. She has a normal-looking conjunctiva, and the cornea looks clear in both eyes. She has good red reflexes.

Because of her ocular abnormalities, the patient is referred to an ophthalmologist, who performs an eyeglass prescription test (refraction), formal visual acuity testing, and a full ophthalmic examination. Her visual acuity was found to be reduced at 20/60 in both eyes, as measured by specialized preverbal acuity cards. The ophthalmologist comments that the patient's anterior segment findings are normal, but the results of dilated funduscopy reveal bilateral pigment clumps in the peripheral retina (Figure 74-1).

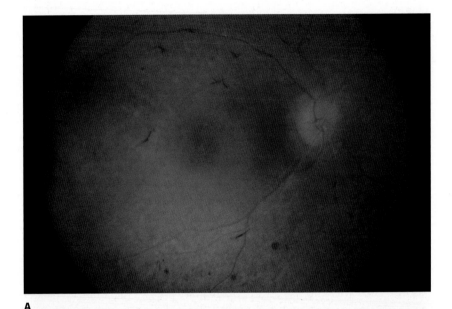

A

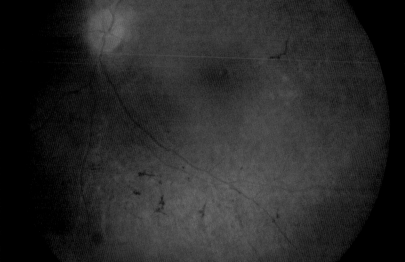

B

Figure 74-1. Optic nerve pallor, macular granularity, arteriolar sheathing, and peripheral retinal pigment clumping, right (A) and left (B) eyes. Courtesy of Anthony J. Vivian, FRCS, FRCOphth.

Diagnosis

The ophthalmologist diagnoses pigmentary retinopathy. Given the patient's hearing loss and generalized weak muscle tone, the pediatrician arranges for a battery of tests looking for systemic associations of pigmentary retinopathy. Following referral to a pediatric endocrinologist, the patient receives a diagnosis of a variant of Zellweger (cerebrohepatorenal) syndrome, a rare disorder of peroxisomal metabolism known to cause pigmentary retinopathy.

This condition belongs to a group of inherited metabolic disorders in which the fundus has pigmentary changes known as retinitis pigmentosa. Zellweger syndrome presents in early infancy, and a majority of infants die within the first 2 years of life. Those who survive with the complete syndrome have severe mental deficiency. Facial deformities, such as a high forehead, underdeveloped eyebrow ridges, and deformed earlobes, are typical. Other abnormalities may include hypotonia, mental retardation, seizures, renal cysts, hepatosplenomegaly, and hearing impairment.

More frequent metabolic causes of pigmentary retinopathies in children can be roughly divided into errors of lipid metabolism, peroxisomal function, lysosomal function, mitochondrial function, and glycogen storage (see "Differential Diagnosis" on pages 512–513). Most inherited metabolic disorders are autosomal recessive, but other modes of inheritance (eg, X-linked, mitochondrial) have been implicated. They are a clinically heterogeneous group of disorders, with variable presentation within each disorder. Thus, clinical manifestations described in "Differential Diagnosis," although comprehensive, are not always present. Presentation is usually in the neonatal period or infancy but can occur at any time, even in adulthood.

Diagnosis of an inherited metabolic disorder does not require extensive knowledge of biochemical pathways or individual metabolic diseases. An understanding of major clinical manifestations of inborn errors of metabolism provides the basis for knowing when to consider the diagnosis.

There may be general symptoms that raise suspicions about systemic disease. These include poor feeding, vomiting, failure to thrive, and lethargy. Developmental delay with loss of developmental milestones is an important warning sign. Routine illnesses may produce severe and rapidly developing symptoms, and recovery periods may be more protracted.

When present, clinical features (including dysmorphism; abnormalities of hair, skin, skeleton, and muscle tone; and abnormalities of vision and hearing) provide important clues to the presence and category of an inborn error of metabolism.

Unusual visual behavior suggesting poor visual acuity as well as night blindness and nystagmus are typical ocular presenting signs, but the retina may appear normal early on in this condition. Children with a normal retina have a shiny reflex to their retina. Loss of this reflex may be an early sign of retinitis pigmentosa, but this is a difficult sign to identify without a specialist's equipment. The characteristic black-bone spicule pigmentation (see Figure 74-1) may vary in intensity but is usually seen in the retinal midperiphery beyond the central retinal location usually viewed with the direct ophthalmoscope used by most pediatricians. In more advanced retinopathy, the optic disc may appear pale, retinal arteries will look attenuated, and patients have constricted peripheral visual fields.

Inherited metabolic disorders can cause irreversible damage early in the course of the disease; thus, it is crucial that patients receive a correct diagnosis and are referred to a tertiary care center without delay. Initial screening tests can be performed (Table 74-1) before the child is referred to a metabolic specialist, who can then coordinate more targeted testing. Imaging and more invasive testing, such as lumbar puncture and biopsy, should be reserved unless the child is very unwell or a specialist's advice has been sought.

Electrodiagnostic testing is critical for diagnosing pigmentary retinopathy because it provides an objective measure of retinal function and is sensitive to mild impairment. An electroretinogram measures the response of different aspects of retinal circuitry. Visual evoked potential

Table 74-1. Initial Screening Tests for Inherited Metabolic Disorders

Test	Name	Findings
Blood		
	Complete blood cell count, including blood film; lipid profile, including lipoproteins and vitamins A and E; liver function and clotting profile, glucose and pyruvate levels, ketone bodies; very-long-chain fatty acids, phytanic acid, amino acids; lactate dehydrogenase, aldolase, and creatinine kinase levels	Vacuolated lymphocytes: Batten Acanthocytes, ↓ vitamins A and E: abetalipoproteinemia ↑ phytanic acid: Refsum Deranged liver and kidney function, long-chain fatty acids: Zellweger Increased serum lactate and pyruvate, moderately raised creatinine kinase: Kearns-Sayre
Urine	pH, acetone and ketone bodies, myoglobin and amino acid levels	Myoglobinuria
CSF	Lactate, pyruvate	Raised CSF lactate and pyruvate: Kearns-Sayre
Audiology	Audiogram, bone conductive testing	Sensorineural deafness: Refsum, Zellweger, Kearns-Sayre
Cardiac	Echocardiography, ECG	Heart block: Kearns-Sayre
Visual	ERG, VEP	ERG readings are reduced and eventually extinguished: advanced retinopathy
Enzyme	Enzyme assay or DNA analysis may be indicated in leukocytes, erythrocytes, skin fibroblasts, liver, or other tissues	Missing lysosomal enzymes: Batten; reduced aldehyde dehydrogenase: Sjögren-Larsson
Imaging and others	Brain CT/MRI, ultrasonography, EEG, nerve conduction studies, and electromyelography may be useful but should be left for a specialist's request; histologic evaluation of skeletal muscle.	Ragged red muscle fibers: Kearns-Sayre

Abbreviations: CSF, cerebrospinal fluid; CT, computed tomography; ECG, electrocardiogram; EEG, electroencephalogram; ERG, electroretinogram; MRI, magnetic resonance imaging; VEP, visual evoked potential.

assesses integrity of the visual pathway leading from the optic nerve to the visual cortex. Components of these tests may also be used to estimate level of vision in young children or children unable to communicate.

Differential Diagnosis

There are a number of metabolic conditions associated with pigmentary retinopathy; differentiating between them involves assessing phenotypic changes and analyzing biochemical and genetic abnormalities. Following are some of the diagnoses other than Zellweger syndrome that include a metabolic condition and pigmentary retinal changes:

Kearns-Sayre Syndrome (Mitochondrial DNA Abnormality)

Proximal muscle weakness, deafness, heart block, diabetes, and short stature are common. Other ocular features include limitation of ocular movements in all directions of gaze (external ophthalmoplegia) and bilateral symmetrical eyelid ptosis. These may develop in the first or second decade of life. Cardiac conduction block can be life-threatening; therefore, an electrocardiogram is essential to workup.

Abetalipoproteinemia (Lipid Metabolism Disorder)

Failure to thrive, steatorrhea, and protruding abdomen may occur in the first few months of life in abetalipoproteinemia (Bassen-Kornzweig syndrome). In infancy, retinitis pigmentosa and signs of spinocerebellar degeneration, such as ataxia and dyspraxia, may develop.

Refsum Disease (Lipid Metabolism Disorder)

Onset is usually in childhood or early adulthood with polyneuropathy, cerebellar ataxia, sensorineural deafness, anosmia, and ichthyosis. Ocular features other than pigmentary retinopathy may include cataracts and small pupils.

Sjögren-Larsson Syndrome (Lipid Metabolism Disorder)

Neonates with Sjögren-Larsson syndrome are often born several weeks premature. In most patients with this syndrome, generalized ichthyosis (usually itchy and face-sparing) is apparent at birth; however, some patients do not have cutaneous disease until later in life. Mental retardation and spastic diplegia or tetraplegia develop during the first 2 years of life. Seizures occur in about 40% of patients with Sjögren-Larsson syndrome. Diagnosis can be made with cultured fibroblast enzyme analysis.

Batten Disease (Lysosomal Storage Disorder)

Batten disease is part of a group of disorders called neuronal ceroid-lipofuscinoses (NCLs) that result from excessive accumulation of lipopigments in the body's tissues. Batten disease is the juvenile form of NCL and usually arises between 4 and 10 years of age. Symptoms include seizures, psychologic disturbances, and mental regression. Ocular signs include visual loss with fundus changes that can include a bull's-eye maculopathy and pigmentary or atrophic patches. Enzyme assays have been developed as diagnostic tests.

When to Refer

If a metabolic condition known to be associated with pigmentary retinopathy is being considered, routine referral to a pediatric ophthalmologist should be made. Even if pigmentary changes in the retina are not obvious, electroretinography may detect changes that can aid in differential diagnosis.

It is essential that doctors promptly diagnose an inherited metabolic disorder and refer these patients to a tertiary care center for treatment. Early treatment can prevent or delay the pathologic processes that cause symptoms.

Treatment

This patient developed a refractive error and was prescribed glasses. She had moderate visual impairment and has been under the care of a low-vision aid specialist to help with near-vision tasks. She has been registered with moderate visual impairment and receives assistance from educational specialists.

In general, as Zellweger syndrome tends to be fatal in early infancy, treatment is supportive and involves medical treatment of seizures and liver and kidney dysfunction.

Although there is no cure for metabolic retinopathies, dietary restriction and early therapy can prevent onset or progression of disability. Treatment focuses on symptomatic therapy and may include hearing aids, vitamin supplementation (as in abetalipoproteinemia), and feeding support to provide adequate calories (ie, gastrostomy). In addition, physical, occupational, and speech therapy can assist with comfort and daily activities. Early spectacle prescription with monitoring and treatment of amblyopia (lazy eye) and strabismus are crucial to normal visual development in these conditions.

In selected cases with cataract, cataract operations may be advocated. Occasionally strabismus surgery is required.

Low-vision aids and educational support can make a difference in the successful development and education of visually impaired children. This support can come in the form of large-type or audio textbooks, magnifying devices, technologic equipment, classroom assistance, or assessment for placement in schools for children with special needs.

The value that local and national support groups can play should not be underestimated. Professional and peer support groups exist for many metabolic disorders. Ophthalmologists should assist families in registering a child as visually impaired and ensure specialist educational support. Or they should refer them to groups such as the American Foundation for the Blind so that they may receive additional support.

Genetic counseling is vital in providing individuals and their families with information on the nature, inheritance, and implications of inherited metabolic disorders to help them make informed medical and personal decisions. Family planning may be assisted by carrier testing and prenatal diagnosis using amniocentesis and chorionic villus sampling.

Advances in medical technology and genetics have resulted in major developments in the diagnosis, classification, and treatment of inherited metabolic disorders. Enzyme replacement, gene transfer, and organ transplantation have become available and are beneficial for many previously untreatable disorders.

Discussion

Although individual metabolic disorders are rare, as a group, their collective incidence has been reported to be 1 in 784 live births.

Key Points

- Metabolic syndromes may present atypically without all systemic manifestations presenting simultaneously. Therefore, it is important to maintain a high index of suspicion by eliciting symptoms and signs through interview and examination.
- Early, full systemic investigation is pertinent to support and improve quality of life for children with inherited metabolic disorders.
- It is essential that doctors promptly diagnose inherited metabolic disorders and refer patients to a tertiary care center for treatment, which, if commenced early, can often reduce morbidity and mortality.
- A multidisciplinary team, including pediatrician, ophthalmologist, metabolic specialist, and medical geneticist, is essential in the management of these patients.
- Most treatments are symptomatic and supportive, but simple interventions such as eyeglasses and hearing aids can dramatically improve quality of life.

Suggested Reading

al-Khaier A, Nischal KK. The eye in metabolic disease. *Hosp Med.* 2003;64(10):609–612

Biswas J, Nandi K, Sridharan S, Ranjan P. Ocular manifestation of storage diseases. *Curr Opin Ophthalmol.* 2008;19(6):507–511

Fraser JA, Biousse V, Newman NJ. The neuro-ophthalmology of mitochondrial disease. *Surv Ophthalmol.* 2010;55(4):299–334

Staretz-Chacham O, Lang TC, LaMarca ME, Krasnewich D, Sidransky E. Lysosomal storage disorders in the newborn. *Pediatrics.* 2009;123(4):1191–1207

Chapter 75

No Ocular Complaints in a Patient With Sickle Cell Disease

Sorath Noorani Siddiqui, FCPS
Alex V. Levin, MD, MHSc

Presentation

A 5-year-old African American boy with known sickle cell hemoglobin-opathy, SS genotype (Figure 75-1), arrives for a routine follow-up visit. He was hospitalized once because of fever and bone crisis and on another occasion because of severe vomiting and dehydration. He has never had

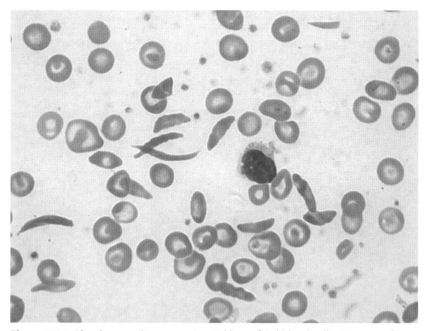

Figure 75-1. Blood smear demonstrating sickling of red blood cells. Courtesy of Gene Gulati, PhD, SH(ASCP).

any ocular complaints. At present he is well. The pediatrician finds normal vision and wonders when to refer him to a pediatric ophthalmologist for screening of ocular manifestations of sickle cell disease.

Diagnosis

The vaso-occlusive process of sickle cell disease caused by abnormal sickling of erythrocytes affects the small vessels of the retina, resulting in ischemia and peripheral retinal neovascularization. Arteriolar closure is the initiating event in development of sickle cell retinopathy.

There are 2 stages of sickle cell retinopathy, nonproliferative retinopathy (NPR) and proliferative sickle cell retinopathy (PSR). In the former, retinal examination may show salmon-patch hemorrhage, iridescent spots, black sunburst spots (changes in retinal pigment epithelium), and arteriovenous anastomoses. Less common findings are cotton-wool spots (areas of superficial retinal ischemia) and abnormal capillaries on the optic nerve head caused by chronic sludging of blood. Similar comma-shaped vessels can also occasionally be seen in inferior bulbar conjunctival capillaries. Peripheral retinal sea-fan neovascularization (Figure 75-2) is the classic sign of PSR. Usually PSR is insidious, with patients remaining asymptomatic until visual loss results from vitreous hemorrhage or retinal detachment.

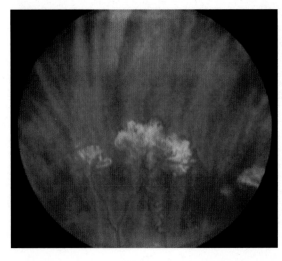

Figure 75-2. Peripheral retinal sea-fan neovascularization in sickle cell disease. Courtesy of Wills Eye Institute Resident Slide Collection.

When to Refer

Examination of a patient with sickle cell disease by a non-ophthalmologist using direct ophthalmoscope is insufficient, as the most likely involved parts of the retina are beyond the view of this instrument. Although there are no consensus guidelines on when to refer children with sickle cell disease to an ophthalmologist, the American Academy of Pediatrics states: "Screening for proliferative retinopathy with periodic retinal examinations beginning at 10 years of age is often recommended, especially for patients with HbSC [sickle cell–hemoglobin C disease]." Additionally, several studies advocate routine screening by an ophthalmologist starting at 10 years of age. Others recommend starting screening with dilated funduscopy at 9 years of age for patients with the SC genotype and 13 years of age for those with the SS genotype.

Children with normal results of a retinal examination performed by an ophthalmologist may be followed up once every 1 or 2 years for serial examinations, whereas those with abnormal retinal findings should undergo fluorescein angiography and be followed up as necessary.

Children with sickle cell disease should be referred to an ophthalmologist for an initial retinal examination beginning at age 10 years. If symptoms of visual loss occur or the child fails a routine vision screening in the pediatric office at a well-child visit, prompt referral for ophthalmic examination is indicated.

Treatment

The asymptomatic child presented here with the SS genotype carries less risk of PSR developing than does a child with SC hemoglobinopathy, according to the medical literature. Because of the rarity of PSR before age 9 years, the authors recommend that this patient have his first ophthalmology consultation at 10 years of age, followed by an ophthalmologic examination every 1 to 2 years if his vision remains stable. Should symptoms of visual loss or change occur, or should the child fail a routine vision screening in the pediatric office, a prompt referral for ophthalmic examination is indicated.

Among patients in whom retinal neovascularization develops, spontaneous regression may occur in up to 60% of cases. Laser treatment is recommended for patients with more severe PSR to prevent bleeding or retinal detachment.

Discussion

One study showed that the prevalence of PSR was 13 times higher in patients with SC than SS hemoglobinopathy. In this study, mean age at onset of NPR was 12.8 years (range, 7 to 18 years). For PSR it was 14 years (range, 9 to 18 years). Only 8.8% of patients with homozygous SS disease went on to have PSR, and vitreous hemorrhage developed in only 3% of these patients. According to another study, PSR developed in up to 72% of patients heterozygous for hemoglobin C and in 33% of patients heterozygous for thalassemia.

Peak onset of PSR has been reported in one study to be between 15 and 24 years of age for the SC genotype versus 20 to 30 years for the SS type, whereas another study found that PSR occurred at 8 years of age in the SC group and at age 16 years in the SS group. Observations from a Jamaican cohort study showed that peripheral retinal vessel closure seen on retinal fluorescein angiography was present in 50% of children with the SC and SS genotypes at 6 years of age and increased to affect 90% of children by age 12 years, but PSR was rare.

Key Points

- Sickle cell disease affects the small vessels of the retina, resulting in ischemia and peripheral retinal neovascularization.
- Proliferative sickle cell retinopathy (PSR) is rarely seen before 9 years of age.
- The authors recommend that the first ophthalmology consultation be performed at 10 years of age, followed by eye examinations once every 1 or 2 years.
- The prevalence of PSR is 13 times higher in patients with SC than SS hemoglobinopathy.

Suggested Reading

Al-Abdullah NA, Haddock TA, Kerrison JB, Goldberg MF. Sickle cell disease presenting with extensive peri-macular arteriolar occlusions in a nine-year-old boy. *Am J Ophthalmol.* 2001;131(2):275–276

American Academy of Pediatrics Section on Hematology/Oncology and Committee on Genetics. Health supervision for children with sickle cell disease. *Pediatrics.* 2002;109(3):526–535. http://aappolicy. aappublications.org/cgi/content/full/pediatrics;109/3/526. Accessed May 22, 2012

Babalola OE, Wambebe CO. When should children and young adults with sickle cell disease be referred for eye assessment? *Afr J Med Med Sci.* 2001;30(4):261–263

Condon PI, Serjeant GR. Ocular findings in homozygous sickle cell anemia in Jamaica. *Am J Ophthalmol.* 1972;73(4):533–543

Downes SM, Hambleton IR, Chuang EL, Lois N, Serjeant GR, Bird AC. Incidence and natural history of proliferative sickle cell retinopathy: observations from a cohort study. *Ophthalmology.* 2005;112(11):1869–1875

Eruchalu UV, Pam VA, Akuse RM. Ocular findings in children with severe clinical symptoms of homozygous sickle cell anemia in Kaduna, Nigeria. *West Afr J Med.* 2006;25(2):88–91

Feist RM, Blodi CF, Spiegel PH. Retinal vascular disorders. In: Wright KW, Spiegel PH, eds. *Pediatric Ophthalmology and Strabismus.* 2nd ed. New York, NY: Springer-Verlag New York; 2003:566–575

Fox PD, Dunn DT, Morris JS, Serjeant GR. Risk factors for proliferative sickle retinopathy. *Br J Ophthalmol.* 1990;74(3):172–176

Gill HS, Lam WC. A screening strategy for the detection of sickle cell retinopathy in pediatric patients. *Can J Ophthalmol.* 2008;43(2): 188–191

Hayes RJ, Condon PI, Serjeant GR. Haematological factors associated with proliferative retinopathy in sickle cell-haemoglobin C disease. *Br J Ophthalmol.* 1981;65(10):712–717

Acknowledgment

The authors gratefully acknowledge being supported in part by the Foerderer Fund.

Chapter 76

Infant With Red, Painful Eye

Brian J. Forbes, MD, PhD
Gil Binenbaum, MD, MSCE

Presentation

A 10-month-old girl is brought to the pediatrician's office with a red right eye. The pediatrician's partner had seen her one week prior to the current visit and started a topical antibiotic regimen for treatment of presumed bacterial conjunctivitis. The mother states that the infant's eye is still red, and she appears to have become increasingly sensitive to light and seems crankier. The child has been otherwise well, without a fever, rash, or symptoms of a viral upper respiratory tract infection. There is no history of known ocular trauma or anyone else at home with red eyes. She is developing normally and her immunizations are up to date. She was a full-term baby without prior medical problems.

On examination, she appears developmentally normal, alert, and afebrile but in some level of distress. Results of the pediatrician's head, neck, and chest evaluation are unremarkable except for her right eye, which is partly closed and ptotic, or droopy (Figure 76-1). Her left eye looks normal externally and has a clear red reflex.

The right eye is very difficult to examine because it is extremely photo-phobic (sensitive to light). The pediatrician can determine that the conjunctiva is very injected, cornea is partially cloudy, and iris is obscured by corneal clouding and some sort of substance inside the eye, which appears brownish-red (Figure 76-2). Fluorescein dye is placed on the cornea, and there is no sign of staining or corneal abrasion. On palpation of the closed eye, the eye feels firmer than the pediatrician might expect.

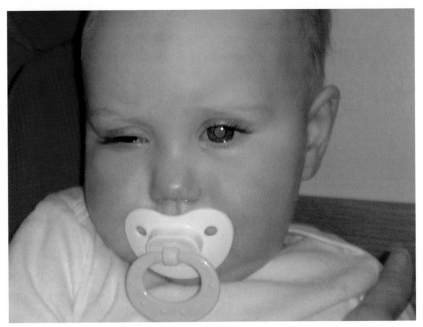

Figure 76-1. Right eyelids are mostly closed with marked photophobia. Conjunctiva is red. Courtesy of Brian J. Forbes, MD, PhD.

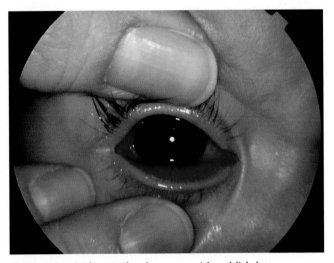

Figure 76-2. Right eye cloudy cornea with reddish-brown material in the anterior chamber obscuring the iris. Courtesy of Brian J. Forbes, MD, PhD.

Diagnosis

Close inspection is key to diagnosis whenever the pediatrician is presented with a red eye. This infant has only one eye involved, even a week after onset of symptoms. Unilateral ocular redness is much less likely to be typical allergic, bacterial, or viral conjunctivitis, which, although often asymmetric in severity and course, does usually involve both eyes eventually. The infant's eyelid is not swollen or particularly red, so there is no cellulitic process.

The patient's cornea is cloudy, which indicates that something is going on beyond simple conjunctivitis. Such a sign should immediately alert the pediatrician to a potentially vision-threatening condition.

Presence of a visible substance within the eye (behind the cornea) is equally concerning. If it were white, it could be a collection of white blood cells (hypopyon) in an infectious endophthalmitis or noninfectious uveitis, or it could be a collection of tumor cells (pseudohypopyon) such as in retinoblastoma. The brownish-red material in this child's eye is hyphema, blood in the anterior chamber of the eye, which is the space between the cornea anteriorly and the iris posteriorly.

Finally, the pediatrician's palpation of the eyes through closed eyelids reveals a hard eye, which can occur when the intraocular pressure is greatly elevated.

It is very important to determine the cause of the hyphema. If the hyphema is related to an ocular injury (the most common cause), any detail about the nature of the trauma is helpful. However, this child has no history of ocular trauma. Non-accidental injury should be considered in a patient with hyphema of uncertain cause. However, spontaneous hyphema can occur with neovascularization of the iris, certain ocular neoplasms, juvenile xanthogranuloma (JXG), and fragile vascular tufts that exist at the pupillary border.

The pediatrician refers the infant to a pediatric ophthalmologist. Blood obscures any view of posterior eye structures. Thus, an ultrasound scan of the eye is obtained to rule out intraocular neoplasm; no mass is identified (Figure 76-3). On further history and physical examination by the

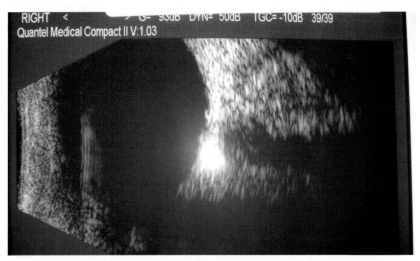

Figure 76-3. Ocular ultrasound done through a closed eyelid performed gently to not exert additional pressure on the eye. Findings show normal vitreal cavity. No mass is identified. Courtesy of Brian J. Forbes, MD, PhD.

ophthalmologist, a solitary orange papule consistent with a xanthogranuloma is discovered on the upper part of the child's buttocks (Figure 76-4). The likely diagnosis of JXG is made. The baby's intraocular pressure is found to be elevated above 35 mm Hg, causing her pain, which has been manifesting as general irritability and poor sleep.

Juvenile xanthogranuloma is the most common form of non–Langerhans cell histiocytosis. This disorder is characterized by smooth, round, orange or red-to-yellowish papules or nodules that are typically asymptomatic. The benign, self-healing lesions appear in infancy and childhood, with one-third of patients presenting with lesions at birth, two-thirds by 1 year of age, and only a small proportion presenting in adulthood. Juvenile xanthogranuloma is more common in whites (10:1) and boys (4:1).

The iris is the most common noncutaneous site in JXG. Eye lesions are present in only a small number of patients, typically those with multiple skin lesions. Visceral lesions do occur but are rare. An important association has been described between juvenile chronic myelogenous leukemia and multiple-lesion JXG, particularly in the presence of concurrent neurofibromatosis.

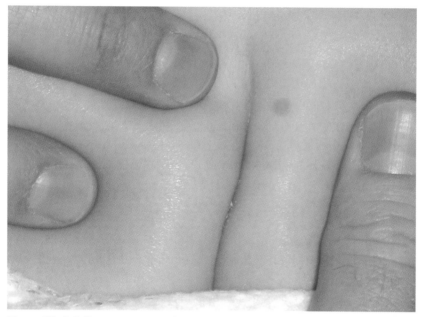

Figure 76-4. Solitary orange papule (raised) on the upper buttocks. Courtesy of Brian J. Forbes, MD, PhD.

Biopsy, which can be diagnostic and cosmetically therapeutic, reveals collections of differentiated non–Langerhans cell histiocytes with late appearance of giant and foam cells. Serum lipid levels are normal in these patients.

Differential Diagnosis

Diagnoses besides JXG that should be considered in the presence of spontaneous hyphema include the following:

Iris Neovascularization

Neovascularization of the iris can occur with conditions such as diabetic retinopathy and retinal vascular occlusion. Bleeding from neovascular growth can lead to hyphema.

Retinoblastoma

The most common malignant intraocular tumor of childhood, retinoblastoma may uncommonly present with hyphema or hypopyon. It often presents with leukokoria (white pupil), glaucoma, strabismus (eye misalignment), or vision loss.

Vascular Tufts at Papillary Border

These congenital vascular malformations can occasionally bleed spontaneously.

When to Refer

A hyphema is considered an ocular emergency because of the risk of high intraocular pressure and should be evaluated by an ophthalmologist as soon as possible. Likewise, corneal cloudiness is a sign of a potentially vision-threatening condition and warrants prompt referral to an ophthalmologist.

Treatment

The infant with JXG is managed successfully as an outpatient with topical corticosteroids and cycloplegic agents for treatment of hyphema, and topical and systemic medications to lower intraocular pressure. (For more information about hyphema management, see Chapter 48.) Figure 76-5 shows the eye 4 weeks after presentation. There are now only small amounts of the blood clot visible through the inferior cornea, and there is some blood on the surface of the lens (visible as an opacity in the middle of the red reflex) and the surface of the iris (causing iris heterochromia, or a difference in iris color).

The patient's hyphema eventually resolves fully. No clear JXG lesion of the iris can be identified, so it is likely situated on the posterior surface of the iris.

Children who have multiple xanthogranulomas are usually referred to an ophthalmologist for periodic screening.

Discussion

Etiology of JXG is not known. Cells of origin have been thought to be dermal dendrocytes involved in a granulomatous reaction to an unidentified stimulus, but recent evidence suggests a $CD4^+$ plasmacytoid monocyte origin.

Hyphema is an uncommon manifestation of JXG and occurs when iris vessels bleed into clear aqueous fluid. Blood typically pools and is visible to the naked eye as bright-red or brownish-red material behind

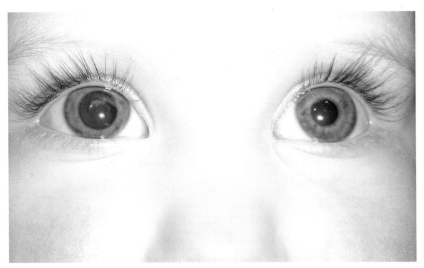

Figure 76-5. Clearing of intraocular hyphema. Small residual blood clot is seen as red curved line in front of inferior iris of right eye with small amount of blood on lens seen as central grayish area. Right pupil is pharmacologically dilated. Courtesy of Brian J. Forbes, MD, PhD.

the cornea. However, red blood cells of smaller hyphemas are visible only with magnification at a slit-lamp biomicroscope. Even the slightest amount of blood in the anterior chamber will cause decreased vision when mixed into clear aqueous. Layered hyphemas are described by the amount of anterior chamber they occupy, and the greater the amount of blood, the higher the risk of vision-threatening complications.

Blood in the anterior chamber is not in and of itself necessarily harmful. However, if quantities are sufficient, it may obstruct the outflow of aqueous humor from the eye, resulting in a rise in intraocular pressure. High intraocular pressure can cause pain, which in a young child may present with generalized symptoms, as in this case. More importantly, prolonged high pressures within the eye can cause corneal blood staining and optic nerve damage with permanent vision loss (glaucoma). Severity and duration of the rise in intraocular pressure are important. Very high pressures can result in irreversible damage in a matter of hours.

Glaucoma associated with hyphema may result from direct obstruction of the trabecular meshwork aqueous drainage structures by fresh blood (hemolytic glaucoma), degrading hemoglobin, or skeletons of the disintegrating red blood cells (ghost cell glaucoma). In addition, any external force strong enough to produce internal bleeding may also directly damage adjacent trabecular meshwork, resulting in sluggish aqueous drainage.

Key Points

- An index of suspicion for juvenile xanthogranuloma (JXG) should be raised in the scenario of nontraumatic ocular hyphema.
- Ocular manifestations of JXG are more typical in patients with multiple cutaneous lesions.
- An important association has been described between juvenile chronic myelogenous leukemia and multiple-lesion JXG, particularly in the presence of concurrent neurofibromatosis.

Suggested Reading

Hernandez-Martin A, Baselga E, Drolet BA, Esterly NB. Juvenile xanthogranuloma. *J Am Acad Dermatol.* 1997;36(3 Pt 1):355–369

Piggott CDS. Dermatologic manifestations of juvenile xanthogranuloma. *Medscape Reference.* http://emedicine.medscape.com/article/1111629-overview. Accessed May 30, 2012

Walton W, Von Hagen S, Grigorian R, Zarbin M. Management of traumatic hyphema. *Surv Ophthalmol.* 2002;47(4):297–334

Zvulunov A, Barak Y, Metzker A. Juvenile xanthogranuloma, neuro-fibromatosis, and juvenile chronic myelogenous leukemia. World statistical analysis. *Arch Dermatol.* 1995;131(8):904–908

Chapter 77

Port-wine Stain and Red Eye

Edel M. Cosgrave, FRCOphth
Anthony J. Vivian, FRCS, FRCOphth

Presentation

A mother brings her 6-year-old son to the pediatrician's office. He has a port-wine stain in the distribution of the ophthalmic and maxillary divisions of the trigeminal nerve (forehead and cheek) on the left side (Figure 77-1). The pediatrician has treated this boy for seizures over the past few years. The mother is concerned because her son's left eye has become increasingly red and caused him discomfort over the past couple of weeks despite being treated with topical antibiotic for conjunctivitis. He also complains of blurred vision and has become photophobic (light sensitive).

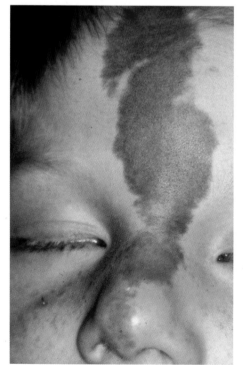

Figure 77-1. Port-wine stain in trigeminal nerve distribution. Courtesy of Anthony J. Vivian, FRCS, FRCOphth.

The pediatrician checks his visual acuity in the office using a Snellen chart and finds it to be 20/20 in the right eye and 20/60 in the left eye. The left eye has always looked redder than the right, but this time it is "angry" looking, and the cornea looks a little hazy (figures 77-2 and 77-3). There is no discharge and no staining of the cornea on instillation of 2% fluorescein drops. The pupil reacts normally to light, although the boy is quite photophobic. The pediatrician assesses intraocular pressure by gently palpating each globe between 2 index fingers. The left globe feels much firmer than the right.

Diagnosis

The pediatrician suspects that this boy has glaucoma and therefore contacts a pediatric ophthalmologist for an urgent opinion. The pediatric ophthalmologist performs a slit-lamp examination, visual field assessment, dilated fundus examination, and refraction. The ophthalmologist notes that the corneal edema on the left eye is caused by a very high intraocular pressure of 45 mm Hg. Corneal diameter is measured in each eye and found to be normal (11 mm). The left optic disc has an

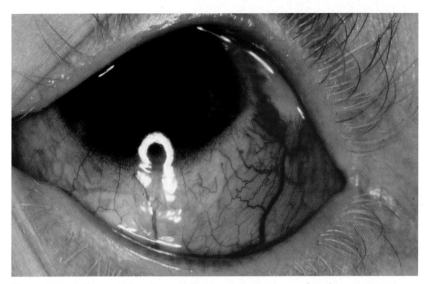

Figure 77-2. Left eye with enlarged blood vessels. Courtesy of Anthony J. Vivian, FRCS, FRCOphth.

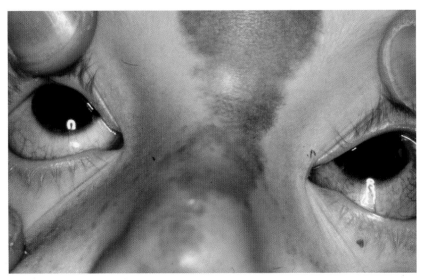

Figure 77-3. Asymmetric redness—left eye more than right eye. Courtesy of Anthony J. Vivian, FRCS, FRCOphth.

enlarged central cup. Diagnosis is glaucoma secondary to the vascular malformation of Sturge-Weber syndrome.

Sturge-Weber syndrome is a rare, congenital neuro-oculocutaneous disorder. This hamartomatous syndrome is characterized by the following:

- Venous angiomatosis of the leptomeninges best visualized by magnetic resonance imaging with contrast.
- Facial angiomatosis that often follows distribution of the first division of the trigeminal nerve (V1). This can be unilateral or bilateral and frequently involves the upper eyelid.
- Ipsilateral gyriform calcification of the cerebral cortex usually visible on plain skull radiograph but visualized best on computed tomography scan.
- Epileptic convulsions or other seizures, which develop in the first year in two-thirds of children.
- Ocular involvement including glaucoma and vascular malformations of the conjunctiva, episclera, choroid, and retina. Other ocular manifestations include iris heterochromia (different colored irides), retinal detachment, strabismus, and homonymous hemianopia (visual field defect involving the right or left half of the visual field of each eye).

Glaucoma develops in a reported 30% of patients with Sturge-Weber syndrome. Approximately 60% of cases present as congenital glaucoma with photophobia and obvious enlargement of the globe (buphthalmos), whereas 40% present in later childhood or adulthood, when globe enlargement is uncommon. Increased corneal diameter and tendency toward myopia suggest globe enlargement. In cases of glaucoma the upper eyelid is usually involved by the hemangioma. Glaucoma most commonly presents before the age of 2 years, with photophobia and enlargement of the globe on the side of the angioma. Neovascular glaucoma also has been reported in Sturge-Weber syndrome.

Differential Diagnosis

Diagnoses besides Sturge-Weber syndrome that should be considered include the following:

Klippel-Trenaunay-Weber Syndrome

This syndrome shares many of the features of Sturge-Weber syndrome, and there may be some overlap between the 2. The important feature of Klippel-Trenaunay-Weber syndrome is facial hemangioma associated with facial hemihypertrophy. The importance of this distinction is that patients with Klippel-Trenaunay-Weber syndrome are at risk of developing visceral tumors of the kidney, adrenal gland, or liver.

Beckwith-Wiedemann Syndrome

This is an overgrowth syndrome characterized by enlarged tongue (macroglossia), central abdominal hernia (omphalocele), visceral hyperplasia, and with the risk of life-threatening hypoglycemia due to pancreatic islet-cell hyperplasia and childhood cancer. Facial hemangiomas occur in some children, allowing a misdiagnosis of Sturge-Weber syndrome.

When to Refer

All patients with suspected diagnosis of Sturge-Weber syndrome should be referred to an ophthalmologist for visual acuity assessment, slit-lamp examination including funduscopy, intraocular pressure measurement, and refraction. Any patient with suspected glaucoma should be urgently referred to an ophthalmologist.

Treatment

Treatment of Sturge-Weber syndrome by a pediatrician and pediatric ophthalmologist involves management of seizures, controlling glaucoma, and the possibility of cosmetic treatment of facial hemangioma with laser. This condition is frequently associated with learning difficulties requiring educational support.

The pediatric ophthalmologist explains the diagnosis of Sturge-Weber syndrome to the mother. Topical antiglaucoma medication is prescribed. The requirement for long-term treatment and follow-up examination, along with the possibility of future surgical interventions to control glaucoma, is explained to the family.

Management of glaucoma associated with Sturge-Weber syndrome is difficult. Medical treatment alone often fails to control intraocular pressure, and most patients require a combination of treatment modalities. Surgical procedures include creating openings in the native drainage system (goniotomy, trabeculotomy); creating a new opening into the anterior chamber to drain intraocular fluid (trabeculectomy); and implantation of external drainage devices (ie, Ahmed valves or Molteno tubes). All these surgical procedures carry a substantial risk of choroidal bleeding, very low intraocular pressure (hypotony), and retinal detachment, which can lead to subsequent loss of vision. Procedures to decrease aqueous production by destruction of the ciliary processes using cryotherapy or diode laser are useful adjuncts to surgery or in managing selected patients in whom surgery is undesirable because of a high risk of surgical complications.

Repeated intraocular interventions can lead to the development of cataract, which may require further surgery.

Discussion

Sturge-Weber syndrome is a sporadic congenital condition caused by failure of regression of a primitive vascular plexus in the cephalic portion of the neural tube during the ninth week of intrauterine life, resulting in angiomatosis of related tissues. Early seizures are associated with developmental and intellectual impairment. When glaucoma occurs, the cause is a combination of elevated episcleral venous pressure and an immature, abnormal drainage angle. It is difficult to control.

Key Points

- All patients with Sturge-Weber syndrome should be referred to an ophthalmologist at time of diagnosis.
- Visual loss can occur through retinal detachment or glaucoma.
- Patients have risk of glaucoma at any time in their lives.
- Follow-up is lifelong, and treatment can be challenging.

Suggested Reading

Comi AM. Presentation, diagnosis, pathophysiology, and treatment of the neurological features of Sturge-Weber syndrome. *Neurologist.* 2011;17(4):179–184

Sami D, Vivian AJ, Taylor D, Saunders D. The phakomatoses. In: *Duane's Ophthalmology.* Philadelphia, PA: Lipincott Williams and Wilkins; 2006

Chapter 78

Chronic Red Eye With Photophobia

John W. Simon, MD

Presentation

A 4-year-old girl recently has been a patient in the pediatrician's office because of conjunctivitis (pinkeye) in both eyes. The pediatrician has treated her with three 10-day courses of various topical antibiotics over the past 6 weeks without improvement. She lately has begun to complain to her parents that she cannot see well and is sensitive to bright lights (photophobic). She has not had a recent respiratory tract infection, and no other family members have had conjunctivitis. The pediatrician has known the child since birth. She has been healthy, her immunizations are up to date, and there is no family history of importance.

Visual acuity measures 20/100 in the right eye and 20/60 in the left eye. There is no discharge, and the eyes are only slightly injected. The pediatrician's examination shows small white specks in the cornea and slightly hazy media in both eyes (Figure 78-1). Because the patient is sensitive to the light of the pediatrician's ophthalmoscope, it is difficult to visualize ocular fundi.

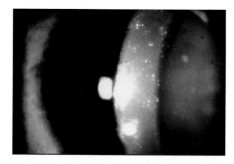

Figure 78-1. View of the cornea showing endothelial (inner layer) deposits and a hazy anterior chamber. Courtesy of John W. Simon, MD.

Diagnosis

The apparent "conjunctivitis" is relatively mild in its external manifestations (ie, minimal injection, no discharge), but the chronicity of the condition and the patient's lack of response to topical antibiotics, along with visual loss, photophobia, and media opacities, are all red flags. (A good rule of thumb is that infectious conjunctivitis that does not respond to topical antibiotics during the first week is not likely bacterial, and a second or third antibiotic drop is more likely to delay diagnosis than effectively treat an infection.) Because of the red flags, the pediatrician refers the girl to an ophthalmologist.

The ophthalmologist's slit-lamp examination demonstrates that there is turbidity in the aqueous humor (or flare), associated with inflammatory cells floating in the anterior chamber. The white specks represent coalescences of these cells, called keratic precipitates, on the posterior corneal surface. This child has iritis, or anterior uveitis, an inflammation of the internal part of the eye. The ophthalmologist will treat the inflammation, usually with topical steroid and cycloplegic drops, and may ask the pediatrician to help identify an underlying diagnosis (see "Differential Diagnosis" on the next page).

About 6% of uveitis cases arise in children. In chronic cases, inflammation can cause stickiness of the iris, which can bind to the underlying lens centrally, causing posterior synechiae (adhesions). In severe cases, these adhesions can be difficult to break with pharmacologic dilation. Sticking of the iris to the overlying cornea peripherally, or anterior synechiae, can also occur. Both can cause secondary glaucoma by blocking the usual fluid dynamics. Other causes of poor vision include cataracts, cystoid macular edema, and deposition of calcium in the cornea, or band keratopathy.

The most common cause in children is juvenile idiopathic arthritis (JIA). Chronic iritis occurs in 10% to 20% of all patients with JIA, and most cases are bilateral. The condition usually causes only minimal symptoms, leading to insidious but progressive morbidity and possible blindness. Involved eyes often are white and quiet appearing, yet 30% to 40% of patients with JIA-associated uveitis experience severe loss of vision. When symptoms are present, they may include mild conjunctival injection, photophobia, and poor vision. In some cases, the joint mani-festations of JIA may be evanescent, or even preceded by the iritis, making diagnosis particularly difficult. As is the case in this patient, children are often mistakenly thought to have conjunctivitis.

Highest risk of iritis occurs in patients with oligoarticular (pauciarticular) JIA, involving fewer than 5 joints, especially in young girls and in asso-ciation with positive antinuclear antibody titer. Polyarticular-onset JIA presents a somewhat smaller risk of iritis, which is distinctly rare in systemic-onset JIA.

Differential Diagnosis

Diagnosis besides JIA that should be considered is viral conjunctivitis. Although viral conjunctivitis can involve the cornea and take several weeks to clear, vision is generally preserved. Itching, tearing, and dis-charge are commonly associated with this condition (see Chapter 2).

When to Refer

Patients with chronic conjunctivitis, especially if associated with vision loss, should be referred to an ophthalmologist.

Treatment

Treatment of iritis begins with intensive topical corticosteroids (eg, prednisolone acetate 1%), typically every hour. Most patients respond to this initial treatment, and the dose can then be tapered. Approximately 20% of patients with JIA-associated uveitis have little or no response to topical corticosteroid therapy. Ironically, risk of long-term treatment with topical corticosteroids includes cataract (especially posterior sub-capsular cataract) and glaucoma. The goal of medical treatment is to eliminate cells in the anterior chamber. Pupils are usually dilated with cycloplegics (eg, atropine 1%) to minimize photophobia, risk of glaucoma, and scarring. The presence of vitreous inflammation may require regional or systemic administration of corticosteroids or additional nonsteroidal anti-inflammatory drugs.

Systemic immunomodulatory agents may be useful for patients with limited or no response to systemic corticosteroids or those in whom unacceptable side effects develop. This treatment is generally given in conjunction with a pediatric rheumatologist.

If necessary, surgical treatment of band keratopathy, cataracts, or glaucoma may be performed.

Discussion

After diagnosis of JIA and initial eye examination, uveitis screening is performed at intervals of 3 to 12 months, depending on risk, which is stratified by age at onset of disease, duration of disease, and immunologic and serum markers. The American Academy of Pediatrics has published recommendations to guide pediatric ophthalmologists. Risk is greatest within the first 4 years of onset of the disease. After intraocular inflammation is noted, more frequent examinations will be necessary. Most children with JIA-associated uveitis have a fairly good visual outcome if they receive early diagnosis and treatment.

Key Points

- Patients with chronic conjunctivitis, especially if associated with vision loss, should be referred to an ophthalmologist.
- Repeated or prolonged treatment with topical antibiotics may delay diagnosis and effective treatment, thus increasing risk of severe ocular morbidity.
- Uveitis, a common complication of some forms of juvenile idiopathic arthritis (JIA), may occasionally be the first sign of JIA.

Suggested Reading

Cassidy J, Kivlin J, Lindsley C, Nocton J; American Academy of Pediatrics Section on Rheumatology and Section on Ophthalmology. Guidelines for ophthalmic examinations in children with juvenile rheumatoid arthritis. *Pediatrics*. 2006;117(5):1843–1845. http://pediatrics.aappublications.org/content/117/5/1843.full. Accessed May 30, 2012

Chapter 79

Poor Vision in a Child With Cerebral Palsy

M. Edward Wilson, MD

Presentation

A 16-year-old boy presents to the pediatrician's office for continued care of his cerebral palsy. The pediatrician has known him since infancy (Figure 79-1). He is nonverbal but has been making progress with gross motor, fine motor, as well as orientation and mobility since restarting occupational therapy and orientation and mobility training. He has a history of seizures but has not required medication for seizures in several years. He takes diazepam for treatment of spasticity.

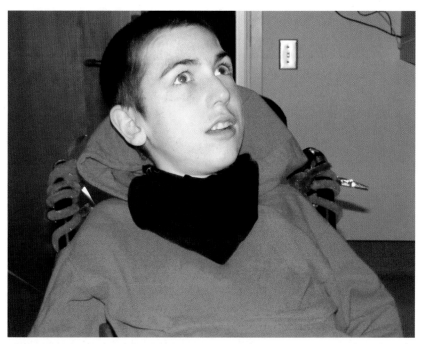

Figure 79-1. Teenaged patient with cerebral palsy who exhibits poor vision. Courtesy of M. Edward Wilson, MD.

His therapists complain that he cannot see very well. His parents tried glasses in the past, but he never wore them consistently. The pediatrician attempts to do standard vision screening, but the patient does not respond to letters or pictures. He is noted to have intermittent drifting outward in either eye. His parents indicate that the drifting is worse when he is tired or inattentive. He had surgery for strabismus (ocular misalignment) when he was 5 years old for crossing of the eyes and again at age 12 for out-turning. He has not seen a pediatric ophthalmologist in the past 3 years. The pediatrician's review of the boy's past records indicates that he has been noted to have mild optic nerve atrophy. It is unclear if this is the reason for poor visual responses during therapy and with his schoolwork.

On examination, the pupils are large in both eyes but are responsive to light. The patient is visually attentive, but his eye tracking is jerky and he loses interest quickly. He seems to see well in his peripheral vision using bright toys brought in from the side, indicating that his visual field is reasonably full.

Diagnosis

The pediatrician correctly refers this boy to the local pediatric ophthalmologist for a complete eye evaluation. The pediatrician has noted that the patient has a history of optic nerve atrophy, strabismus, and refractive error. However, he has never worn glasses consistently and has residual strabismus despite 2 previous surgeries. His visual acuity cannot be tested in the conventional way because he is nonverbal.

In the pediatric ophthalmology office, this teenaged boy (Figure 79-2) is able to match letters presented on the eye chart using a placard placed on his lap containing the letters H, O, T, and V. This test is a way for a nonverbal child to point to the letter presented on the chart rather than verbalize it. He does not need to know the alphabet; he merely matches what he sees. The letters H, O, T, and V are used because they avoid any right-to-left confusion the child may have. The patient tests at 20/160 in each eye and improves to 20/80 with glasses corrected for marked astigmatism and farsightedness (hyperopia). His optic nerve atrophy is mild and has not changed since early childhood.

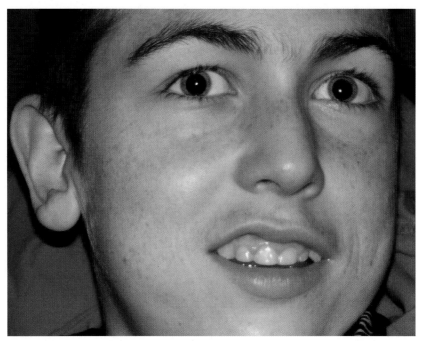

Figure 79-2. Close-up of patient showing exotropia and poor visual attentiveness. Courtesy of M. Edward Wilson, MD.

His exotropia-type strabismus is intermittent and variable, and it is controlled better when his spectacle prescription is placed over his eyes. A test that allows rapid assessment of accommodative ability, called dynamic retinoscopy, reveals that he has inconsistent focusing a bility on near targets.

Differential Diagnosis

Diagnoses besides mild optic nerve atrophy, refractive error (substantial improvement with glasses), and accommodative insufficiency (substantial improvement with bifocals for near work) that should be considered include severe optic nerve atrophy (glasses may not be beneficial when the optic nerve damage is severe) and cortical visual impairment (this may produce severe visual impairment but can improve over time).

When to Refer

Patients with cerebral palsy should be examined by a pediatric ophthalmologist as soon as the diagnosis is made or with any new-onset vision problem.

Treatment

Glasses are prescribed for the boy's hyperopia and astigmatism. The parents are informed that glasses with a large astigmatism correction take some time to get accustomed to. The patient does not like anything on his face but will soon notice the change in his vision and will accept the glasses if the parents are persistent enough to keep them on him during the initial transition. Some children with cerebral palsy will benefit from the addition of a bifocal in the glasses because their focusing for up-close viewing is inconsistent. This may be tried after the patient gets used to wearing glasses.

The ophthalmologist will reassess the intermittent out-turning of the patient's eyes once a year throughout the childhood years and even in adulthood. If it progresses to constant misalignment despite glasses, additional surgery can be performed.

A referral is made to the local vision rehabilitation center, and direct communication is made with therapists involved in the patient's overall care plan. Because the patient is a teenager, his therapy is directed toward areas of daily living and occupational skills. Orientation and mobility instruction and occupational therapy skills are critical as he approaches adulthood. The vision rehabilitation team will take an integral role in the activities of daily living training. He will need in-office and at-home training to maximize use of the vision he has.

Discussion

The ophthalmic findings in this case are not unusual in children with cerebral palsy. Optic atrophy from perinatal hypoxia is common and usually nonprogressive. Strabismus is common, and multiple surgeries are sometimes needed to maintain some degree of binocularity. With early surgery, however, some children with cerebral palsy gain considerable binocular vision, stereovision, and stability over time. As infants, these children need the services of early interventionists. Early surgery for constant strabismus should not be withheld from cerebral palsy patients simply because they may require multiple surgeries. Glasses should be prescribed for any significant refractive error, and bifocals can help when near focusing is inconsistent or insufficient. Near-focusing difficulty (accommodative insufficiency) is a common and underdiagnosed problem associated with cerebral palsy.

In addition to these considerations, occupational therapy, physical therapy, orientation and mobility instruction, and visits to a vision rehabilitation center can vastly improve the functional vision of patients with cerebral palsy. Because every child is different, these treatments are customized to the findings and needs of the child.

Key Points

- Patients with cerebral palsy should be examined by a pediatric ophthalmologist as soon as the diagnosis is made.
- Static encephalopathy from perinatal hypoxia usually includes some damage to the optic nerve or optic pathways.
- Ocular motor control and alignment are commonly affected, and eyeglasses are also commonly needed.
- In addition to the therapies offered through public schools as part of the US Department of Education Individualized Education Program, comprehensive vision rehabilitation centers can assist by offering visual aids and occupational therapy specific to the visual needs of the child.

Suggested Reading

Jacobson LK, Dutton GN. Periventricular leukomalacia: an important cause of visual and ocular motility dysfunction in children. *Surv Ophthalmol.* 2000;45(1):1–13

Lawrence L, Wilson ME. Pediatric low vision. In: Wilson ME, Saunders RA, Trivedi RH, eds. *Pediatric Ophthalmology: Current Thought and a Practical Guide.* Berlin, Germany: Springer-Verlag Berlin Heidelberg; 2009:461–470

Chapter 80

Blistering Rash After Eye Infection

Sharon S. Lehman, MD

Presentation

A 9-year-old boy is prescribed sulfacetamide eyedrops for conjunctivitis at an urgent care center. Three days later he presents to the pediatrician's office with malaise, fever, and erythematous rash on his trunk spreading to his extremities (Figure 80-1). There are some early bullae, which separate from the underlying dermis with pressure. The pediatrician's examination of the patient's oral cavity shows blistering lesions of his mouth and lips. The boy is unable to take anything by mouth.

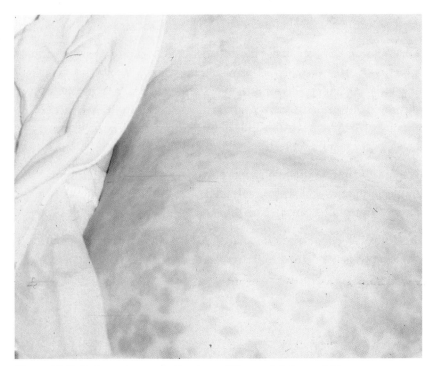

Figure 80-1. Erythematous rash. Courtesy of Sharon S. Lehman, MD.

The pediatrician admits him to the hospital for further evaluation and treatment.

Diagnosis

The patient's medical course after drug administration suggests an adverse cutaneous drug reaction. Although this reaction is related to an eyedrop, severe reactions can occur anywhere. Because the conjunctiva is a mucous membrane, it is subject to the same reactions as tissue anywhere else in the body.

The patient is evaluated by various specialists, including those in dermatology, infectious disease, and ophthalmology. Diagnoses considered include Stevens-Johnson syndrome (SJS)/toxic epidermal necrolysis (TEN) (SJS and TEN are on a spectrum of severity, with SJS having less and TEN having more skin involvement), staphylococcal scalded skin syndrome, or exanthematous drug reaction (see "Differential Diagnosis" on the next page). The rash progressing to bullae as well as the mucositis and ocular involvement after drug exposure are most consistent with SJS/TEN.

This syndrome is potentially life-threatening. It acutely presents with fever and malaise; erythematous rash that progresses to bullae, which may separate epidermis from dermis; significant mucosal involvement; and conjunctival redness. Life-threatening complications may occur because of skin loss, which can lead to volume and electrolyte imbalances, overwhelming infection, sepsis, and shock.

The most common inciting agents are medications, mainly sulfonamide antibiotics and anticonvulsants. *Mycoplasma pneumoniae* is a known infectious cause.

A cytotoxic T-lymphocyte–mediated disease, SJS/TEN causes keratinocyte apoptosis with epidermal necrosis and formation of subepidermal bullae (Figure 80-2).

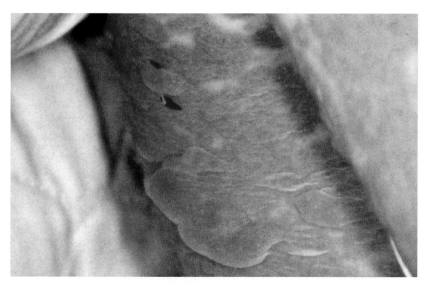

Figure 80-2. Skin bullae seen in Stevens-Johnson syndrome/toxic epidermal necrolysis. Courtesy of Sharon S. Lehman, MD.

Differential Diagnosis

Diagnoses besides SJS/TEN that should be considered include the following:

Exanthematous Drug Reaction

Exanthematous maculopapular rash is the most common skin drug reaction. Many medications, especially penicillin, as well as viruses may be inciting factors. Concurrent viral infection may increase the occurrence of drug reactions. Skin reaction occurs within 2 weeks after drug exposure and resolves in 1 to 2 weeks without complications. Itching occurs, along with central to peripheral spread with eventual confluence of maculopapular lesions. Eosinophils are seen on skin biopsy.

Staphylococcal Scalded Skin Syndrome

This syndrome occurs most commonly in children younger than 5 years. It presents with fever, reddening of the skin, and pain and blistering around the mouth. Toxins produced by the bacteria cause epidermolysis in a superficial plane. In contrast with SJS/TEN, there is a lack of mucous membrane involvement.

When to Refer

If SJS/TEN is suspected, the patient should be urgently admitted to the hospital because the disease is potentially fatal.

Treatment

Initial systemic therapy is discontinuation of the offending agent. Admission to an intensive care unit (ICU) or burn unit that is able to supply acute systemic support and skin care is imperative. Improved survival has been shown to correlate with rapid admission to an ICU. Use of antibiotics should be based on culture results. Use of systemic steroids and other adjunctive therapies such as intravenous immuno-globulin remains controversial.

Daily ophthalmologic examination is necessary acutely. Use of anti-biotics should be based on culture results. Use of systemic steroids is controversial. Disruption of symblepharon (scarring of the conjunc-tival sac) is performed and sedation is frequently necessary. Continued frequent lubrication is necessary. Preservative-free ocular lubricant is suggested. Topical cyclosporine may be useful in managing the inflam-matory component of the chronic dry eye. Topical steroids may also be necessary to aid in the control of inflammation. Eyelid surgery may be necessary to help with eyelid position and trichiasis. Ocular surface reconstruction with amniotic membrane transplantation may eventually be indicated.

Discussion

Skin lesions in SJS/TEN usually heal within days or weeks. The most common skin complication is changes in pigmentation. There can be a loss of nails. Strictures and adhesions may form during the healing process.

Ocular complications may be vision threatening. Early ocular prob-lems include exposure with epithelial defects, secondary infection with corneal ulcers, and adhesions of de-epithelialized conjunctival surfaces of the globe and eyelid (symblepharon). Late ocular complications include chronic dry eye with vascularization and scarring of the cornea (Figure 80-3). Eyelid malposition and misdirected lashes (trichiasis)

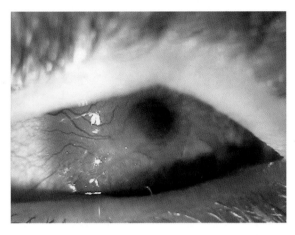

Figure 80-3. Ocular complication of corneal scarring in Stevens-Johnson syndrome/toxic epidermal necrolysis. Courtesy of Sharon S. Lehman, MD.

may further aggravate ocular surface problems. Chronic irritation and photophobia (light sensitivity) may limit a patient's ability to use his or her eyes.

Key Points

- A high level of suspicion for Stevens-Johnson syndrome/toxic epidermal necrolysis is imperative because of the possibility of life-threatening disease.
- Early diagnosis and treatment with special attention to drug discontinuation and rapid admission to an intensive care unit may improve survival.
- Daily ophthalmologic care is necessary while the disease is acute.
- For those patients who survive, ocular complications often require long-term ophthalmologic care.

Suggested Reading

Lehman SS. Long-term ocular complication of Stevens-Johnson syndrome. *Clin Pediatr (Phila).* 1999;38(7):425–427

McKenna JK, Leiferman KM. Dermatologic drug reactions. *Immunol Allergy Clin North Am.* 2004;24(3):399–423

Pereira FA, Mudgil AV, Rosmarin DM. Toxic epidermal necrolysis. *J Am Acad Dermatol.* 2007;56(2):181–200

Chapter 81

Tall Boy With Nearsightedness

Fay Charmaine Cruz, MD

Presentation

A 12-year-old boy is brought into the pediatrician's clinic because of bruises after playing basketball. He is tall for his age group and on further investigation can perform several "tricks" (due to his joint laxity). He has large hands with unusually long fingers (Figure 81-1). He wears thick prescription lenses. There are no other medical problems, and he has an unremarkable family medical history.

Diagnosis

The pediatrician suspects Marfan syndrome based on 2 factors: body habitus and joint laxity. The patient is referred to ophthalmology, cardiology, and genetics. An ophthalmologic consultation reveals high myopia and lens subluxation via slit-lamp examination (Figure 81-2). These eye findings further confirm the diagnosis of Marfan syndrome.

Marfan syndrome is associated with dilatation of the ascending aorta as a principal cause of mortality (with or without aortic regurgitation or dissection of the ascending aorta). The patient undergoes imaging studies to detect anomalies such as protruding acetabulums or dural ectasia.

Marfan syndrome is an autosomal-dominant disorder involving fibrillin mutation, more specifically the *FBN1* locus on the long arm of chromosome 15. It is a connective tissue disorder that primarily affects the cardiovascular system, skeletal system, and eyes. The most common ophthalmic findings are myopia and lens subluxation; less common eye findings include flat cornea, small pupils, strabismus (ie, misalignment), glaucoma, and retinal detachment. Besides joint laxity, these patients can have scoliosis and pectus deformities.

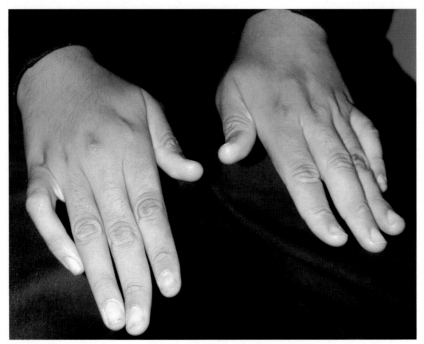

Figure 81-1. Unusually long fingers. Courtesy of Shira L. Robbins, MD.

Differential Diagnosis

The following diagnoses should be considered when presented with an unusually tall young individual with refractive error:

Homocystinuria

Significant findings would be widening of epiphyses and metaphyses of long bones. Osteoporosis is present at a young age with vertebral involvement. Lens subluxation can also be seen in this condition.

Congenital Contractual Arachnodactyly (Beals Syndrome)

Eyes are not affected and gene mutation is of *FBN2* rather than *FBN1*.

Ehlers-Danlos Syndrome

Similar to Marfan syndrome, Ehlers-Danlos syndrome is a disorder that affects soft connective tissue. It is a multisystemic disease associated with skin hypersensitivity, joint hypermobility, and generalized tissue fragility. There can be many associated eye findings including cataract and lens subluxation.

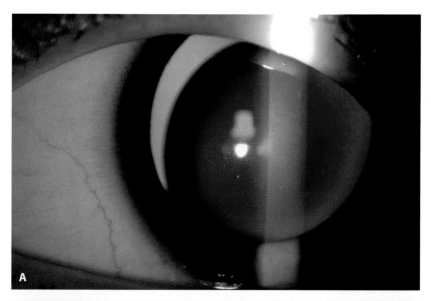

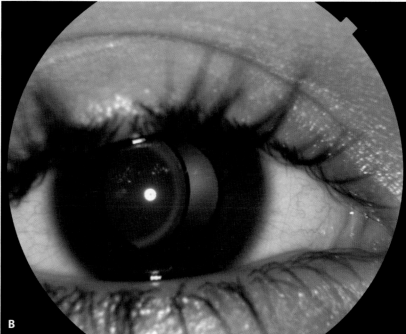

Figure 81-2. Natural lens dislocation secondary to loose zonules in a patient with Marfan syndrome. **A,** The lens is dislocated inferotemporally, allowing the superior and nasal edge to be seen through the pupil, left eye. Courtesy of Shira L. Robbins, MD. **B,** The lens is dislocated temporally, allowing the nasal edge to be seen through the pupil, right eye. Courtesy of David B. Granet, MD.

Mitral Valve, Aorta, Skin, Skeletal Phenotype

Another connective tissue disorder similar to Marfan syndrome, mitral valve, aorta, skin, skeletal (MASS) phenotype has the skeletal features of Marfan syndrome. *However, it does not affect the eyes.*

Stickler Syndrome

This syndrome can present with mitral valve prolapse—cardiac involvement similar to Marfan sydrome. Eye problems include cataract, glaucoma, large retinal detachment secondary to vitreoretinal degeneration, and severe myopia.

Isolated Medial Necrosis of Aorta (Erdheim Disease)

This is associated with lesions of the elastic fiber. Usually patients present with a dissecting aortic aneurysm.

When to Refer

A multispecialty approach is used to treat patients with Marfan syndrome. To arrive at an accurate clinical diagnosis, an ophthalmologic referral is warranted. However, eye findings in this syndrome are progressive. Any normal eye findings do not exclude the diagnosis; therefore, repeat examinations are required. If patients are myopic, giving prescription glasses will provide an improvement in visual acuity. If patients have a subluxated lens, prescription glasses can be the solution to blurring of vision until surgery.

Treatment

Pediatricians play a primary role in prevention of any complications that occur in patients with Marfan syndrome. As mentioned earlier, a multispecialty approach will greatly benefit these patients. The ophthalmologist can refract the patient and provide the best corrected visual acuity. Individuals with severe subluxation of the lens are candidates for surgery. This lens surgery requires an experienced surgeon because of the difficulty in technique (it is more complicated than the usual cataract surgery). Implantation of a replacement lens sometimes requires suture fixation and is not always possible. There is also an increased risk of retinal detachment and glaucoma associated with this condition and subsequent surgery.

Any patient with Marfan syndrome who is active in sports should wear protective eyewear. The laxity of the natural lens makes it prone to dislocation.

The inheritable nature of the disease makes genetic counseling mandatory. An affected parent has a 50% risk of having an affected child with chromosome 15 mutations.

Discussion

Marfan syndrome has a large variety of clinical manifestations. Although the syndrome is potentially fatal, patients can still have a life span comparable to the general population. Visual outcome is improved by early detection, early treatment, and prevention of accompanying amblyopia.

Key Points

- An ophthalmic evaluation may help make or confirm diagnosis because of the lens dislocation commonly seen in Marfan syndrome.
- Ocular clinical findings associated with Marfan syndrome may arise with age, thus necessitating annual eye examinations.
- Surgery to treat lens dislocation is technically difficult and requires an experienced ophthalmologist.

Suggested Reading

American Academy of Pediatrics Committee on Genetics. Health supervision for children with Marfan syndrome. *Pediatrics.* 1996;98(5):978–982

Behrman RE, Kleigman RM, Janson HB. *Nelson's Textbook of Pediatrics.* 16th ed. Philadelphia, PA: Elsevier Saunders; 2000

Dean JC. Marfan syndrome: clinical diagnosis and management. *Eur J Hum Genet.* 2007;15(7):724–733

Jones KL. *Smith's Recognizable Patterns of Human Malformation.* Philadelphia, PA: Elsevier Saunders; 2006

Chapter 82

Decreased Vision in a Child With Leukemia History

Donald P. Sauberan, MD
Scott E. Olitsky, MD

Presentation

The pediatrician is seeing a 6-year-old boy in whom acute lymphoblastic (lymphocytic) leukemia (ALL) was diagnosed 9 months ago. The boy received an appropriate chemotherapy regimen to achieve remission and is currently undergoing maintenance chemotherapy. He comes to the pediatrician's office today complaining of visual disturbances in his right eye. He does not report any pain in the eye but does believe that the vision in that eye has worsened. He denies increased fatigue, weight loss, fever, joint pain, easy bruising, or bleeding gums.

On examination, there are no bruises, petechiae, or lymphadenopathy. The pediatrician finds the visual acuity to be 20/20 in the left eye and 20/40 in the right eye. The pediatrician tries to look at the retina with the direct ophthalmoscope but is unable to achieve a view. The pediatrician is concerned, given the boy's history of leukemia, and therefore calls the pediatric ophthalmologist, who agrees to see the patient that afternoon.

Diagnosis

The pediatric ophthalmologist examines the boy and finds a swollen and elevated right optic nerve with surrounding retinal hemorrhages.

Most patients will already have a diagnosis of leukemia when their ocular manifestations are noted. However, it is possible for the eye to show the first symptom or sign of the disease. Initial signs that could suggest a diagnosis of leukemia include hyphema (bleeding in the anterior chamber of the eye), retinal hemorrhages seen on a dilated pupil examination (Figure 82-1), or a mass noted on the iris. Ocular manifestations of leukemia occur most commonly in the acute manifestations of the disease process and are more common in ALL as opposed to acute myelogenous leukemia.

There are several broad categories of ocular sequelae, including direct infiltration of leukemia into the eye, infectious disease related to leukemia, and ophthalmic side effects of treatment. The first category is the appearance of actual leukemic infiltrates occurring in the ocular tissues. Leukemic infiltrates can occur in any part of the eye but are most often clinically apparent in the retina. These infiltrates often look like whitish, feathery areas in the retina. Often these infiltrates mimic an infectious cause. They are most common surrounding the optic nerve and macula.

Optic nerve infiltration can also occur during the leukemic process. These patients have an elevated nerve, often with hemorrhages (Figure 82-2). They may have an afferent pupillary defect as well as abnormalities

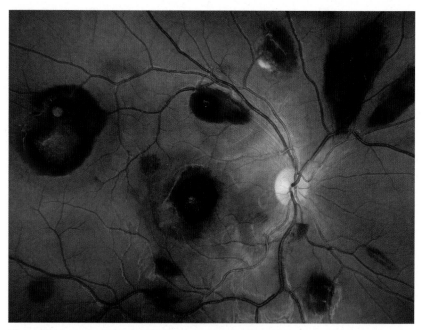

Figure 82-1. Retinal leukemic infiltrates with associated hemorrhages. Courtesy of Debra Brown, COT, CRA, University of California, San Francisco.

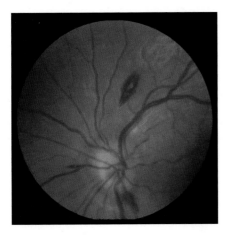

Figure 82-2. Leukemic optic nerve infiltration seen by elevated optic nerve with associated hemorrhages. Courtesy of Alex V. Levin, MD, MHSc.

in visual acuity and visual fields. Optic nerve infiltration must be differentiated from elevated optic nerves secondary to increased intracranial pressure from relapse affecting the central nervous system (CNS). This can be definitively diagnosed with a lumbar puncture, confirming the presence of leukemic cells in the cerebrospinal fluid (CSF) or opening CSF pressure. Documentation of intraocular extension of leukemia represents a relapse.

Less common is an actual orbital deposition of leukemic cells, which presents as an orbital mass. This often presents with proptosis (bulging of the eye) and can also resemble a cellulitis-type picture. Interestingly, it is more common to see histologic involvement of the eye than clinical involvement of the ocular structures.

Another large category of leukemia-induced ocular sequelae is infectious-related disease. This often appears in a similar fashion to a retinal leukemic infiltrate, usually showing a whitish lesion present in the retina. However, compared with leukemic retinal infiltrates, there is usually an overlying vitreous inflammation (vitreitis) present. This vitreitis is seen as a diffusely cloudy vitreous or hazy vitreous overlying the retinal lesion.

Fungal infections are not uncommon given these patients' level of immunosuppression. Aspergillosis, for example, although rare in the general population, is a common fungal eye infection seen in immunocompromised patients. Cytomegalovirus retinitis is also a common opportunistic infection seen in immunocompromised patients. This retinitis classically presents with large amounts of retinal hemorrhages and associated white inflammatory areas. Cytomegalovirus retinitis can be visually devastating; thus, prompt recognition of this entity is required to allow for adequate antiviral treatment.

Leukemic retinal infiltrates and infectious retinal infiltrates can look very similar. Leukemic retinal infiltrates are most often seen in patients with blast crisis or those who are not in remission. Infectious infiltrates tend to occur in patients who are in clinical remission but remain immunocompromised.

Lastly, ocular side effects can occur from the treatment used to combat leukemia. Bone marrow transplant and chemotherapy have the potential to cause multiple ocular sequelae. Bone marrow transplantation has been shown to cause cataracts, graft-versus-host (GVH) disease, and retinopathy. Cataract formation is believed to occur in about one-fourth of patients who underwent bone marrow transplantation. Ocular GVH disease has effects on the corneal surface, leading to keratoconjunctivitis sicca (dry eye), corneal epithelial defects, and secondary infections.

Differential Diagnosis

Differential diagnoses that should be considered include optic neuritis, increased intracranial pressure from any cause, or an unrelated bleeding disorder.

When to Refer

Patients with a history of leukemia should be referred to an ophthalmologist if a change in vision occurs. In addition, patients with pain, photophobia, or tearing should be referred as well because this could suggest changes in the cornea secondary to the disease itself or its treatment.

Treatment

This boy underwent radiotherapy to rapidly treat the direct involvement of the optic nerve.

Treatment of intraocular extension of ALL must be treated systemically. Treatment of optic nerve involvement frequently involves radiotherapy to the involved optic nerves in addition to chemotherapy for systemic relapse.

Treatment of leukemic infections involves systemic therapy for the presumptive organism, not only because topical ocular treatment does not penetrate into the eye very well but also because of the possibility of systemic infection.

Patients with ocular GVH disease require aggressive management of symptoms, including liberal use of artificial tears for dry eye. Long-term use of corticosteroids in immunosuppression also increases the likelihood of cataract and glaucoma development; the pediatrician must be aware of this. In addition, one must always be concerned with the development of amblyopia, as any side effect that affects visual acuity can lead to amblyopia.

Discussion

Ocular involvement in ALL is rare but can have long-lasting and devastating effects on vision. Therefore, monitoring of vision in patients with leukemia or a history of the disease is suggested.

Key Points

- Ocular manifestations of leukemia are not uncommon, although overt clinical manifestations may be.
- Any ocular involvement by leukemic infiltrates should be considered central nervous system leukemia and treated accordingly.
- The development of secondary infections can occur at any stage of disease and must be considered.
- Treatment of leukemia may lead to various ocular side effects, which may lead to severe and potentially vision-threatening complications.
- Continual monitoring of visual status in patients with leukemia or a history of the disease is mandatory to minimize a poor outcome.

Suggested Reading

Bradfield YS, Kushner BJ, Gangnon RE. Ocular complications after organ and bone marrow transplantation in children. *J AAPOS.* 2005;9(5):426–432

Sharma T, Grewal J, Gupta S, Murray PI. Ophthalmic manifestations of acute leukaemias: the ophthalmologist's role. *Eye (Lond).* 2004;18(7):663–672

Suh DW, Ruttum MS, Stuckenschneider BJ, Mieler WF, Kivlin JD. Ocular findings after bone marrow transplantation in a pediatric population. *Ophthalmology.* 1999;106(8):1564–1570

Chapter 83

Floaters and Light Sensitivity

Yasmin Bradfield, MD

Presentation

A 15-year-old Hispanic boy presents to the pediatric clinic complaining of light sensitivity and floaters in his right eye for the past week. He states that there has been no change in his symptoms since they began. He denies decreased vision, eye pain, eye trauma, or prior eye problems. He also denies fever, rash, joint or back pain, abdominal pain, or recent illnesses. He moved from El Salvador 5 years ago and has not traveled recently. He is in foster care and has an unknown family history. He is taking no medications and has no drug allergies.

On examination, the pediatrician finds a healthy-appearing male adolescent in no acute distress. He is able to read 20/20 in each eye on the Snellen visual acuity chart at distance and with a near card. His eye movements look normal, but his right pupil appears sluggish in reacting to light compared with his left. There is no afferent pupillary defect. He has diffuse redness of his right conjunctiva without any discharge. He also seems to have some haziness to his right cornea inferiorly. His left eye looks normal when examined with a penlight.

The pediatrician sends the patient to a local pediatric ophthalmologist the same day. The ophthalmologist calls the pediatrician after the examination is completed to let the pediatrician know that the patient has white blood cells in his anterior chamber on slit-lamp biomicroscopy. He also has keratic precipitates on his cornea, which led to its hazy appearance. The ophthalmologist agrees that the patient's right pupil is less reactive but did not see any posterior synechiae (attachments between iris and lens). The patient's eye pressure is elevated in the right eye. In addition, on dilated retinal examination, there is a white retinal lesion in the right inferior retina, with surrounding satellite lesions, retinal hemorrhages, and vascular sheathing (Figure 83-1). His left eye appears normal.

Diagnosis

The ophthalmologist diagnoses panuveitis of unclear cause. An evaluation is performed to rule out toxoplasmosis, sarcoidosis, Lyme disease, syphilis, and Wegener granulomatosis. A chest radiograph, complete blood cell (CBC) count with differential, chemistry panel, and toxoplasmosis antibody titers are ordered, along with tests of angiotensin-converting enzyme level, cytoplasmic antineutrophil cytoplasmic antibodies, perinuclear antineutrophil cytoplasmic antibodies, fluorescent treponemal antibody absorption, and antinuclear antibodies.

The pediatrician speaks with the ophthalmologist a few days later, who informs the pediatrician that the patient has had no change in his floaters but has less photophobia (light sensitivity). His chest radiograph is normal, and all of his laboratory results are negative except for IgG titers positive for *Toxoplasma gondii*. His IgM titer results are negative for *T gondii*.

A diagnosis of toxoplasmosis chorioretinitis with uveitis is given.

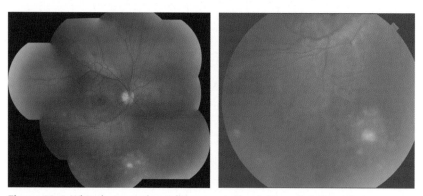

Figure 83-1. White lesion with satellite areas in the right eye inferior retina. Courtesy of David Gamm, MD, PhD.

T gondii is an obligate intracellular parasite. Sources of human infection include cat feces and raw meat, in which there is exposure to oocysts and tissue cysts, respectively. Other risk factors include eating raw vegetables outside the home, contact with soil, poor hand hygiene, and drinking water from a contaminated reservoir.

Toxoplasmosis can be congenital or acquired, and the presentation varies with age. Infants and young children frequently present with strabismus (eye misalignment), leukocoria (white pupil), nystagmus (rapid, rhythmic eye movements), and reduced vision because of bilateral involvement. Teenagers often present with unilateral floaters, photophobia, decreased vision, and conjunctival hyperemia.

Lesions in the retina and choroid can be solitary, multiple, or adjacent to a pigmented scar. They are usually located in the posterior pole of the retina. Active lesions present as grayish-white focal areas of retinal necrosis with associated vasculitis, hemorrhage, and vitreitis. Anterior uveitis is common, with keratic precipitates, white blood cells in the anterior chamber, and iris synechiae.

Laboratory diagnosis of toxoplasmosis is based on detection of serum *T gondii*–specific antibodies, or in atypical cases, aqueous humor or vitreous *T gondii* DNA by polymerase chain reaction. In congenital infections, a brain computed tomography scan should be performed to look for hydrocephalus and periventricular calcifications.

Differential Diagnosis

Diagnoses besides ocular toxoplasmosis that should be considered include the following:

Tuberculosis

Pulmonary symptoms with fever and weight loss, lymphadenopathy, choroidal tubercles (nodule) with retinal detachment, granulomatous uveitis and keratitis, choroidal neovascular membrane

Toxocariasis

Exposure to dog or cat feces parasite, unilateral, leukocoria, macular granuloma with exudates, serous retinal detachment, retinal scarring

Sarcoidosis

Iris nodules, conjunctival yellowish lesions, dry eyes, erythema nodosum, facial nerve palsy, myositis

Lyme Disease

Associated with tick bites, optic nerve swelling, conjunctivitis, Bell palsy

Syphilis

Interstitial keratitis with corneal edema, infiltrates and neovascularization (salmon patch), scleritis, optic nerve swelling, pseudo-retinitis pigmentosa

Wegener Granulomatosis

Peripheral ulcerative keratitis, orbital involvement leading to proptosis and eye muscle restriction, scleritis

Cytomegalovirus Retinitis

Immunocompromised patient, retinal hemorrhages along perivascular pattern beginning in the periphery, brush-fire appearance to retinal hemorrhages and necrosis, eye appearing white and quiet anteriorly

Candida Endophthalmitis

Immunocompromised patient, fluffy vitreous balls, creamy retinal infiltrates surrounded by hemorrhage (Roth spot), bilateral, choroidal neovascular membrane

When to Refer

Cloudiness of the cornea, new-onset photophobia that is not accompanied by an infectious presentation, and new-onset multiple floaters can be signs of a potentially vision-threatening condition and warrant referral to an ophthalmologist.

Treatment

Initially the teenager is prescribed prednisolone and atropine eyedrops, as well as glaucoma eyedrops to help lower his intraocular pressure. After obtaining the correct diagnosis, the patient is started on a regimen of clindamycin (300 mg orally 4 times a day) and oral trimethoprim and sulfamethoxazole (once daily).

He is examined by his ophthalmologist every 2 to 3 days for the first week, with improvement of the uveitis and retinal toxoplasmosis lesion (Figure 83-2). Topical atropine therapy is discontinued after the first week because there is less inflammation and photophobia. He continues taking the antibiotics; prednisolone dosage is tapered off over the next 3 weeks. His intraocular pressure improves and glaucoma drops are discontinued. Over the treatment course, he notices the floaters becoming less bothersome, and he has complete resolution of his conjunctival redness and light sensitivity. The retinal lesion becomes inactive.

Therapy for ocular toxoplasmosis includes various combinations of oral antibiotics with corticosteroids. Commonly used antibiotics include pyrimethamine, sulfadiazine, clindamycin, trimethoprim-sulfamethoxazole, azithromycin, and tetracycline.

In congenital infections, treatment involves triple therapy with pyrimethamine, sulfadiazine, and leucovorin. Leucovorin (folinic acid) should be administered in conjunction with pyrimethamine to provide for the synthesis of nucleic acids. Monitoring by CBC and platelet counts is required weekly because of the reversible bone marrow suppression possible with pyrimethamine. Current standard treatment of congenital toxoplasmosis is to continue triple therapy for up to 1 year after birth.

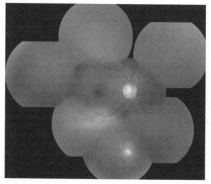 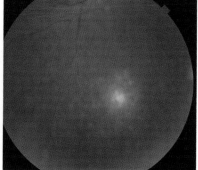

Figure 83-2. More discrete white lesions of the right eye inferior retina. Retinal blood vessel sheathing is noted as the whitened focal areas of the inferior vasculature. Courtesy of David Gamm, MD, PhD.

Discussion

Toxoplasmosis is the most common cause of posterior uveitis in immunocompetent children. The name of the causative parasite, *T gondii*, derives from the Greek word toxon, meaning bow, and gondii for a rodent indigenous to North Africa, from which the organism was first isolated.

Visual prognosis after treatment in immunocompetent individuals is usually good, as long as the central macula is not affected. Surgical treatment with a vitrectomy may be required in cases of retinal detachment secondary to vitreous traction or persistent vitreous opacities. Because children with a history of toxoplasmosis retinal infection can have a reactivation of their lesion, they need an annual dilated eye examination.

Key Points

- Symptoms of ocular toxoplasmosis in children include strabismus, leukocoria, nystagmus, and reduced vision. Teenagers often present with floaters, photophobia, decreased vision, and conjunctival hyperemia.
- Children with an history of toxoplasmosis retinal infection can have a reactivation of their lesion.
- These children need to have an annual dilated eye examination and be aware of visual symptoms that may indicate active chorioretinitis and uveitis.

Suggested Reading

Bonfioli AA, Orefice F. Toxoplasmosis. *Semin Ophthalmol.* 2005;20(3):129–141

Commodaro AG, Belfort RN, Rizzo LV, et al. Ocular toxoplasmosis: an update and review of the literature. *Mem Inst Oswaldo Cruz.* 2009;104(2):345–350

Smith JR, Cunningham ET Jr. Atypical presentations of ocular toxoplasmosis. *Curr Opin Ophthalmol.* 2002;13(6):387–392

Chapter 84

Letters Are Backwards

David B. Granet, MD

Presentation

Parents bring their 9-year-old son to the pediatrician's office because of "reading issues." He has been evaluated by an occupational therapist, physical therapist, educational psychologist, special education teacher, and developmental vision therapist. As they hand the packet of evaluations to the pediatrician, the parents report on how smart their son is. However, he cannot read as well as they think he should. He does not like to read out loud and never reads for fun. Although he reads at grade level, the parents believe he should be more advanced. They note that he reverses letters at times, but this is improving slowly. His older sister was always a great reader and they want to know why he is not.

History reveals that the father experienced difficulty with reading before law school, when it seemed to improve. The mother did not experience problems with reading. The patient's handwriting has not come along very well but according to his parents, he is a fast runner, great at soccer, and playing video games.

The patient thinks everything is "fine." He has no complaints when asked but does report that reading is "boring" and that he extremely dislikes reading aloud. He says he is in the middle level of his class in reading.

Physical examination is unremarkable. Diagnoses of visual motor integration deficit from the occupational therapist and tracking issues from the vision therapist are recorded in the evaluation paperwork.

The pediatrician recognizes that this child's issues are more related to education rather than health concerns but wants to address the parents' worries and make sure a vision problem is not missed. The boy is referred to a pediatric ophthalmologist for evaluation.

Diagnosis

At the pediatric ophthalmologist's office, the child has a complete examination including relevant developmental history, school history, and medical history (including medications). Ability of the eyes to work individually and together (ductions, versions, convergence, and fusional amplitudes) as well as ocular structures are evaluated. Focusing ability of the eye, in dynamic and static fashion, is detected and in part requires the use of dilating drops.

Generally a discussion ensues, educating the parents as to the scientific basis for understanding of the way people read. Although the eyes seem an obvious target for creating reading difficulties, it turns out they are uncommonly involved. There are many examples of misalignment of eyes that create poor ocular coordination yet leave the child reading with no difficulty; these include Brown and Duane syndrome. Most children with nystagmus (repetitive wiggling of the eyes) and good vision read just fine. Children who are monocular have not been demonstrated to have decreased reading skills. Thus, rushing to blame the ocular system for reading difficulties must be avoided.

However, there are some ocular-related conditions that do make the physical act of reading more difficult. They include mostly refractive errors and problems with convergence or accommodation. These do not impair comprehension.

A special discussion of tracking eye problems is warranted. Typically this is the term used when someone seems to have difficulty smoothly following a moving target horizontally across field of gaze. While interesting, this is not the system of eye movements used in reading. We jump (or saccade) from word to word, with occasional reversals until the end of the line, and then jump to the start of the next. These systems, smooth pursuit and saccadic, are very different. There is evidence that enhanced expertise at a task improves pattern of saccades but not the other way around; ie, working on eye movements does not improve reading skills, but as we read better our eye movements become more precise.

Convergence difficulty at near is termed convergence insufficiency. This problem is complex but does respond to eye exercises. These orthoptic exercises can be done inexpensively at home or in someone's office at greater cost. Improving convergence insufficiency does not necessarily make one a better reader or improve comprehension, but it does reduce a physical barrier to reading.

Dyslexia represents a completely different reading issue and is beyond the scope of this chapter. However, dyslexia is a neurobiologic disorder and is not characterized by reversals of letters. Typical reading remediation programs contain extra practice time and use of oral guided reading, with the student alternating reading out loud with a parent or teacher, as their central components. In simplistic terms, getting sound components of decoding print to connect to the language center in the brain is the goal.

This patient had a healthy eye examination and was diagnosed with developmental delay of reading skills with no underlying pathology.

Differential Diagnosis

Diagnoses besides developmental delay of reading skills with no underlying pathology that should be considered include
- Dyslexia
- Convergence insufficiency
- Large refractive error including high hyperopia or high astigmatism
- Learning disability

When to Refer

Children should be referred to an ophthalmologist who has experience with the care of children when they do not pass a pediatric vision screening or have an ocular abnormality. Ophthalmologic referral also is warranted when a child has severe development delay or suspected learning disabilities that may result from near-vision problems such as convergence insufficiency, accommodative insufficiency, or severe hyperopia (farsightedness).

Treatment

Successful treatment of reading problems uses multifactorial intervention from multiple disciplines, including physicians, educators, special education teachers, counselors, and other professionals as needed.

Discussion

Educating parents whose children underperform in school is the responsibility of every physician who cares for these families. This situation is an emotional one that goes to the core of parenting. Education and information greatly assist these families in navigating the many emotional issues and therapies that are available.

The American Academy of Pediatrics, along with other organizations, has developed in-depth resources on this topic for physicians and parents.

Key Points

- Dyslexia is a neurobiologic disorder not characterized by reversals of letters.
- Subtle ocular deficits do not cause reading problems; nor do tracking problems.
- Successful reading programs use multifactorial intervention.

Suggested Reading

American Academy of Pediatrics, American Academy of Ophthalmology, American Association for Pediatric Ophthalmology and Strabismus, American Association of Certified Orthoptists. Learning disabilities, dyslexia, and vision. *Pediatrics.* 2009;124(2):837–844

Gomi CF, Granet DB. Learning disabilities and vision. In: Garg A, Prost ME, Azad R, et al, eds. *Surgical and Medical Management of Pediatric Ophthalmology.* New Delhi, India: Jaypee Brothers Medical Publishers; 2007:99–105

Granet DB. Learning disabilities, dyslexia, and vision: the role of the pediatric ophthalmologist. *J AAPOS.* 2011;15(2):119–120

Handler SM, Fierson WM, American Academy of Pediatrics, American Academy of Ophthalmology, American Association for Pediatric Ophthalmology and Strabismus, American Association of Certified Orthoptists. Learning disabilities, dyslexia, and vision. *Pediatrics.* 2011;127(3):e818–e856

Shein J, Gomi CF, Granet DB. Learning disorders and vision therapy. In: *Albert and Jakobiec's Principle and Practice of Ophthalmology.* Philadelphia, PA: Saunders; 2008:4301–4303

Section 12

Incidental Findings

Chapter 85

Failed Vision Screen

Robert W. Arnold, MD

Presentation

A family comes to the pediatrician's office with no visual concerns but requesting a prekindergarten physical examination for their older son. He and his younger brother seem very healthy and athletic.

Neither boy was adequately cooperative during attempts to screen their vision at their respective 3-year-old well-child checkups despite using the seemingly child-friendly umbrella/sailboat eye chart at 20 feet. By age 4 years, however, both passed the pediatric nurse's visual acuity screening. At that visit their mother commented that she thought the older boy seemed to cross his eyes at times. Because a prominent inner eyelid fold (epicanthus) was evident without overt crossing, the pediatrician reassured the mother that it was "pseudostrabismus," in which eyes falsely appear misaligned (see Figure 54-1 on page 376).

During the vision screening portion of his prekindergarten physical examination, the older brother is unable to see even large letters while his mother covers his right eye. Previously the pediatric nurse had allowed the child to hold his own hand or a black plastic occluder over the non-tested eye. Because the boy fails the vision screening, he is referred to the local eye doctor.

The eye doctor's examination shows that the patient is almost legally blind (20/125) in the left eye. Visual acuity in his right eye is 20/25.

Diagnosis

The eye doctor diagnoses unequal farsightedness (hyperopia). Glasses are prescribed, and patching of the right eye with good vision (20/25) is started in an attempt to improve vision in the almost legally blind left eye.

The mother mentions that she occasionally sees her younger son crossing his eyes as well, which prompts the eye doctor to recommend bringing both boys back for the follow-up visit.

Indeed, at the follow-up visit 1 month later, it becomes apparent that both brothers have vision problems, suggesting that they had peeked with their better-seeing eye during the 4-year well-child vision screenings. Vision in the left eye of the older boy has improved to 20/100 with eyeglasses alone. Although patching was previously prescribed, the family did not want to start until their son "got used" to his glasses. The eye doctor educates the family on the necessity of starting a patch regime of the right eye to treat his left eye amblyopia (lazy eye).

The younger brother is also found to have amblyopia during his confirmatory eye examination. His visual acuities are 20/30 in the right eye and 20/50 in the left eye, with intermittent esotropia (crossing) on the cover test (see Figure 55-1 on page 379). Unlike his brother, who had one very hyperopic eye, the younger brother has bilateral severe hyperopia, as found during his full eye examination by cycloplegic retinoscopy. Glasses for his full amount of hyperopia are prescribed. The eye doctor wants to know the effect of eyeglasses alone, so patching is held off for now.

When to Refer

A child who fails a vision screening should be referred to an eye care specialist for a confirmatory eye examination. A full dilated eye examination is required to rule out other forms of eye disease that can lower vision.

Treatment

Both boys consistently wear their glasses, and eyeglass frames broken during sports activities are promptly replaced by the conscientious parents, even though their insurance covers only 1 pair per year.

After 6 months of eyeglass therapy, the younger brother has much straighter eyes while wearing glasses but more profound crossing when the glasses are removed, demonstrating accommodative esotropia (see figures 56-1 and 56-2 on pages 386 and 388). His visual acuity is now 20/25 in his right eye and 20/30 in his left eye.

After 6 months of frequent follow-up visits, the older brother is reluctantly but consistently tolerating patching of his better sighted eye. He still has essentially straight eyes. He has normal visual acuity of 20/20 in the sound eye but visual acuity of 20/50 in the other eye due to persistent anisometropic (asymmetric) amblyopia. The vision in his amblyopic eye is no longer improving with patching. This news saddens everyone but prompts the pediatrician to do some research on recent advances in pediatric vision screening.

Discussion

Much recent information about amblyopia has come from multicenter, carefully controlled, randomized research from the Pediatric Eye Disease Investigator Group (PEDIG). The PEDIG amblyopia treatment studies enroll children capable of performing a standardized, patched visual acuity test and have demonstrated that part-time patching (2 hours daily) is as effective for some forms of amblyopia as blurring the sound eye with 1% atropine penalization on weekends or daily. Newly diagnosed amblyopic patients often have profound visual acuity improvements with eyeglass therapy alone. Eyeglasses gradually improve vision in patients with bilateral amblyopia due to high hyperopic and astigmatic refractive errors. Amblyopia therapy can be moderately effective even when started as late as the early teenage years; however, a PEDIG long-term follow-up study showed that patients achieved better visual acuity when starting amblyopia therapy before age 5 years. Despite prolonged therapy in some of America's larger eye centers, mean posttreatment visual outcome of amblyopic eyes when therapy began as early as 3 or 4 years was still slightly less than the sound eye by about 2 lines.

Although most conventional vision screening has involved eye charts, new technology called photoscreening identifies children with anatomic risk factors for amblyopia such as strabismus (eye misalignment) or abnormal refractive error. Photoscreening evaluates abnormal reflections from the retina (red and Brückner reflex) (Figure 85-1) using a special camera or video system. Photoscreening can reliably be performed in children with actual or developmental age as young as 1 year. Long-term community studies have demonstrated that treatment outcomes may be

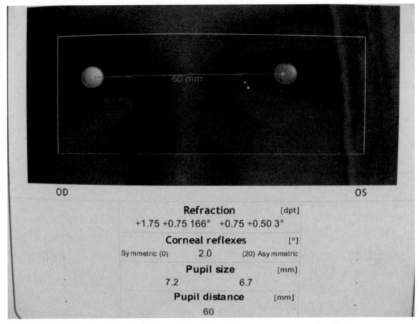

Figure 85-1. Example of photoscreening. This demonstrates a red reflex asymmetry that is quantified as a difference of hyperopia on this photoscreening device. Courtesy of Robert W. Arnold, MD.

30% to 40% better for children whose amblyopia is detected by photoscreening before the age of 2 years.

The American Academy of Pediatrics (AAP) recommends that a series of vision screening tests be performed in all children, starting with red reflex in newborns to detect cataract and infant cover test to detect constant strabismus. Photoscreening at younger ages should be followed by patched, visual acuity testing with Lea or HOTV acuity charts (see Figure 65-1 on page 446). Pediatricians are ideally suited to be the continuous medical home for vision screening because recognition of additional risk factors requires communication and clinical knowledge. Some parents will observe warning signs of eye disease such as strabismus, nystagmus (eye wiggling), large tearing eyes, or white pupil. Children with developmental delays and syndromes are at increased risk of amblyopia. Children with a family history of amblyopia and excess farsightedness are at particularly high risk of amblyopia, just like the family in this chapter.

To improve office-based vision screening, the pediatrician in this case carefully instructed nursing staff about AAP guidelines for vision screening, put into use updated acuity charts, and implemented use of adhesive patches during screening, to ensure monocular testing and no cheating with a better-sighted eye. Photoscreening seemed very expensive at first; however, *Current Procedural Terminology* code **99174** became available with sufficient relative value units to justify the technology, particularly in a group practice.

Two years later the brothers have been treated for almost 3 years. The younger boy still has a visual acuity of 20/25 and 20/30 with spectacles and is looking forward to wearing contact lenses some day, especially for sports. After glasses and patching did not create additional improved vision in the older boy's amblyopic eye, he reluctantly underwent a summer of intensive therapy with patching 6 to 10 hours daily and 1% atropine eyedrops every day. His acuity improved to 20/20 in the sound eye and 20/40 in the amblyopic eye. Currently, with a lesser schedule of 2 hours of daily patching during school, he has regressed to 20/50 visual acuity in the amblyopic eye with evidence of a small-angle strabismus. Even though he has not attained "perfect vision" he has improved greatly from being almost legally blind initially. It may now be possible for him to obtain an unrestricted driver's license when the time comes.

His mother is now wearing no-line (progressive) bifocals full time at age 36 years and has an 18-month-old daughter. At her 18-month well-child visit, a computer-interpreted photoscreening is performed, and results suggest the need for referral because of unequal farsightedness (Figure 85-1). A confirmatory eye examination finds fairly equal fixation and minimal esodeviation on the cover test, but a cycloplegic refraction shows moderately high hyperopia, more so in the right eye. She is prescribed spectacles but no patching therapy. One year later, she is able to match 20/30 visual acuity in each eye. By age 4 years her patched visual acuity measured with the HOTV chart is 20/20 in each eye.

Key Points

- During visual acuity screening, techniques such as covering one eye with a patch should be used to ensure monocular testing and no cheating with a better-sighted eye.
- Increased risk of amblyopia is present in children with developmental delays, syndromes , family history of amblyopia, and excess farsightedness.
- Photoscreening is a useful tool to screen for amblyogenic risk factors in children who are difficult to screen for visual acuity.
- Photoscreening can reliably be performed in children with actual or developmental age as young as 1 year.
- The photoscreening procedure qualifies for non-investigational *Current Procedural Terminology* code **99174.**

Suggested Reading

Alaska Blind Child Discovery. Vision screen and amblyopia. https://vimeo.com/album/1877048. Accessed June 6, 2012

American Academy of Pediatrics Committee on Practice and Ambulatory Medicine, Section on Ophthalmology. Use of photoscreening for children's vision screening. *Pediatrics.* 2002;109(3):524–525

American Academy of Pediatrics Committee on Practice and Ambulatory Medicine and Section on Ophthalmology, American Association of Certified Orthoptists, American Association for Pediatric Ophthalmology and Strabismus, American Academy of Ophthalmology. Eye examination in infants, children, and young adults by pediatricians. *Pediatrics.* 2003;111(4):902–907

Cotter SA; Pediatric Eye Disease Investigator Group, Edwards AR, et al. Treatment of anisometropic amblyopia in children with refractive correction. *Ophthalmology.* 2006;113(6):895–903

Kirk VG, Clausen MM, Armitage MD, Arnold RW. Preverbal photoscreening for amblyogenic factors and outcomes in amblyopia treatment: early objective screening and visual acuities. *Arch Ophthalmol.* 2008;126(4):489–492

Pediatric Eye Disease Investigator Group. A randomized trial of atropine vs patching for treatment of moderate amblyopia in children. *Arch Ophthalmol.* 2002;120(3):268–278

Pediatric Eye Disease Investigator Group, Repka MX, Kraker RT, et al. A randomized trial of atropine vs patching for treatment of moderate amblyopia: follow-up at age 10 years. *Arch Ophthalmol.* 2008;126(8):1039–1044

Salcido AA, Bradley J, Donahue SP. Predictive value of photoscreening and traditional screening of preschool children. *J AAPOS.* 2005;9(2):114–120

Scheiman MM, Hertle RW, Beck RW, et al. Randomized trial of treatment of amblyopia in children aged 7 to 17 years. *Arch Ophthalmol.* 2005;123(4):437–447

Wallace DK, Chandler DL, Beck RW, et al. Treatment of bilateral refractive amblyopia in children three to less than 10 years of age. *Am J Ophthalmol.* 2007;144(4):487–496

Head Tilted or Turned to See

Richard W. Hertle, MD

Presentation

The parents of a 3½-year-old boy tell the pediatrician they have noticed that their child has a "funny look" when he is watching television or looking across the room, out the car window, or across an open space outdoors. He has had this "funny" head position on and off since he was a little more than 1 year old. The child is otherwise growing, developing, and behaving normally, and there is no remarkable medical history. The parents both began wearing glasses at an early age.

The boy does not have any neuromuscular abnormalities that the pediatrician can detect on examination. He turns his head as he is visually challenged by distance (Figure 86-1). The boy has decreased vision in both eyes on vision screening examination. For that reason, the patient is referred to a pediatric ophthalmologist for a comprehensive eye examination.

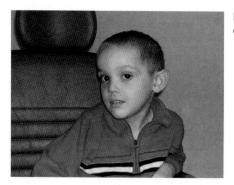

Figure 86-1. Child with ocular torticollis. Courtesy of Richard W. Hertle, MD.

Diagnosis

The pediatric ophthalmologist conducts a detailed examination, including visual acuity testing and a full ocular motor and binocular examination with microscopic and ophthalmoscopic examinations to identify any structural abnormality of the eyes or orbits. Electrophysiologic testing, including eye movement recording, is performed to evaluate for childhood forms of nystagmus, or involuntary, rapid eye movements (Figure 86-2). Appropriate imaging to rule out structural abnormalities of the adnexa, orbits, and central nervous system (CNS) is performed. The pediatric ophthalmologist diagnoses infantile nystagmus syndrome (congenital nystagmus) as the cause of this ocular torticollis.

Torticollis in childhood is most commonly the result of abnormalities of the CNS, visual system, or neck musculature. Besides benign muscular tightness of the sternocleidomastoid muscle leading to the classic head position, or a baby "packaged" funny in utero, differential diagnosis of wryneck includes sequelae to inflammatory, ocular, neurologic, or orthopedic diseases. Abnormalities of the CNS resulting in torticollis include spinal syrinx, posterior fossa abnormalities, and cervical spinal cord tumors. A distant fourth potential diagnosis is Sandifer syndrome, a congenital condition characterized by gastroesophageal reflux disease (GERD) and anomalous head posture with CNS symptoms and signs, including dystonia, developmental retardation, dysphagia, seizures, and extreme irritability.

Head posturing associated with abnormalities of the visual system is usually compensatory and serves to enhance binocular vision (eliminate diplopia, or double vision) or improve visual acuity. The visual system

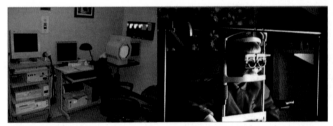

Figure 86-2. Electroretinography testing (left) and eye movement recording (right). Courtesy of Richard W. Hertle, MD.

can be a strong cause of torticollis. Ocular causes of anomalous head posture include strabismus, nystagmus, refractive errors, dissociated ocular deviations, and eyelid anomalies. Clinical differentiation of these disorders is accurately accomplished after a thorough history and examination of the visual system. However, cause of the head posture can be elusive in patients with a combination of ocular and systemic abnormalities, such as strabismus, nystagmus, and cerebral palsy. In these situations, additional special testing is required. This includes electrophysiologic testing (ie, electroretinography, visual evoked potentials, and eye movement recordings) and neuroimaging.

Strabismus is a misalignment of the visual axis that interferes with binocular vision and in children can lead to monocular vision loss in the less preferred eye. Children with forms of strabismus in which the deviation is constant in all positions of gaze (comitant strabismus) and there is alternating fixation with monocular suppression and no diplopia do not usually adopt a head posture to improve binocular function. In forms of strabismus in which ocular deviation changes as a function of gaze (incomitant strabismus), such as cranial nerve palsy, there is a position of gaze in which the eyes can be used together. Children with incomitant strabismus will often posture their head to use this position of gaze to obtain singular binocular vision. This indicates the ability to use the eyes in a binocular fashion.

About 50% of children with the infantile form of nystagmus have an eccentric position of gaze in which their nystagmus is least and their vision, and thus visual function, is greatest (ie, an eccentric null position). These children often cleverly posture their head so that their null zone is straight ahead, thus optimizing vision (Figure 86-3).

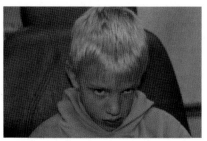

Figure 86-3. Child with torticollis caused by nystagmus and an upgaze null. Courtesy of Richard W. Hertle, MD.

Unusual or high refractive errors, usually hyperopia and astigmatism, can be optically minimized with an anomalous head posture by turning the head and using the eyelids to change refraction of light. This maneuver is much the same way a child with myopia (nearsightedness) will squint to see in the distance. Eyelid anomalies, masses, and malposition (ie, ptosis, or droopy eyelid) result in image deprivation to one or both eye(s), and children will position their head to look under or around the eyelid anomaly or mass. Most often this results in a chin-up position to view below a ptotic eyelid (Figure 86-4).

A history of complicated pregnancy, labor and delivery, or birth; abnormal growth and development; familial occurrence; and timing of onset, duration, and exacerbations of torticollis will help in differentiating nonocular causes of torticollis. Important neurologic history includes developmental delay, seizures, and meningitis. Neurologic and genetic examination will rule out an obvious neurologic or orthopedic cause of anomalous head posture and help identify any genetic syndrome.

Differential Diagnosis

Diagnoses besides nystagmus that should be considered include orthopaedic torticollis (neck and spine disorders), CNS torticollis (eg, tumors, inflammation, cranial pressure abnormalities), gastrointestinal torticollis (GERD), ocular torticollis, eyelid anomalies (ptosis and tumors), refractive errors (astigmatism and hyperopia), strabismus (horizontal, vertical, restrictive, paralytic), and nystagmus (infantile and acquired with eccentric gaze null position).

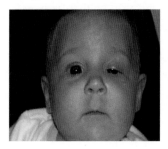

Figure 86-4. Infant with left upper lid ptosis with chin elevation. Courtesy of Richard W. Hertle, MD.

When to Refer

Ophthalmologic referral is warranted if any portion of the vision screening evaluation is abnormal or if no obvious abnormalities are found during routine primary care evaluation (as in this patient).

Treatment

Treatment of CNS lesions, neck musculature abnormalities, and GERD, if they are causing the torticollis, will improve head position. Ophthalmic treatments are geared to decrease the ocular cause of torticollis. These treatments include correcting structural anomalies of the globe, such as cataracts, and then addressing amblyopia (lazy eye) by providing glasses, patching, and atropine eyedrop penalization of the better-seeing eye. Correction of refractive errors with glasses or contact lenses is very important for improving vision, visual function, ocular alignment, and head position.

Surgery on the extraocular muscles, eyelids, or ocular adnexa is indicated to correct strabismus unresponsive to treatment with eyeglasses and amblyopia. It may be necessary to surgically move the eccentric null zone in patients with infantile nystagmus to the primary (straight-ahead) gaze position, remove adnexal lesions, or repair ptosis that is depriving the eye of vision.

Discussion

Torticollis is the third most common pediatric orthopedic diagnosis in childhood.

Key Points

- Any anomalous head posture warrants a thorough evaluation.
- Torticollis in childhood is most commonly the result of abnormalities of the central nervous system, visual system, or neck musculature.
- In some cases, the cause may be a life-threatening or sight-threatening condition (eg, malignant mass), for which early treatment can be of paramount importance.

Suggested Reading

Bray PF, Herbst JJ, Johnson DG, Book LS, Ziter FA, Condon VR. Childhood gastroesophageal reflux. Neurologic and psychiatric syndromes mimicked. *JAMA.* 1977;237(13):1342–1345

Do TT. Congenital muscular torticollis: current concepts and review of treatment. *Curr Opin Pediatr.* 2006;18(1):26–29

Hertle RW, Zhu X. Oculographic and clinical characterization of thirty-seven children with anomalous head postures, nystagmus, and strabismus: the basis of a clinical algorithm. *J AAPOS.* 2000;4(1):25–32

Kumandaş S, Per H, Gümüş H, et al. Torticollis secondary to posterior fossa and cervical spinal cord tumors: report of five cases and literature review. *Neurosurg Rev.* 2006;29(4):333–338

Chapter 87

Droopy Eyelids and Wandering Eyes

David Stager, Jr, MD

Presentation

An 11-year-old girl presents to the pediatrician's office with a 3-month history of droopy eyelids and outward drifting of the eyes. The parents note that the droopiness tends to worsen toward the end of the day. There is no other muscle weakness noted by the child or family. The child is otherwise healthy with no pertinent family ocular history. She reports intermittent horizontal diplopia (double vision), which is better in the morning. Her medical record reveals no prior evidence of any eye problems.

Systemic physical examination is unremarkable except her eyes. She has excellent visual acuity of 20/20 in both eyes. Ocular rotations are full. A moderate-angle exotropia (drifting out) is present, with the corneal light reflex displaced nasally in the right eye. The external eye examination demonstrates bilateral upper eyelid ptosis of 4 mm in the right eye and 3.5 mm in the left (Figure 87-1). Her pupils are briskly reactive with no afferent pupillary defect. The results of direct ophthalmoscopy are normal with no evidence of optic nerve edema.

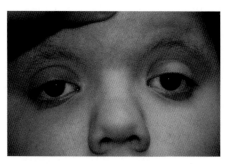

Figure 87-1. Marked ptosis with exotropia. Courtesy of David Stager, Jr, MD.

Because of the strabismus (ocular misalignment) and eyelid ptosis, the pediatrician decides to consult a pediatric ophthalmologist. While the physician leaves the examination room to call this colleague, the patient takes a nap. When the pediatrician returns, she awakens and the pediatrician immediately notices substantial improvement in her ptosis (Figure 87-2).

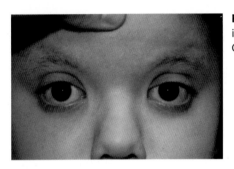

Figure 87-2. Marked improvement in eyelid ptosis with right exotropia. Courtesy of David Stager, Jr, MD.

Diagnosis

The improvement in ptosis with rest confirms the pediatrician's suspicion of ocular myasthenia gravis (MG). After examination by the pediatric ophthalmologist, this diagnosis is confirmed.

Further diagnostic testing may include an edrophonium test, ice pack or rest test, and acetylcholine receptor antibody titer test. An edrophonium test is highly sensitive but not always practical in children. In this test, a rapid, short-acting acetylcholinesterase agent (edrophonium chloride) that improves muscle function is administered intravenously. The patient is observed for improvement in signs and symptoms, indicating a positive test. Although edrophonium testing is usually performed by a neurologist or an ophthalmologist, the other tests can be performed by a pediatrician. An ice pack test (Figure 87-3) is a quick and easy office test that will frequently show improvement in eyelid ptosis and ocular motility after 5 minutes of covering the eyes with a cold pack. Similar findings will often be present after napping or resting, as in this patient. Although these 2 tests are highly specific, they are not as sensitive as a negative result. Negative results of ice pack and rest tests do not exclude the disease entirely. Acetylcholine receptor antibody testing is highly specific, but in children with ocular MG, up to 50% may be seronegative.

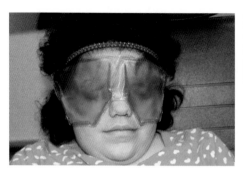

Figure 87-3. Ice pack test for eyelid ptosis. Ptosis improves in most patients with ocular myasthenia gravis. Courtesy of David Stager, Jr, MD.

Young female patients are affected by ocular MG more than young males. Eyelid ptosis is the most common clinical abnormality seen (present in more than 75% of patients), and exotropia is the most common form of strabismus in these patients. Variability, fatigability, and sparing of the pupil are key features that distinguish ocular MG from other forms of strabismus and ptosis.

Differential Diagnosis

Other diagnoses besides ocular MG that should be considered include

Oculopharyngeal Dystrophy

Oculopharyngeal dystrophy is an autosomal-dominant form of progressive myopathy including eyelid ptosis and less commonly, paralytic strabismus. However, this condition lacks the variability of ocular MG and almost always occurs after age 45 years.

Mitochondrial Myopathy

Mitochondrial myopathy may present with ptosis in children, but findings are rarely restricted to the eyes.

Bilateral Third Cranial Nerve Palsy

Bilateral third cranial nerve palsy will involve ptosis and strabismus, but findings are not variable and a history of trauma or intracranial disease is common.

Botulism

Botulism is a rare condition that results from an exotoxin produced by the gram-positive anaerobic bacillus *Clostridium botulinum*. It may present with ophthalmoplegia but is frequently generalized to involve hypotonia and descending weakness.

When to Refer

A prompt referral to a pediatric ophthalmologist is indicated when there is suspicion of ocular MG.

Treatment

This patient underwent treatment with oral pyridostigmine, and within several weeks her ptosis and exotropia resolved. Although not life-threatening, ocular MG may be severely debilitating. In younger patients, amblyopia resulting from strabismus or ptosis becomes a major concern because it may threaten normal visual development (see Chapter 65). A neurologist should be involved in guiding treatment. The most common treatment modalities include oral pyridostigmine (anacetyl-cholinesterase inhibitor) and corticosteroids. Plasmapheresis and thymectomy have also been used successfully.

Surgical management of ptosis and strabismus should be considered for refractory cases in which medical management fails. The prognosis for children with ocular MG is generally good, with many patients going into remission with medical management alone.

Discussion

Pediatric ocular MG is an acquired autoimmune disorder characterized by unilateral or bilateral variable ptosis and ophthalmoplegia. Auto-antibodies binding to proteins at the level of the neuromuscular junction have been implicated as the mechanism that disrupts normal neuromuscular transmission.

Clinical involvement is confined to the levator muscle of the upper eyelid, ocular orbicular muscle, and extraocular muscles. It should be noted that in some patients with ocular involvement generalized MG may develop, although the risk is lower in children than adults with ocular MG.

Key Points

- Pediatric ocular myasthenia gravis (MG) is an acquired autoimmune disorder characterized by unilateral or bilateral variable eyelid ptosis and ophthalmoplegia that worsen with fatigue and improve with rest.
- Children with ocular MG have a relatively low risk of progressing to generalized MG.
- Treatment should focus on relieving symptoms and preventing the development of amblyopia and generalized MG.
- Prognosis for children with ocular MG is generally good, with many patients going into remission with medical management alone.

Suggested Reading

Porter NC, Salter BC. Ocular myasthenia gravis. *Curr Treat Options Neurol.* 2005;7(1):79–88

Weinberg DA, Lesser RL, Vollmer TL. Ocular myasthenia: a protean disorder. *Surv Ophthalmol.* 1994;39(3):169–210

Chapter 88

Headache and Visual Loss

Edel M. Cosgrave, FRCOphth
I. Christopher Lloyd, MB, BS, DO, FRCS, FRCOphth

Presentation

An 11-year-old girl presents with a 2-month history of headache and blurred vision. The headaches occur on most days, feel like a tight band across her head, and are throbbing in nature. They are worse in the mornings and sometimes radiate to the back of her head. Her vision is intermittently blurred, and she experiences transient double vision (diplopia), which has lasted up to 10 minutes on several occasions. She has some nausea in the mornings, with vomiting on a couple of occasions, and also has increasing sensitivity to light (photophobia). She has sometimes been aware of a rhythmic whistling sound in her ears (pulsatile tinnitus).

The mother reports that her daughter has become more lethargic recently, and she has been sent home from school on 2 occasions because of her headache and dizziness. Three weeks before the onset of these symptoms, she had completed a course of penicillin for treatment of a pharyngeal (paratonsillar) abscess. The mother had migraines in her teens and wonders if this might be the cause of her daughter's symptoms.

The girl's height and weight are in the 50th percentile for her age. Menstruation has not yet started. Her blood pressure, temperature, and pulse are normal. Results of the physical examination, including ear, nose, and throat and neurologic assessment, appear normal. Urinalysis shows that the urine is clear with no hematuria or proteinuria.

Visual acuity is reduced to 20/40 in both eyes. Pupil reactions appear normal in each eye, and there is no anisocoria (difference in pupil size).

With direct ophthalmoscope, optic discs appear swollen to the pediatrician. Visual fields are full on confrontation testing (patient able to identify the correct number of fingers held in each quadrant of peripheral vision with each eye individually).

The combination of recent-onset headaches, reduced vision, and optic nerve edema (swollen optic discs) prompts an urgent magnetic resonance image (MRI) of the orbits and brain to rule out intracranial and intraorbital disease. The MRI result is reported as normal.

Diagnosis

The pediatrician considers the differential diagnosis of swollen optic discs in the presence of a normal MRI result. This includes venous sinus thrombosis, idiopathic intracranial hypertension (commonly termed pseudotumor cerebri), postinfectious papillitis, and pseudopapilledema (optic nerves that appear swollen in the absence of raised intracranial pressure). The pediatrician considers ordering magnetic resonance (MR) venography to look for venous sinus thrombosis and stenosis. The pediatrician refers the patient to pediatric ophthalmology colleagues for further investigation of her visual symptoms before ordering a lumbar puncture.

The ophthalmologists' examination confirms bilateral reduced visual acuity, but this improves to 20/20 with a small myopic correction. Ocular motility findings are normal, as are pupil reactions. There is no evidence of intraocular inflammation. However, both optic nerve heads are confirmed as grossly elevated and imaged as a baseline (Figure 88-1). B-scan ultrasound examination of optic nerves shows a distended optic nerve sheath (Figure 88-2). There is no evidence of optic disc drusen. Retinal findings are otherwise normal. Visual fields are formally assessed using automated perimetry and show bilateral, enlarged blind spots (Figure 88-3). Color vision is tested and found to be slightly subnormal in each eye.

Given the optic nerve appearance, the patient was admitted to the hospital for lumbar puncture. The result confirms raised intracranial pressure with an opening pressure of 40 cm H_2O. In light of her recent history of pharyngeal infection, an MR venogram is ordered. This

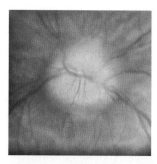

Figure 88-1. Swollen optic nerve, elevated appearance with blurring of superior and right-sided margins as seen by haze to blood vessel detail. Courtesy of I. Christopher Lloyd, MB, BS, DO, FRCS, FRCOphth.

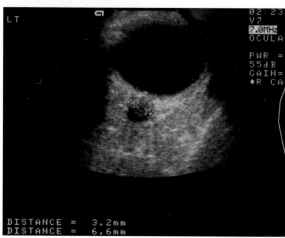

Figure 88-2. Ultrasound showing swollen optic nerve, (area between hatch marks). Courtesy of I. Christopher Lloyd, MB, BS, DO, FRCS, FRCOphth.

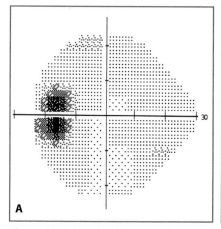
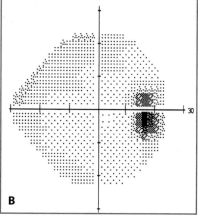

Figure 88-3. Visual field testing showing enlarged blind spot (dark areas temporally) consistent with bilateral optic nerve pathology. **A,** Left eye; **B,** right eye. Courtesy of I. Christopher Lloyd, MB, BS, DO, FRCS, FRCOphth.

shows a filling defect in the sagittal sinus—evidence of sinus thrombosis—and the cause of her raised intracranial pressure and optic nerve edema. Optic nerve edema in the presence of raised intracranial pressure is termed papilledema.

Patients with cerebral venous thrombosis may present with throbbing, band-like, or thunderclap-like headache. Sigmoid sinus thrombosis often causes pain in the occipital and neck region. Patients may present with a syndrome similar to pseudotumor cerebri. Cranial nerve syndromes are often seen with venous sinus thrombosis. These include vestibular neuropathy, pulsatile tinnitus, unilateral deafness, double vision (particularly horizontal due to cranial sixth nerve palsy), facial weakness, and transient obscuration of vision.

The cause is usually infection extending from sinuses or the pharynx. Rarely, sphenoid sinusitis may be associated with cavernous sinus thrombosis. Other causes include trauma, pregnancy, inflammatory bowel conditions, hypercoagulable states, hyperhomocysteinemia, hematologic conditions, collagen vascular conditions, nephrotic syndrome, and dehydration.

Several medications are reported to increase the risk of cerebral venous thrombosis. Among these are oral contraceptives, corticosteroids, aminocaproic acid, thalidomide, tamoxifen, erythropoietin, phytoestrogen, and asparaginase.

Assessment of a patient with headache and visual disturbance may require an extensive history and physical examination along with testing. The patient should be asked to describe the headache in terms of duration, intensity and frequency, location, type of pain, and associated symptoms.

Differential Diagnosis

Diagnoses besides venous sinus thrombosis that should be considered include the following:

Space-Occupying Lesions

Headache is almost never the first or only sign of a tumor. Changes in personality and mental functioning, vomiting, seizures, and other symptoms are more likely to appear first. Photophobia can be a feature of space-occupying lesions as well as of migraine and meningitis. Craniopharyngioma is the most common intracranial tumor in childhood, with an incidence of 1 to 2 cases per million. The most common presenting symptoms of craniopharyngioma are headache (55%–86%), endocrine dysfunction (66%–90%), and visual disturbances (37%–68%). Most young patients present with growth failure and delayed puberty. Optic pathway dysfunction on presentation is noted in 40% to 70% of patients. Children rarely become aware of visual problems (only 20%–30%) and often present with severe visual damage. Three major clinical syndromes have been described and relate to the anatomic location of the craniopharyngioma. Prechiasmal localization typically results in associated findings of optic atrophy (eg, progressive decline of visual acuity and constriction of visual fields). Retrochiasmal location commonly is associated with hydrocephalus with signs of increased intracranial pressure (eg, papilledema, horizontal double vision). Intrasellar craniopharyngioma usually manifests with headache and endocrinopathy. The most common differential diagnosis is chiasmal glioma.

Hypertension

Severe hypertension can cause blurred vision, headache, and swollen optic discs. Most cases of severe hypertension in childhood are due to renal causes; only occasionally is drug treatment (eg, steroids) or excess catecholamine drive responsible. Hypertensive retinopathy and papilledema are often seen at presentation. Chronic hypertension leads to protective cerebral vasospasm; a rapid fall in blood pressure can result in acute underperfusion of the brain, presenting clinically as seizures, encephalopathy, and sudden blindness. Any child with severe hypertension should be discussed urgently with a pediatric nephrologist at a tertiary care center, and most of these patients need to be transferred.

Idiopathic Intracranial Hypertension

Idiopathic intracranial hypertension describes signs and symptoms of raised intracranial pressure without evidence of a mass lesion or hydrocephalus. Opening cerebrospinal fluid (CSF) pressures greater than 20 cm H_2O in a child older than 5 years suggest the diagnosis (see Chapter 37). Because of its dynamic nature, instant CSF pressure measurement using height of a fluid column via lumbar puncture may be misleading and can be falsely elevated if a child is upset during the procedure. Overnight monitoring of CSF pressure is invasive but provides an optimal standard.

Papillitis

This term describes inflammation restricted to the optic nerve head. In children, most cases are caused by an immune-mediated process. These cases may be associated with infection (eg, viral) or immunization. Children typically present with bilateral subacute visual deterioration, headache, periorbital pain or painful eye movements, and swollen optic nerves.

Pseudopapilledema

In the presence of a normal MRI and normal CSF pressures, pseudopapilledema caused by optic nerve head drusen or hyperopia should be considered. These are typically identified on initial ophthalmic examination with confirmatory ancillary tests of B-scan ultrasound and fluorescein angiogram.

When to Refer

The pediatrician should refer to an ophthalmologist any child with headache and associated visual signs and symptoms such as blurred vision, visual field defects, diplopia, or swollen optic nerves. These features should also prompt urgent neuroimaging.

Treatment

The patient is admitted to the hospital and treated with intravenous antibiotics and acetazolamide, and is anticoagulated by the hematologists. After 6 months of treatment, she makes a full recovery.

The mainstay of treatment for infective cerebral venous sinus thrombosis is early and aggressive intravenous antibiotic administration for a period of 3 to 4 weeks. Acetazolamide is used to reduce intracranial pressure. Anticoagulation is used to arrest the thrombotic process and prevent septic emboli. Heparin is used in the acute phase and usually followed by 6 to 12 months of oral anticoagulation.

Discussion

Headaches are rare before 4 years of age but increase in prevalence throughout childhood, reaching a peak in the teens.

Tension-type headaches are the most common. Pain is usually mild to moderate in intensity, with a steady pressing or tightening quality. Many children with tension-type headache episodes also have other disorders, such as disturbed sleep, anxiety and depression, school problems, and family stress. These headaches are not associated with visual symptoms.

Migraine headaches are typically throbbing and preceded or accompanied by visual aura. The most commonly experienced visual phenomena include teichopsia (ie, bright, shimmering jagged lines that begin centrally and spread out across the visual field). Alice in Wonderland syndrome, or metamorphopsia, describes the distortion of visual images in size, shape, and color. Other visual effects include photopsia (flashing lights), scotoma (blind spot), or partial loss of vision.

Headache associated with ocular disease is generally localized around orbital and retro-orbital or brow area. Causes may include inflammation such as uveitis, preseptal or orbital cellulitis, raised intraocular pressure, or ocular surface disease such as keratitis or recurrent erosion syndrome. Additional signs may include periorbital swelling and tenderness, red eye, discharge, and irregular pupils.

Sinus headache can result from infective or allergic inflammation of the sinuses leading to increased mucus and fluid secretion. Optic neuropathy may accompany sinus disease caused by infective, inflammatory, compressive, neoplastic, or vascular processes secondary to destruction of the bony wall and optic nerve compression.

Key Points

- New-onset headache, visual disturbance, and optic nerve swelling all point toward an intracranial mass until proved otherwise, and urgent neuroimaging should be undertaken.
- Cerebral venous sinus thrombosis may present like idiopathic intracranial hypertension.
- A history of head trauma or infection of the sinuses in the case of a child with significant headaches should prompt investigation.

Suggested Reading

Awad AH. Headaches. In: Taylor D, Hoyt CS, eds. *Pediatric Ophthalmology and Strabismus.* 3rd ed. Philadelphia, PA: Elsevier; 2005:1065–1069

Friedman DI, Frishberg B. Neuro-ophthalmology and its contribution to headaches: a case-based approach. *Expert Rev Neurother.* 2010;10(9):1467–1478

Appendix A

Table of Contents by Condition

Appendix B

General Resources

American Academy of Pediatrics Guidelines and Policies

American Academy of Pediatrics Committee on Practice and Ambulatory Medicine, Section on Ophthalmology. Use of photoscreening for children's vision screening. *Pediatrics.* 2002;109(3):524–525

American Academy of Pediatrics Committee on Practice and Ambulatory Medicine and Section on Ophthalmology, American Association of Certified Orthoptists, American Association for Pediatric Ophthalmology and Strabismus, American Academy of Ophthalmology. Eye examination in infants, children, and young adults by pediatricians. *Pediatrics.* 2003;111(4):902–907

American Academy of Pediatrics Section on Ophthalmology, American Academy of Ophthalmology, American Association for Pediatric Ophthalmology and Strabismus. Screening examination of premature infants for retinopathy of prematurity [published correction appears in *Pediatrics.* 2006;118(3):1324]. *Pediatrics.* 2006;117(2):572–576

American Academy of Pediatrics Section on Ophthalmology, American Association for Pediatric Ophthalmology and Strabismus, American Academy of Ophthalmology, American Association of Certified Orthoptists. Red reflex examination in neonates, infants, and children. *Pediatrics.* 2008;122(6):1401–1404

American Academy of Pediatrics Section on Ophthalmology and Council on Children with Disabilities, American Academy of Ophthalmology, American Association for Pediatric Ophthalmology and Strabismus, American Association of Certified Orthoptists. Learning disabilities, dyslexia, and vision. *Pediatrics.* 2009;124(2):837–844

Cassidy J, Kivlin J, Lindsley C, Nocton J; American Academy of Pediatrics Section on Rheumatology, Section on Ophthalmology. Ophthalmologic examinations in children with juvenile rheumatoid arthritis. *Pediatrics.* 2006;117(5):1834–1845

Handler SM, Fierson WM; American Academy of Pediatrics Section on Ophthalmology and Council on Children with Disabilities, American Academy of Ophthalmology, American Association for Pediatric Ophthalmology and Strabismus, American Association of Certified Orthoptists. Learning disabilities, dyslexia, and vision. *Pediatrics.* 2011;127(3):e818–e856

Levin AV, Christian CW; American Academy of Pediatrics Committee on Child Abuse and Neglect, Section on Ophthalmology. The eye examination in the evaluation of child abuse. *Pediatrics.* 2010;126(2): 376–380

Lueder GT, Silverstein J; American Academy of Pediatrics Section on Ophthalmology, Section on Endocrinology. Screening for retinopathy in the pediatric patient with type 1 diabetes mellitus. *Pediatrics.* 2005;116(1):270–273

Basic Eye Conditions

Wright KW. *Pediatric Ophthalmology for Primary Care.* 3rd ed. Elk Grove Village, IL: American Academy of Pediatrics; 2008

General Overview of Pediatric Eye Examination

LaRoche GR. Examining the visual system. In: Goldbloom RB. *Pediatric Clinical Skills.* 4th ed. Philadephia, PA: Elsevier Saunders; 2011:101–121

Vision Testing Techniques

Robbins SL, Christian WK, Hertle RW, Granet DB. Vision testing in the pediatric population. *Ophthalmol Clin North Am.* 2003;16(2):253–267

Index